LIFE CHANGE EVENTS RESEARCH 1966–1978

AN ANNOTATED BIBLIOGRAPHY OF THE PERIODICAL LITERATURE

Edited by

Thomas H. Holmes
and
Ella M. David

PRAEGER

PRAEGER SPECIAL STUDIES • PRAEGER SCIENTIFIC

New York • Philadelphia • Eastbourne, UK
Toronto • Hong Kong • Tokyo • Sydney

Library of Congress Cataloging in Publication Data

Holmes, Thomas H.
  Life change events research, 1966–1978.

  Includes index.
  1. Medicine, Psychosomatic—Bibliography. 2. Stress
(Psychology)—Bibliography. 3. Stress (Physiology)—
Bibliography. 4. Change (Psychology)—Bibliography.
5. Adjustment (Psychology)—Bibliography. I. David,
Ella M. II. Title
Z6665.5.H64   1984   016.61607′1   83-19281
[RC49]
ISBN 0-03-070287-9

Published in 1984 by Praeger Publishers
CBS Educational and Professional Publishing
a Division of CBS Inc.
521 Fifth Avenue, New York, New York, 10175 U.S.A.

456789 ·   052   987654321

Printed in the United States of America
on acid-free paper

PREFACE

Life change events research is the branch of stress research that attempts to identify, measure, and study the consequences of discrete life experiences. Although the life events can be rare and dramatic experiences, they are most often familiar, and sometimes predictable, occurrences in the course of human life: changing schools, getting married, being fired from a job, losing a family member or friend by death, retiring, taking a vacation. The first questions researchers asked about such life events concerned their effect on health: can life events make people sick? But it was not long before others began to ask questions about the effect of life events on performance, as well. Do life events influence our ability to work, play, function as parents and spouses, cope with daily life? And so today the study of life change events is the shared domain of investigators in both the health and social sciences.

The research literature is international and appears in journals of many disciplines: internal medicine, clinical and social psychiatry, psychosomatic medicine, clinical and community psychology, sociology, public health, nursing, environmental health, social work. This bibliography surveys that varied literature in English for the period 1966-1978, the years before one could easily search the literature with the now-standard indexing term, "Life Change Events."

Researchers and scholars continue to debate the questions asked, the issues raised, the methodologies developed, and the findings discussed in the publications we list in this bibliography. And the debate widens as new applications of life events research are explored. We offer this bibliography as a guide not only for investigators who plan to do life events research, but also for those interested in applying the research to their own work as clinicians, counselors, educators, and policymakers.

We gratefully acknowledge the contribution made by the librarians and staff of the Reference Division, the Online Services Center, and the Circulation Department of the University of Washington Health Sciences Library. They provided cheerful and reliable assistance in searching the literature and locating these materials.

This project was supported in part by the Margaret O'Donnell Psychiatry Research Fund and by the Holmes Psychiatry Fund.

We thank Marion E. Amundson for her great help in the production of this manuscript.

Seattle, Washington

T.H.H.
E. M. D.

HOW TO USE THIS BOOK

We have divided life change events research into nine major subject areas (A through I) shown in the Table of Contents. Entries in Part A deal primarily with illness, those in Part B focus on kinds of performance, entries in Part C emphasize psychological measures, and so on. We assigned entries to subject areas according to the main orientation of the research report, and then we grouped entries into subsections by specific topics. Browsing through a section designated in the Table of Contents will acquaint the reader with the primary research on a given topic.

Each entry in this bibliography appears in only one place. Because many studies deal with more than one topic or contain data relevant to secondary topics, we have fully indexed each entry in the Subject Index. The Subject Index complements and amplifies the Table of Contents, allowing the reader to trace secondary as well as primary research interests. It also guides the reader to information that overlaps the topical boundaries of the Table of Contents, such as populations of special interest (by age, sex, occupation, nationality, kind of activity) and the use of specific research instruments (named life events inventories, standardized symptom questionnaires, various personality measures). Recurring research issues and themes also appear in the Subject Index.

The Author Index allows readers to trace the work of specific research investigators and teams. All authors are fully indexed in the Author Index.

TABLE OF CONTENTS

INTRODUCTION

Three publication dates serve as convenient markers in the chronology of life change events research. In 1957 Hawkins, Davies, and Holmes reported the first use of a standardized questionnaire, the Schedule of Recent Experience (SRE), to study the frequency of life events preceding the onset of tuberculosis. In 1967 Holmes and Rahe reported the development of a ratio scale of values, the Social Readjustment Rating Scale (SRRS), to quantify the life event reports collected by the SRE. And in 1977 the subject heading "Life Change Events" entered the list of index terms used by the National Library of Medicine in its computerized Medical Literature Analysis and Retrieval System (MEDLARS), the primary bibliographic reference tool of the health sciences.

During the 1957-1966 decade, independent research teams both in and outside the United States—Seattle, St. Louis, New York, London, and Israel—conducted systematic studies of the relation of life events to the onset of a number of illnesses. The scientists reported their preliminary findings to each other at research meetings, through correspondence, and in a few early publications. Their work culminated in a burst of publications at the beginning of the second decade. In 1967-1968 alone, three major methodological approaches to life events research were reported in scientific journals. Antonovsky and Kats described the development of their Life Crisis History tool, Holmes and Rahe explained their scaling method to quantify perceptions of life events, and Brown and Birley outlined their life events interview method. By the end of the 1967-1976 decade, the nature and effects of life change events had become a prominent topic in research literature.

The designation of "Life Change Events" as a Medical Subject Headings term used by MEDLARS signaled its coming of age as a research field. For a decade, life change events research had been indexed under the more general heading of "Stress, psychological." But in 1977 the National Library of Medicine recognized the need for a separate index term to accommodate the growing number of publications and to facilitate information retrieval in the future. Judging from our own experience, that expectation of continued research and interest in the field is well founded. The publication of the Social Readjustment Rating Scale study in 1967 brought us a flurry of inquiries about the use of our research instruments and the results of our investigations, and even 15 years later we continue to receive daily requests for information about the Schedule of Recent Experience and the Social Readjustment Rating Scale. The fact that inquiries come from researchers in nonmedical as well as medical disciplines is additional testimony to the growth and expansion of the field.

While retrieval of life change events research published since 1977 has been greatly simplified, finding earlier research remains a problem. The broad category called "Stress, psychological" includes thousands of titles and abstracts, so it is necessary to ferret out the life change research even after a computer search has been run. And that problem is compounded by another obstacle: terminology in the literature itself. Titles and abstracts can be misleading. "Stress," "psychological distress," "social stress," and similar phrases are used by authors to describe a variety of things, sometimes life change events and sometimes not. Take, for example, this title: "Social and psychological correlates of smoking behavior among black women." As it happens, there are no life change data in that article, but there is an even chance there would be in a similarly titled work. If an abstract fails to name the instruments or procedures used to measure "social stress," nothing short of finding and reading the article can resolve the question.

Most of the people who write us ask for two things: information about our work and help finding any life change research related to their particular area of interest. In 1978 we decided to make a systematic effort to answer the recurring question, "Do you know if anyone has studied life change events and my research topic?" This annotated bibliography is the result of that project. Its purpose is to simplify the search for life change events research reported between 1966 and 1978.

OBJECTIVES AND DEFINITION OF TERMS

We set out to find anything that might be of use to a researcher curious about life change events. Our goal was quantitative, rather than evaluative. The rule of thumb in choosing entries for the bibliography has been, "When in doubt, keep it in: let the bibliography user decide the value of the research."

All publications coming from the Holmes and Masuda laboratories since 1966 have purposely refrained from using the word "stress" because it is impossible to govern that word's interpretation. The concepts of "life change" and "social readjustment" were adopted to identify the methodological orientation of work using the Schedule of Recent Experience and the Social Readjustment Rating

Questionnaire. But many of the publications included in this bibliography do not call themselves "life change events" research, preferring to characterize their methodological orientation with other terms such as "stressful life events," "life stress," and "psychosocial crises." We call this a life change events bibliography as a convenience and to establish a link with the MEDLARS indexing term.

Any objective, discrete life situation or experience qualifies as a life change event in this bibliography. We used the life events in the Schedule of Recent Experience as a starting point, but we have not limited the search to those 42 events. The spectrum of events ranges from the minor (change in eating habits) through major and memorable life experiences (getting married, changing jobs) to exceptional and catastrophic events (being caught in a natural disaster, leaving one's country as a refugee). We have, however, excluded personal experiences of an ongoing nature ("problems," "strains," "pressures," "concerns") and less available to documentation as discrete events.

CRITERIA FOR SELECTION OF BIBLIOGRAPHY ENTRIES

All research included in the bibliography deals with human subjects and is written in English. Each entry meets at least one of four criteria: (1) it collects data on the incidence of life change events, using any method; (2) it uses a life change events research instrument, for any purpose; (3) it collects data on the consequences or aftermath of a specific life change event; or (4) it reviews and analyzes a relevant area of the literature. In addition, most entries meet two other criteria: they are found in the periodical literature and they were published between 1966 and 1978.

The exceptions to those last two criteria deserve mention. We limited our search to the periodical literature, primarily because original research generally appears in journal and serial publications. But since our objective is to make life change events research more accessible, it would be wrongheaded to exclude two edited collections of representative reports from major research teams. And so we have included as bibliography entries the chapters from two books devoted entirely to life change events research, Barbara Snell Dohrenwend and Bruce P. Dohrenwend's Stressful Life Events: Their Nature and Effects and E. K. Eric Gunderson and Richard H. Rahe's Life Stress and Illness. For the same reason, we include unpublished student research when it meets the other criteria. There is no good way to track down master's and medical theses, so our coverage is limited to work known to us. Doctoral dissertations can be traced through <u>Dissertation Abstracts International</u> and obtained through interlibrary loan programs, although we relied solely on the abstract listings. And then there is the inevitable handful of miscellaneous documents—the occasional mimeographed paper, a preliminary report of promising research, a copy of a paper read at a meeting—that we cannot resist including. The source of such manuscripts is identified in the bibliography citation.

The time span of the bibliography is 1966 through 1978, corresponding to the available back-file units in the MEDLARS computer searches. But there are several entries dated before 1966 and one or two dated after 1978, again because including the information would better serve users of this bibliography.

EXTENT OF THE SEARCH

We conducted our literature search by two methods, a hand search and a computer search. We began by reviewing the contents of eight scientific journals we considered to be early and prominent publishers of life change events research. We also conducted a search of our files to collect names, titles, abstracts, manuscripts, student theses, and reprints sent to us since 1966. In a final hand search, we used <u>Science Citation Index</u> and <u>Social Sciences Citation Index</u> to find publications that cited the work of Holmes, Rahe, and Masuda. These two reference tools were very useful in providing leads to possible users of the Schedule of Recent Experience and the Social Readjustment Rating Scale. We ordered computer searches run on several reference services: the National Library of Medicine's MEDLARS database, <u>Psychological Abstracts</u>, <u>Sociological Abstracts</u>, and <u>Dissertation Abstracts</u>.

There was, of course, some overlap in the leads generated by the separate searches, but not nearly as much as we expected. By sheer bulk the MEDLARS search would seem exhaustive since we received a printout of over 1,300 items. And yet after eliminating duplicated items in the hand and computer searches, we found more than 400 leads remained from the hand searches. It proved impractical to keep a tally of the actual number of articles we considered for inclusion in the bibliography, because the list of leads grew with every article we read.

We feel confident that we have found most of the life change events research published in periodicals from 1966 through 1978, but equally confident that we have missed some items. Errors of commission and errors of omission—by research authors, publishers, and bibliographers alike—can sometimes be discovered only by chance and rectified only after considerable delay. But we have (with the exception of one thesis and most dissertations) laid hands on every item listed in this bibliography, confirmed its bibliographic citation, and reviewed its contents.

CONTENTS OF THE BIBLIOGRAPHY

This bibliography contains 857 annotated entries: 671 journal and serial publications, 88 doctoral dissertations, 44 master's and medical theses, 37 chapters in books, and 17 unpublished papers and reports.

The 671 published articles, representing 78% of the total number of bibliography entries, appear in 184 journals. The distribution of the articles in the 184 journals is shown in Table 1. Six of the eight journals we selected for our hand search—numbers 1, 2, 3, 4, 7, 8, 17, and 24—proved, indeed, to be prominent publishers of life change events research. (For those interested in studies of the distribution of research articles in journals, see bibliography entry H101.)

ANNOTATION OF BIBLIOGRAPHY ENTRIES

This bibliography is designed to serve as a guide to the research, not as a review of it. The annotations, therefore, report no data, nor are the studies' results discussed. Under "Subjects" we describe the main characteristics of the population under study, and as "Method" we list the primary (but not necessarily all) research instruments and procedures used to collect data. When the article title, description of subjects, and the methods of measurement do not provide adequate information, they have been supplemented to clarify the stated objective of the study. The annotations in this bibliography are not complete abstracts of the articles.

TABLE 1

Distribution of 671 Articles in 184 Journals

		Number of Articles	% Total	
1.	Journal of Psychosomatic Research	99	14.7	
2.	Psychosomatic Medicine	45	6.7	
3.	Archives of General Psychiatry	40	6.0	
4.	Journal of Health and Social Behavior	27	4.0	
5.	Journal of Nervous and Mental Disease	23	3.4	34.8%
6.	British Journal of Psychiatry	19	2.8	
7.	American Journal of Psychiatry	17	2.5	
8.	Journal of Human Stress	16	2.4	
9.	Psychological Reports	15	2.2	
10.	Psychological Medicine	13	1.9	
11.	Social Science and Medicine	11		
12.	American Journal of Community Psychology	10		
13.	Journal of Consulting and Clin. Psychology	10		
14.	Nursing Research	9		
15.	Annals of the N.Y. Academy of Sciences	8		
16.	Military Medicine	8		
17.	Psychosomatics	7		
18.	American Journal of Epidemiology	6		
19.	Archives of Environmental Health	6	17.9	
20.	British Medical Journal	6		
21.	International J. of Health Services	6		
22.	International J. of Psychiatry in Medicine	6		
23.	Medical Journal of Australia	6		
24.	Social Psychiatry	6		
25.	American Journal of Public Health	5		
26.	Australia-New Zealand J. of Psychiatry	5		
27.	Comprehensive Psychiatry	5		29.7%
28. . . . 184.	157 other journals (1-4 articles each)	237	35.3	35.3%

LIFE CHANGE EVENTS
AND ILLNESS

GENERAL ILLNESS:
Incidence, Onset, and Susceptibility
(A1 - A58)

A1   Aakster, C. W.: Psycho-social stress and health disturbances.

PER   Social Science and Medicine 8:77-90, 1974.
        Subjects: 1,552 Dutch citizens, ages 25-65, randomly
        selected in a survey of the normal population.
        Method: Each subject was interviewed at home for socio-
        logical and medical information. Data collection included
        a history of health disturbances (any change warranting ex-
        pert attention), an index of social mobility (life changes
        plus subjective evaluation), and types of adjustment and
        adjustive failures in childhood and adult years.

A2   Anderson, Sister Joan Therese, R. S. M.: Life change units
    and subsequent illness in women in religious life. Unpublished
    master's thesis, State University of New York at Buffalo, 1975.
        Subjects: 380 women in religious life.
        Method: Each subject completed three questionnaires: a
        modified Social Readjustment Rating Questionnaire (SRRQ),
        a similarly modified Schedule of Recent Experience (SRE)
        for the 18-month period from July 1972 through December
        1973, and an 18-month illness history (January 1973 through
        June 1974). The Social Readjustment Rating Scale for
        Women in Religious Life was developed from the SRRQ data,
        and its Life Change Unit item-values were used to quantify
        the SRE data. The Seriousness of Illness Rating Scale
        (SIRS) was used to quantify illness reports.

A3   Andrews, Gavin; Tennant, Christopher; Hewson, Daphne; and
      Schonell, Malcolm: The relation of social factors to physical
      and psychiatric illness. American Journal of Epidemiology
      108:27-35, 1978.
          Subjects: 863 Australian adults randomly selected in a
          community survey of a suburb of Sydney.

          Method: All subjects completed a questionnaire that col-
          lected data on chronic physical symptoms (Belloc Scale)
          and psychiatric health (20-item version of the General
          Health Questionnaire). The two health measures were
          studied in relation to life events (Tennant and Andrews in-
          ventory and scalings), social status, migration experience,
          social support, maturity of coping, and adverse childhood
          experience.

A4   Bedell, Jeffrey R.; Giordani, Bruno; Amour, Judith L.;
      Tavormina, Joseph; and Boll, Thomas: Life stress and the
      psychological and medical adjustment of chronically ill chil-
      dren. Journal of Psychosomatic Research 21:237-242, 1977.
          Subjects: 45 children, ages 6-15, attending a camp for
          children with a chronic illness (diabetes, 19; asthma, 7;
          cystic fibrosis, 5; perceptual motor dysfunction, 4; cleft
          palate, 3; hearing impairment, 3; blindness, 2; burns, 1;
          and crippled, 1).

          Method: Each child was administered three self-report
          measures: Coddington's Schedule of Recent Experience for
          children, the Piers-Harris Self Concept Scale, and the
          State-Trait Anxiety Inventory for Children. Camp coun-
          selors recorded illness-related problems for each child,
          using the Camp Counselor Rating Scale.

A5   Bruhn, John G.; Philips, Billy U.; and Wolf, Stewart: Social
      readjustment and illness patterns: Comparisons between
      first, second, and third generation Italian-Americans living
      in the same community. Journal of Psychosomatic Research
      16:387-394, 1972.
          Subjects: 204 Italian-Americans living in Roseto, Pennsyl-

          vania.
          Method: Each subject completed two questionnaires: the
          Schedule of Recent Experience and an illness history cover-
          ing the same 3-year period. [See also A259.]

A6   Burke, Jon Franklin: Relationship of life changes to illness
      (Doctoral dissertation, University of Oregon, 1970). Disser-
      tation Abstracts International 31:6236-B, 1971.

Subjects: 148 college students in their last semester of course work before graduation.
Method: Each subject completed three questionnaires: the Schedule of Recent Experience, an illness history (for current school year), and a modified Cornell Medical Index. Subjects' medical records were also consulted for illness data, and the Seriousness of Illness Rating Scale was used to quantify illness data.

A7 Cline, David W., and Chosey, Julius J.: A prospective study of life changes and subsequent health changes. Archives of General Psychiatry 27:51-53, 1972.
    Subjects: 134 cadets enrolled in an officer training program.
    Method: Each subject completed the Schedule of Recent Experience and the Multiple Affect Adjective Check List. Subjects then reported all subsequent health changes at intervals of 2 weeks, 4 months, and 8 months.

RC 321A66

A8 Doll, Richard E.; Rubin, Robert T.; and Gunderson, E. K. Eric: Life stress and illness patterns in the U.S. Navy: II. Demographic variables and illness onset in an attack carrier's crew. Archives of Environmental Health 19:748-752, 1969.
    Subjects: 738 crew members on a U.S. Navy attack carrier during a 6-month deployment to Vietnam.
    Method: This is the second part of a six-part prospective study using the Schedule of Recent Experience, records of illness developed during subsequent sea duty, and data concerning environmental and demographic variables. [See Parts I (A52) and III-VI (A48, A49, A50, A51).]

RC963A22

A9 Garrity, Thomas F.; Marx, Martin B.; and Somes, Grant W.: The influence of illness severity and time since life change on the size of the life change–health change relationship. Journal of Psychosomatic Research 21:377-382, 1977.
    Subjects: 314 college freshmen.
    Method: All subjects completed Anderson's College Schedule of Recent Experience at the beginning of the school year. Three waves of health interviews were held, at 3, 6, and 9 months into the school year; each subject participated in one of the three study periods. At the health interview subjects completed Langner's 22-item index of psychophysiological symptoms and then reported the following health data for the preceding 60 days: number of health problems, number of illness episodes, number of days with illness, and number of days of disability.

RC 52. J6

A10   Garrity, Thomas F.; Marx, Martin B.; and Somes, Grant W.:
Langner's 22-item measure of psychophysiological strain as
an intervening variable between life change and health outcome.
Journal of Psychosomatic Research 21:195-199, 1977.
> Subjects: 314 college freshmen.
> Method: This report is a reanalysis of data originally re-
> ported in 1975 (see A24). In the 1975 article, Langner's
> 22-item index was studied as one of five health outcome
> measures. In this article Langner's 22-item index is ex-
> amined as an intervening variable between life change (in-
> dependent variable) and health outcome (the four dependent
> variables).

RC52.J6

A11   Garrity, Thomas F.; Marx, Martin B.; and Somes, Grant W.:
The relationship of recent life change to seriousness of later
illness. Journal of Psychosomatic Research 22:7-12, 1978.
> Subjects: 313 college freshmen.
> Method: All subjects completed Anderson's College Sched-
> ule of Recent Experience (past 12 months). At least three
> months later each subject was interviewed about health
> problems in the preceding 60 days (type, number of days
> duration, number of days of disrupted activity, and self-
> rated seriousness of episode), and each subject was asked
> to rate his or her overall health status on a 10-point scale.
> The Seriousness of Illness Rating Scale was used to quantify
> the reported illness data.

RC52.J6

A12   Garrity, Thomas F.; Somes, Grant W.; and Marx, Martin B.:
Factors influencing self-assessment of health. Social Science
and Medicine 12A:77-81, 1978.
> Subjects: 314 college freshmen.
> Method: All subjects completed Anderson's College Sched-
> ule of Recent Experience (past 12 months) and a question-
> naire concerning demographic characteristics. At follow-
> up interviews at least three months later the following data
> were collected: self-rating of perceived health status (10-
> point scale); self-report of recent health (preceding 60 days);
> perceived current stressfulness of life (4-point scale);
> psychophysiological symptomatology (Langner's 22-item
> index); and socioeconomic status (following Hollingshead's
> method).

PER

A13   Garrity, Thomas F.; Somes, Grant W.; and Marx, Martin B.:
The relationship of personality, life change, psychophysiologi-
cal strain and health status in a college population. Social
Science and Medicine 11:257-263, 1977.

PER

Subjects: 250 college freshmen.
Method: This study is an extension of the research reported in A24. Of the 314 subjects studied in the earlier report, 250 were found to have Omnibus Personality Inventory data on file at the student counseling center. The social conformity, liberal intellectualism, and emotional sensitivity dimensions of the OPI were examined in relation to subjects' life change (Anderson's College SRE) scores, health outcome measures, and scores on Langner's 22-item index of psychophysiological strain.

A14 Gitter-Cohen, Barbara Jo: The relationship of significant life events and physical illness in children (Doctoral dissertation, California School of Professional Psychology, 1976). Dissertation Abstracts International 38:4456-B, 1978.
Subjects: 54 children enrolled in the 4th, 5th, or 6th grade.
Method: Mothers of subjects volunteered to complete three questionnaires about their children: an inventory of demographic variables, the "Significant Life Events Scale for Children" [Coddington's SRE for children?], and an illness history based on a modification of the Seriousness of Illness Rating Scale for use with children.

A15 Gunderson, E. K. Eric; Rahe, Richard H.; and Arthur, Ransom J.: The epidemiology of illness in naval environments: II. Demographic, social background, and occupational factors. Military Medicine 135:453-458, 1970.
Subjects: 2,684 officers and crew members aboard three U.S. Navy cruisers during a 6-8 month deployment overseas.
Method: This is the second of a two-part study using the Schedule of Recent Experience, medical records from ships' dispensaries, and data concerning demographic, social, and occupational variables. [See also Part I (A43).]

A16 Heisel, J. Stephen; Ream, Scott; Raitz, Raymond; Rappaport, Michael; and Coddington, R. Dean: The significance of life events as contributing factors in the diseases of children. III. A study of pediatric patients. Behavioral Pediatrics 83: 119-123, 1973.
Subjects: 34 children with juvenile rheumatoid arthritis, 35 hemophiliac children, 32 newly admitted general pediatrics patients, 31 surgical patients, and 88 children on their first visit to a child psychiatry clinic.
Method: Medical records were reviewed and parents of subjects were interviewed for data on the occurrence of life

events in the year preceding onset of the illness problems in four of the patient groups. For the fifth group, the hemophiliac children, the number of life events and the number of hemorrhages in each of two years were studied and correlations were tested from both low and high bleeders. [See also Parts I and II (H89, H36.)]

A17 Heno, Jan Williams: The relationship of psychosocial stressors (life change), locus of control and field dependence to illness susceptibility (Doctoral dissertation, Texas A & M University, 1976). Dissertation Abstracts International 37:1476-B, 1976.
Subjects: 201 university students.
Method: Each subject completed instruments measuring life change, locus of control, and field dependence. In addition, all subjects filed 8 weekly illness reports. [No instruments are named in this abstract.]

A18 Hinkle, Lawrence E., Jr.: The effect of exposure to culture change, social change, and changes in interpersonal relationships on health. In Stressful Life Events: Their Nature and Effects. Barbara Snell Dohrenwend and Bruce P. Dohrenwend (Eds.), pp. 9-44. New York: Wiley, 1974.
The author summarizes the findings from studies he has carried out over a 20-year period. He describes studies of illness distribution among similar people in relatively unchanging environments (telephone company employees with 20 years of continuous employment) and among people exposed to major cultural and social change (immigrants in exile, refugees, political prisoners, and prisoners of war). He also describes prospective studies of life change and illness manifestation on a short-term basis (colds and acute gastroenteritis in female telephone operators during 6 winter months) and on a long-range basis (a 20-year study of occupational mobility and coronary heart disease and death among male Bell Telephone employees).

A19 Holmes, Thomas H., and Masuda, Minoru: Life change and illness susceptibility. In Separation and Depression. J. P. Scott and E. C. Senay (Eds.), pp. 161-168. Publication No. 94. Washington, D.C.: American Association for the Advancement of Science, 1973. [Reprinted in Stressful Life Events: Their Nature and Effects. Barbara Snell Dohrenwend and Bruce P. Dohrenwend (Eds.), pp. 45-72. New York: Wiley, 1974.]

The authors summarize the development and application of the Schedule of Recent Experience, the Social Readjustment Rating Questionnaire and Social Readjustment Rating Scale, and the Seriousness of Illness Rating Scale. They also describe life event scaling studies for both general and specific populations, cross-cultural scaling studies, retrospective and prospective studies of life change and illness onset, and correlation studies of magnitude of life change and seriousness of illness.

A20   Holmes, T. Stephenson: Adaptive behavior and health change. Unpublished medical thesis, University of Washington, 1970.
     Three studies were reported:
     (1) "Profiles of Life Change"
        Subjects: 199 hospitalized patients from the general medical wards and a comparison group of 80 resident house staff physicians.
        Method: All subjects completed the Schedule of Recent Experience (for previous 10-year period).
     (2) "Long-Term Predictions of Health Change"
        Subjects: 52 medical students.
        Method: In the prospective part of this study, all subjects completed the Schedule of Recent Experience (for past year). At follow-ups 10 and 23 months later, subjects completed health change reports. In the retrospective part of this study, 35 subjects completed a second Schedule of Recent Experience two years after the initial administration of the instrument, to test subjects' recall of the same year's life changes.
     (3) "Short-Term Intrusions into the Life Style Routine"
        Subjects: 55 individuals, ages 16-60, drawn as a sample of convenience.
        Method: The Schedule of Daily Experience (SDE), a modification of the SRE, was developed to record life changes on a daily basis. Each subject completed the SDE daily for at least two weeks (and up to nine weeks) and kept a daily diary of health changes (signs, symptoms, inconveniences) which included notations of possible reasons for symptoms and of subject's general state of mind that day. [See also A364.]

A21   Holmes, T. Stephenson, and Holmes, Thomas H.: Long-range predictions of health change. Psychosomatic Medicine 31:445, 1969. (Abstract)
     This is an abstract of the second study reported above in A20.

A22 Hotaling, Gerald T.; Atwell, Saundra G.; and Linsky, Arnold S.: Adolescent life changes and illness: A comparison of three models. Journal of Youth and Adolescence 17:393-403, 1978.

> Subjects: 118 college freshmen chosen by random sample.
> Method: Subjects were interviewed to obtain medical history for the preceding 12 months (type of illness, days of disability, whether medical care was sought) and to inquire about frequency of contact with subject's family during the past 12 months (as a measure of social support). Subjects also completed Coddington's Schedule of Recent Experience for high school age subjects and a mental health checklist (a modification of Langner's 22-item measure of psychiatric symptomatology). Three models for the life change and illness relationship were investigated: the "direct stress and illness model," the "sick role behavior model," and the "mental health model."

A23 Liao, Winston: Psychological stress, health status, and health behavior: Application of the life changes concept. Psychological Reports 41:246, 1977.

> Subjects: 83 second-year pharmacy students.
> Method: Subjects completed Anderson's College Schedule of Recent Experience and an inventory of sociodemographic items. Two months later subjects completed Langner's 22-item screening index of psychiatric symptomatology and a "health outcome inventory" (number of health problems, number of separate episodes, number of separate days upon which health problem was experienced, disability days, professional consultations and lay consultations).

A24 Marx, Martin B.; Garrity, Thomas F.; and Bowers, Frank R.: The influence of recent life experience on the health of college freshmen. Journal of Psychosomatic Research 19:87-98, 1975.

> Subjects: 314 college freshmen.
> Method: At the beginning of the school year, 1,840 freshmen completed an inventory of demographic variables and a modified version of Anderson's College Schedule of Recent Experience (for the previous 12 months). At least three months later during the academic year 314 of the subjects were personally interviewed for health history data for the 60 days preceding interview: number of different health problems, number of separate illness episodes, number of days upon which illness was experienced, number of days of disrupted activity, and health care utilization. At the health interview subjects also completed Langner's 22-item

index of psychiatric symptomatology and rated the perceived stressfulness of their lives on a 4-point scale. The modification of Anderson's College Schedule of Recent Experience used in the Marx and Garrity studies is appended to this article. [See also A10.]

A25 Matsuda, Karen Joy: An exploratory study of the relationship among life change, anxiety, and illness in a well population. Unpublished master's thesis, University of Washington, 1978.
   Subjects: 57 employees in a governmental agency.
   Method: Each subject completed a survey of demographic variables, the State-Trait Anxiety Inventory (STAI), the Schedule of Recent Experience (two years), and an illness history for the same two years covered in the SRE (number of health changes, number of days lost from work, number of days hospitalized).

A26 Mattila, Vilho J., and Salofangas, Raimo K. R.: Life changes and social group in relation to illness onset. Journal of Psychosomatic Research 21:167-174, 1977.
   Subjects: 165 employees of a large working place, ages
RC52.J6 20-49, who had been employed there for the last three years successively.
   Method: Subjects completed a modified Schedule of Recent Experience (3 years) and a questionnaire concerning social background. Health records for the past 3 years were obtained from the occupational health center.

A27 Mehrabian, Albert, and Ross, Marion: Quality of life change and individual differences in stimulus screening in relation to incidence of illness. Psychological Reports 41:267-278, 1977.
   Two studies were reported:
   (1) "Assessment of Pleasant, Arousing, and Dominance-Eliciting Qualities of Specific Life Changes"
      Subjects: 80 university undergraduates in an introductory psychology course.
      Method: Subjects rated 14 different life changes on semantic differential-type scales: pleasant/unpleasant, arousing/unarousing, dominance-inducing/submissiveness-inducing.
   (2) "Life Change and Personality in Relation to Incidence of Illness"
      Subjects: 175 university undergraduates in an introductory psychology course (none had participated in Study 1).

Method: Each subject completed a modified Schedule of Recent Experience, a questionnaire measure of stimulus screening (Mehrabian, 1977), and an illness history (based on disease items in Wyler's Seriousness of Illness Rating Scale).

A28   Metzner, Helen Low; Harburg, Ernest; and Lamphiear, Donald E.: Early life social incongruities, health risk factors and chronic disease. Journal of Chronic Diseases 30: 225-245, 1977.

Subjects: 1,144 adults (age 35-69) drawn from the Tecumseh Community Health Study population.
Method: As part of a larger study, all subjects were administered health questionnaires and physical examinations to collect data on 9 risk factors (systolic and diastolic blood pressure, blood glucose level, serum cholesterol, serum uric acid, lung function, adiposity, number of cigarettes smoked, current alcohol consumption) and 5 chronic diseases (coronary heart disease, hypertension, diabetes, chronic bronchitis, asthma). Five years later mortality data were collected, and subjects were administered a structured interview to collect data on occurrence of three "life stress" variables before age 17: "residential geographic mobility" (number of dwelling units lived in, number and sizes of communities lived in, length of residence and frequency of moves), "parental deprivation" (living without one or both natural parents for more than a year), and "parental status incongruency" (difference between education and occupation of father and mother). The relation of the "early life stress" variables to adult health status and mortality rates was examined for men (N=529) and women (N=615) by age subgroups.

A29   Michalos, Alex C.: Life changes, illness and personal life satisfaction in a rural population. Sociological Abstracts 26(3): 78S09104 (RSS 1978 1948), 1978. [Full article subsequently published in Social Science and Medicine 13A:175-181, 1979.]

Subjects: 434 adults drawn in a random sample of 220 households in a rural Canadian township.
Method: Two home visits were made to each household. During the initial visit a one-page questionnaire of census-type questions was administered. During the second visit, each household member over 15 years old was interviewed: a modified Schedule of Recent Experience (for past year) was administered, a self-report of general illness was

obtained (6 measures of health status "in last 2 weeks"), and a measure of Personal Life Satisfaction (12-point scale) was made.

A30   Noffsinger, Edward Brallier: Psychosocial stress and illness (Doctoral dissertation, University of California, Berkeley, 1977). Dissertation Abstracts International 38:3855-B, 1978.
Subjects: 179 healthy, married, middle-class Caucasian males.
Method: Subjects were drawn from the rolls of the Kaiser/ Permanente health care organization in Santa Clara, California. Three instruments were completed by all subjects: a measure of recent life change (modified Schedule of Recent Experience for the past 6 months), a measure of anticipated life changes (modified Schedule of Recent Experience for the future 6 months), and a measure of chronic hassles ("Modified Hassle Inventory"). At follow-up investigation three months later, two sources of health outcome were used: subjects' reports on a health change history form and subjects' Kaiser/Permanente medical records.

A31   Orr, Prudie Luther: Life events and health status (Doctoral dissertation, University of Arkansas, 1977). Dissertation Abstracts International 38:2379B-2380B, 1977.
Subjects: 521 case workers in Arkansas, all college graduates.
Method: In Phase 1 of this prospective study, subjects completed the Recent Life Changes Questionnaire, an abbreviated version of the Community Adaptation Schedule, an Interpersonal Checklist, the State-Trait Anxiety Inventory (Form X), and the Eysenck Personality Inventory. Ten months later in Phase 2, subjects completed the Physical Health Status Questionnaire (number of episodes of physical illnesses experienced in past 10 months).

A32   Pesznecker, Betty L., and McNeil, Jo: Relationship among health habits, social assets, psychologic well-being, life change, and alterations in health status. Nursing Research 24:442-447, 1975.
Subjects: 548 residents of Renton, Washington.
Method: A questionnaire mailed to subjects collected data concerning health habits, social assets, psychologic well-being, life change (a modified Schedule of Recent Experience for past 2 years), and health changes. [See also C55.]

RT 1. N 8

A33   Rahe, Richard H.: Life change and subsequent illness reports. In <u>Life Stress and Illness</u>. E. K. Eric Gunderson and Richard H. Rahe (Eds.), pp. 58-78. Springfield, Illinois: Charles C Thomas, 1974. [Following this chapter, on pages 79-89, is Paul D. Nelson's "Comment" on Rahe's presentation.]

    The author reviews his work with colleagues at the U.S. Navy Medical Neuropsychiatric Research Unit in San Diego, California. Studies that gathered recent life change data from nearly 4,000 Navy subjects are used as the basis of discussion of "the utility of a life changes questionnaire for predicting near-future illness." The discussion includes sections on the methodology of studies using the Schedule of Recent Experience and results from both retrospective and prospective studies.

A34   Rahe, Richard H.: Life-change measurement as a predictor of illness. <u>Proceedings of the Royal Society of Medicine</u> <u>61</u>: 1124-1126, 1968.

    <u>Subjects</u>: Nearly 2,500 enlisted men and officers aboard three U.S. Navy cruisers at sea on 6-month deployment (two to Vietnam, one to the Mediterranean).

    <u>Method</u>: At the beginning of each ship's cruise, subjects completed the Schedule of Recent Experience; illness distribution was predicted by assigning subjects to high risk and low risk groups on the basis of their life change scores. At the end of each ship's cruise 6 months later, predictions were tested by reviewing each subject's medical record.

A35   Rahe, Richard H.: Subjects' recent life changes and their near-future illness reports: A review. <u>Annals of Clinical Research</u> <u>4</u>:250-265, 1972.

    The author reviews the life changes and illness research he has carried out over ten years in over 4,000 subjects, including studies of U.S. Navy populations. Topics of discussion include the following: development of a life changes questionnaire, prediction of near-future illness in both retrospective and prospective studies, and a description of ongoing research designs.

A36   Rahe, Richard H.: Subjects' recent life changes and their near-future illness susceptibility. <u>Advances in Psychosomatic Medicine</u> <u>8</u>:2-19, 1972.

    The author reviews the life changes and illness research he has carried out over five years in over 5,000 subjects. Topics of discussion include the following: development of a life changes questionnaire, prospective studies in the prediction of near-future illness, studies using physiologic and psychologic measures of subjects' reactivity to recent life changes, and a description of ongoing studies of subjects prone to coronary heart disease.

A37   Rahe, Richard H., and Arthur, Ransom J.: Life-change patterns surrounding illness experience. Journal of Psychosomatic Research 11:341-345, 1968.

RC52.J6
    Subjects: 3,265 U.S. Navy officers and enlisted men.
    Method: Each subject completed the military version of the Schedule of Recent Experience (covering 4 years, divided into 6-month intervals). Subjects also completed an illness history for the previous 4 years (also divided into 6-month intervals), reporting any health changes, physical and mental, deemed significant by the subject.

A38   Rahe, Richard H.; Floistad, Ivar; Bergan, Thomas; Ringdal, Rasmus; Gerhardt, Rolf; Gunderson, E. K. Eric; and Arthur, Ransom J.: A model for life changes and illness research: Cross-cultural data from the Norwegian navy. Archives of General Psychiatry 31:172-177, 1974.

RC321 A66
    Subjects: 2,485 U.S. Navy enlisted men and 1,058 Norwegian Navy trainees.
    Method: Each subject completed the military version of the Schedule of Recent Experience (for the past 2 years, divided into 6-month intervals); he also completed the Macmillan Health Opinion Survey. Medical records were later reviewed by physicians for new illnesses reported during the 6-12 months subjects were at sea.

A39   Rahe, Richard H.; Gunderson, E. K. Eric; Pugh, William M.; Rubin, Robert T.; and Arthur, Ransom J.: Illness prediction studies: Use of psychosocial and occupational characteristics as predictors. Archives of Environmental Health 25:192-197, 1972.

RC963 A22
    Subjects: 4,463 U.S. Navy enlisted men stationed aboard six large Navy ships.
    Method: At the beginning of the cruise each subject completed the Schedule of Recent Experience, the Macmillan Health Opinion Survey, a questionnaire concerning personal background, and a job description form (including pay grade, number of months in grade, number of men supervised, and job satisfaction). Fourteen significant illness predictors were studied using precruise and cruise (6-8 months) illness reports.

A40   Rahe, Richard H. , and Holmes, Thomas H.: Life crisis and
disease onset: A prospective study of life crises and health
changes. Mimeographed paper, September 1, 1966 (available
from Dr. Holmes, Department of Psychiatry and Behavioral
Sciences RP-10, University of Washington School of Medicine,
Seattle, Washington 98195). [A revised version of this paper
appeared as Part III in Dr. Rahe's chapter, "Life Crisis and
Health Change," in Psychotropic Drug Response: Advances in
Prediction. P. R. A. May and J. R. Wittenborn (Eds.), pp.
106-112. Springfield, Illinois: Charles C Thomas, 1969.]
Subjects: 84 resident physicians.
Method: Subjects completed the Schedule of Recent Experi-
ence (covering past 10 years), and then eight months later
subjects reported health changes which occurred in the interval.

A41   Rahe, Richard H. , and Holmes, Thomas H.: Life crisis and
disease onset: A qualitative and quantitative definition of the
life crisis and its association with health change. Mimeo-
graphed paper, September 1, 1966 (available from Dr. Holmes,
Department of Psychiatry and Behavioral Sciences RP-10,
University of Washington School of Medicine, Seattle, Wash-
ington 98195). [A revised version of this paper appeared as
Part II in Dr. Rahe's chapter, "Life Crisis and Health Change,"
in Psychotropic Drug Response: Advances in Prediction.
P. R. A. May and J. R. Wittenborn (Eds.), pp. 99-106.
Springfield, Illinois: Charles C Thomas, 1969.]
Subjects: 88 resident physicians.
Method: Each subject completed the Schedule of Recent
Experience (covering past 10 years) and an illness history
of major health changes during each of the past 10 years.
Life Change Unit (LCU) totals for each year were plotted on
a graph and health change data were superimposed on each
subject's graph.

A42   Rahe, Richard H.; Mahan, Jack L.; and Arthur, Ransom J.:
Prediction of near-future health change from subjects' preceding life changes. Journal of Psychosomatic Research 14:401-
406, 1970.

Subjects: 2,664 enlisted men and officers aboard three U.S.
Navy cruisers on 6- to 8-month cruises.
Method: At the beginning of the cruises, each subject com-
pleted the military version of the Schedule of Recent Ex-
perience (for past 2 years, divided into 6-month intervals).
At the end of each cruise, subjects' medical records were

examined by a research physician to document the number, type, and severity of new illnesses reported during the cruise.

A43   Rahe, Richard H.; Mahan, Jack L.; Arthur, Ransom J.; and Gunderson, E. K. Eric: The epidemiology of illness in naval environments: I. Illness types, distribution, severities, and relationship to life change. Military Medicine 135:443-452, 1970.

     Subjects: 2,684 enlisted men and officers aboard three U.S. Navy cruisers on 6- to 8-month cruises.
     Method: At the beginning of the cruise, each subject completed a personal history questionnaire (demographic factors, social background, military status and job, and job satisfaction), the Macmillan Health Opinion Survey, and the military version of the Schedule of Recent Experience. At the end of the cruise, each subject's medical record was examined by a research physician to document number, type, and severity of each new illness reported during the cruise. [See also Part II (A15).]

A44   Rahe, Richard H.; McKean, Joseph D., Jr.; and Arthur, Ransom J.: A longitudinal study of life-change and illness patterns. Journal of Psychosomatic Research 10:355-366, 1967.

     Subjects: 50 U.S. Navy and Marine personnel with a mean of 10 years of service who were ultimately discharged for psychiatric illness.

RC52.J6

     Method: The health records and active duty service records of each subject were examined for life changes (using the military version of the Schedule of Recent Experience) and illness experience (number of episodes, severity of illness, frequency and distribution of illnesses). The data were compared to Hinkle's data from a study of the illness experience of 1,527 American working men [see A18].

A45   Rahe, Richard H.; Meyer, Merle; Smith, Michael; Kjaer, George; and Holmes, Thomas H.: Social stress and illness onset. Journal of Psychosomatic Research 8:35-44, 1964.

     Subjects: From six studies: 20 employees in a tuberculosis sanatorium who contracted the disease, matched to

RC52 J6

20 employees who remained well; 40 tuberculosis outpatients, 40 patients with newly diagnosed cardiac disease, and 40 control subjects; 25 subjects consecutively admitted to a hospital for inguinal hernia repair; 39 dermatology

clinic outpatients with newly acquired skin disease; 35 married pregnant women; and 33 unmarried pregnant women.

Method: Subjects in all six studies completed the Schedule of Recent Experience (covering the preceding 10 years).

A46 Rose, Robert M.; Jenkins, C. David; and Hurst, Michael W.: Health change in air traffic controllers: A prospective study. I. Background and description. Psychosomatic Medicine 40: 142-165, 1978.

Subjects: 416 air traffic controllers.

Method: In this 3-year prospective study, nine categories of variables were investigated as possible predictors of psychological or physical health change: (1) endocrine and cardiovascular responsivity at work; (2) behavioral responsivity at work; (3) work environment; (4) sociodemographic background; (5) specific psychological attitudes and orientation; (6) work morale and satisfaction; (7) life change events, as measured by the Review of Life Experiences (ROLE) inventory devised for this study; (8) work competence; and (9) general psychological assessment. Health changes were documented by an extensive schedule of regular examinations, reports, and questionnaires. [See H103 for description of development and application of the ROLE inventory.]

A47 Roskies, Ethel; Iida-Miranda, Maria-Lia; and Strobel, Michael G.: Life changes as predictors of illness in immigrants. In Stress and Anxiety (Vol. 4). Irwin G. Sarason and Charles D. Spielberger (Eds.), pp. 3-21. New York: Wiley, 1977.

Subjects: 303 adult Portuguese immigrants in Montreal.

Method: Each subject was interviewed and individually administered a modified version of the Schedule of Recent Experience, the U.S. National Health Survey checklist, and a modified General Health Questionnaire.

A48 Rubin, Robert T.; Gunderson, E. K. Eric; and Arthur, Ransom J.: Life stress and illness patterns in the U.S. Navy: III. Prior life change and illness onset in an attack carrier's crew. Archives of Environmental Health 19: 753-757, 1969.

Subjects: 687 enlisted men in the crew of a U.S. Navy attack carrier during a 6-month deployment to Vietnam.

Method: This is the third part of a six-part prospective study using the Schedule of Recent Experience, medical records of illnesses developed during subsequent sea duty, and data concerning various environmental and demographic variables. [See also Parts I (A52), II (A8), and IV-VI (A49, A50, A51).]

A49   Rubin, Robert T.; Gunderson, E. K. Eric; and Arthur, Ransom J.: Life stress and illness patterns in the U.S. Navy: IV. Environmental and demographic variables in relation to illness onset in a battleship's crew. Journal of Psychosomatic Research 15:277-288, 1971.

    Subjects: Entire enlisted crew of the USS New Jersey during a 7-month deployment to Vietnam.

RC52.J6   Method: This is the fourth part of a six-part prospective study using the Schedule of Recent Experience, medical records of illnesses developed during subsequent sea duty, and data concerning various environmental and demographic variables. [See also Parts I (A52), II (A8), III (A48), and V-VI (A50, A51).]

A50   Rubin, Robert T.; Gunderson, E. K. Eric; and Arthur, Ransom J.: Life stress and illness patterns in the U.S. Navy: V. Prior life change and illness onset in a battleship's crew. Journal of Psychosomatic Research 15:89-94, 1971.

    Subjects: Entire enlisted crew of the USS New Jersey during a 7-month deployment to Vietnam.

RC52.J6   Method: This is the fifth part of a six-part prospective study using the Schedule of Recent Experience, medical records of illnesses developed during subsequent sea duty, and data concerning various environmental and demographic variables. [See also Parts I (A52), II (A8), III-IV (A48, A49), and VI (A51).]

A51   Rubin, Robert T.; Gunderson, E. K. Eric; and Arthur, Ransom J.: Life stress and illness patterns in the U.S. Navy: VI. Environmental, demographic, and prior life change variables in relation to illness onset in naval aviators during a combat cruise. Psychosomatic Medicine 34:533-547, 1972.

    Subjects: 121 naval aviators flying combat missions from an aircraft carrier during a 6-month deployment to Vietnam.

    Method: This is the sixth and last part of a prospective study using the Schedule of Recent Experience, medical records of illnesses developed during subsequent sea duty, and data concerning various environmental and demographic variables. [See also Parts I (A52), II (A8), and III-V (A48, A49, A50).]

A52 Rubin, Robert T.; Gunderson, E. K. Eric; and Doll, Richard E.: Life stress and illness patterns in the U.S. Navy: I. Environmental variables and illness onset in an attack carrier's crew. Archives of Environmental Health 19:740-747, 1969.
> Subjects: 738 enlisted crew members aboard an attack carrier during a 6-month deployment to Vietnam.
> Method: This is the first part in a six-part prospective study using the Schedule of Recent Experience, medical records of illnesses developed during subsequent sea duty, and data concerning various environmental and demographic variables. [See also Parts II (A8) and III-VI (A48, A49, A50, A51).]

RC963A22

A53 Schless, Arthur P.; Teichman, Alicia; Mendels, J.; Weinstein, Norman W.; and Weller, Kenneth: Life events and illness: A three-year prospective study. British Journal of Psychiatry 131:26-34, 1977.
> Subjects: 87 medical students.
> Method: On a prospective basis for 3 years, each subject reported life events data and health change data. The Recent Life Events (RLE) questionnaire, a modification of the Schedule of Recent Experience for use with a medical student population, was used to collect life change data. Unweighted and weighted scores were calculated for symptoms and for life events (all events vs. undesirable events), and the temporal relations of symptoms to life events were examined.

RC321B856X

A54 Theorell, Tores: Selected illnesses and somatic factors in relation to two psychosocial stress indices—a prospective study on middle-aged construction building workers. Journal of Psychosomatic Research 20:7-20, 1976.
> Subjects: 200 middle-aged male construction building workers, steadily employed and free of major illness in the past year.
> Method: Subjects were screened for two psychosocial risk factors: "discord" (using measures of irritability and life dissatisfaction variables) and "life change" (using a modified Schedule of Recent Experience). Each was assigned to one of five study groups (high discord/high life change, high discord/low life change, etc.). Two years after the initial psychosocial screening, subjects participated in a clinical examination that gathered data on blood pressure, serum lipids, serum transaminases, and illness patterns (coronary heart disease, psychiatric illness, and "other illness") during the 2-year follow-up period.

RC52.J6

A55   Thurlow, H. John: Illness in relation to life situation and sick-
      role tendency. Journal of Psychosomatic Research 15:73-88,
      1971.

RC52.J6
         Subjects: 165 workers in a Canadian brewery.
         Method: Subjects completed a questionnaire concerning
         their life changes during the past five years (modified
         Schedule of Recent Experience) and their attitudes, outlook,
         and tendency to adopt the "sick role" (using the MMPI and
         a locus of control measure). Employee medical records
         were examined for the preceding five years (number of ill-
         ness episodes, number of days off work). The illness ex-
         perience of 111 of the subjects was studied prospectively
         for the following two years.

A56   Tutone, Robert M.: Correlates of illness susceptibility.
      British Journal of Medical Psychology 50:79-86, 1977.
         Subjects: 55 male undergraduate students.
         Method: Each subject completed three questionnaires: a
         modified Schedule of Recent Experience (for past 4 years),
         the Profile of Mood States instrument, and a 4-year illness
RC321B83 history (based on disease items in the Seriousness of Ill-
         ness Rating Scale). Measures of systemic activity (auto-
         nomic indices of pulse rate, respiration, peripheral circu-
         lation, and skin resistance) were obtained while subject
         was at rest and when he was under threat of electric shock
         ("Black box" test).

A57   Wyler, Allen R.; Masuda, Minoru; and Holmes, Thomas H.:
      Magnitude of life events and seriousness of illness. Psycho-
      somatic Medicine 33:115-122, 1971.
         Subjects: 232 patients with illness of recent onset or ex-
         acerbation representing 42 disease categories.
         Method: Each subject completed the Schedule of Recent
         Experience (for the preceding 2 years). The Seriousness
         of Illness Rating Scale was used to quantify the seriousness
         of the 42 disease categories. [See H31 for development of
         the SIRS.]

A58   Zaleznik, Abraham; Kets de Vries, Manfred, F. R.; and
      Howard, John: Stress reactions in organizations: Syndromes,
      causes and consequences. Behavioral Science 22:151-162,
      1977.
B453X   Subjects: 2,000 high status members of a large organiza-
         tion in Canada.

Method: Subjects completed a series of questionnaires including a health survey to identify five "stress syndromes": emotional distress, medication use, cardiovascular disturbance, gastrointestinal disturbance, and allergy respiratory disturbance. Subjects also completed an organizational survey and a personal history survey which contained a modified Schedule of Recent Experience to measure life changes.

GENERAL ILLNESS:
Hospitalization
(A59-A70)

A59   Aagaard, Jorgen: Admission to hospital: An analysis of the social anamnesis of children admitted to a paediatric department. Publication No. 18, Institute of Social Medicine. Aarhus, Denmark: University of Aarhus, 1978. [Summary, tables, figures, and description of computer program are in English; the text is in Danish. An English version of the report was subsequently published in Acta Paediatrica Scandinavica 68:531-539, 1979.]
   Subjects: 361 Danish children over one year old who were admitted to the pediatric department of a hospital during the course of one year.
   Method: Children were assigned to diagnostic groups for analysis of data provided by their parents. Parents of each child completed questionnaires concerning the family's social background and selected life events. The life events data were collected and evaluated using a modification of Coddington's Schedule of Recent Experience for children.

A60   Aagaard, Jorgen: Psychosocial stress and illness in children. Discussion of a method. Ugeskrift for Laeger 139:2961-2965, 1977. [Abstract in English; text in Danish.]
   The author reviews the development of Coddington's Schedule of Recent Experience for children and discusses the modifications of that method used in the author's pilot study of Danish children admitted to a hospital. Findings from the pilot study are reported in a companion article below (A61).

A61   Aagaard, Jorgen, and Bro, Poul: Psychosocial stress and illness in children. A preliminary report. Ugeskrift for Laeger 139:2966-2970, 1977. [Abstract in English; text in Danish]

RJ 1A 382 X

Subjects: 140 Danish children, age one or older, admitted to the pediatric department of a hospital during a period of $3\frac{1}{2}$ months.

Method: Children were assigned to diagnostic groups for analysis of data provided by their parents. Parents of patients completed a questionnaire concerning the family's social background and life events in the past year. A modification of Coddington's Schedule of Recent Experience for children was used to measure life changes. [See also A59, the report of the larger study which was modelled on this pilot study.]

A62   Goldberg, Evelyn L., and Comstock, George W.: Life events and subsequent illness. American Journal of Epidemiology 104:146-158, 1976.

Subjects: 83 matched pairs of cases and controls drawn from a large-scale prospective study of two general populations.

RA421A37   Method: All subjects were interviewed by questionnaire concerning demographic, health, and psychosocial variables. Included was a life events checklist (modified Schedule of Recent Experience) on which subjects indicated whether an event had occurred during the previous year. Six to twelve months later, subjects were reinterviewed: a shortened version of the first questionnaire was used, and detailed questions about illnesses, disability, and hospitalization were asked. A "case" was defined as "any person who died or was hospitalized during the follow-up interval for an illness starting after the first interview." Individually matched controls had not reported any new illnesses or hospitalizations during the interval. A number of scoring methods for life events data were examined.

A63   Mutter, Arthur Z., and Schleifer, Maxwell J.: The role of psychological and social factors in the onset of somatic illness in children. Psychosomatic Medicine 28:333-343, 1966.

Subjects: 45 children hospitalized for an acute disease process and 45 well children who had no illness during the previous six months.

Method: Subjects and their parents were interviewed using a semistructured, clinically oriented interview schedule; medical records were also reviewed. Data were collected in the following areas: the number, quality, and impact of changes in the child's psychosocial setting in the six months prior to illness onset (or interview for well children); the child's ability to cope with change; and the psychological and social organization of child and family.

A64   Rundall, Thomas G.: Life change and recovery from surgery. Journal of Health and Social Behavior 19:418-427, 1978.
> Subjects: 5,858 adult surgical patients in one of six disease-operation categories (gastric ulcer surgery, biliary surgery, appendectomy, abdominal hysterectomy, vaginal hysterectomy, and prostatectomy).
> Method: The day before surgery each subject completed a 16-item life events checklist (for the previous 3 months). Forty days after surgery each patient completed a health status questionnaire concerning patient's perception of his or her recovery from surgery. The patient's nurse, surgeon, and anesthetist completed forms documenting each patient's preoperative physical status, the stage of his or her disease, seventh-day postoperative health status, and day-of-discharge status. Medical records were also consulted.

A65   Rundall, Thomas Gene: Life change and recovery from surgery (Doctoral dissertation, Stanford University, 1976). Dissertation Abstracts International 37:6775A-6776A, 1977.
> This is the original study upon which publication A64 (above) was based. Included in the dissertation are experiments in different ways to analyze life change data: total number of events vs. weighted values, number of personal failures, number of achievements, number of losses.

A66   Tolsdorf, Christopher C.: Social networks, support, and coping: An exploratory study. Family Process 15:407-417, 1976.
> Subjects: 10 recently hospitalized, first-admission psychiatric patients and 10 recently hospitalized medical (non-psychiatric) patients, all of whom were male veterans (matched for age, marital status, education, and socioeconomic status).
> Method: An interview (2-6 hours) based on a 66-question interview guide was conducted with each subject. Data were collected on subjects' social networks (size, membership, qualities, expectations, attitudes), coping styles, and the presence and type of "recent life stresses."

A67   Volicer, Beverly J.: Hospital stress and patient reports of pain and physical status. Journal of Human Stress 4(2):28-37, 1978.

Subjects: 535 medical and surgical patients in a community hospital.

Method: Each patient completed Volicer's Hospital Stress Rating Scale [see G57 and H54], rated the pain he or she experienced on a pain thermometer, and provided reports of physical status both during hospitalization and after discharge.

A68 Volicer, Beverly J., and Burns, Mary W.: Preexisting correlates of hospital stress. Nursing Research 26:408-415, 1977.

Subjects: More than 450 general medical and surgical patients in a community hospital.

RTI. N8 Method: Subjects completed the Schedule of Recent Experience and the Hospital Stress Rating Scale [see G57 and H54]. Data collection also included demographic variables, information about prior hospitalizations, and diagnosis. The Seriousness of Illness Rating Scale was applied to the diagnosis data.

A69 Volicer, Beverly J.; Isenberg, Marjorie A.; and Burns, Mary W.: Medical-surgical differences in hospital stress factors. Journal of Human Stress 3(2):3-13, 1977.

Subjects: 535 medical and surgical patients in a community hospital.

Method: All subjects completed the Hospital Stress Rating Scale [see G57 and H54]. Differences between medical and surgical patients in the nine dimensions of stress measured by the HSRS were examined. Controlled variables were age, education, number of previous hospitalizations, number of years since last hospitalization, and seriousness of illness (using the Seriousness of Illness Rating Scale).

A70 Wershow, Harold J., and Reinhart, George: Life change and hospitalization—a heretical view. Journal of Psychosomatic Research 18:393-401, 1974.

Subjects: 88 male patients newly admitted to the medical service of a VA hospital who had not been hospitalized in the past 2 years.

RC52.J6 Method: All subjects were interviewed for demographic background data, and the Schedule of Recent Experience was administered in the form of a "highly structured interview schedule." [See also H85 for a response to this report by Robert D. Caplan.]

GENERAL ILLNESS:
Chronic Pain
(A71-A74)

A71   Branch, Susan Hollister: The types, incidence, and magnitude
of premorbid stress in chronic pain patients. Unpublished
master's thesis, University of Minnesota at Minneapolis, 1976.
   Subjects: 42 patients (23 male, 19 female) currently or
   previously hospitalized with chronic pain of at least 6 months
   duration.
   Method: Each subject completed the Social Readjustment
   Rating Questionnaire and the Schedule of Recent Experience.
   A Social Readjustment Rating Scale for this chronic pain
   population was developed from the SRRQ data and was used
   to quantify the SRE data.

A72   Duncan, Gary H.; Gregg, John M.; and Ghia, Jawahar N.:
The pain profile: A computerized system for assessment of
chronic pain. Pain 5:275-284, 1978.
   The authors describe the development of the Pain Profile,
   a computer-based system which provides a mathematical
   comparison of three aspects of the chronic pain experience:
   pathophysiology, psychology, and behavior. It is composed
   of an Organic Index, a Psychosocial Index (including a 2-
   year Schedule of Recent Experience and periodic monitoring
   of "current stress" during treatment), and a Pain Behavior
   Index.

A73   Ghia, Jawahar N.; Mao, Willie; Toomey, Timothy C.; and
Gregg, John M.: Acupuncture and chronic pain mechanisms.
Pain 2:285-299, 1976.
   Subjects: 40 patients with chronic pain below the waist and
   not amenable to conventional medical and/or surgical
   treatment.
   Method: Subjects were administered the Schedule of Recent
   Experience as part of a battery of instruments expected to
   be relevant to treatment outcome. A Multidisciplinary Pain
   Clinic approach and the differential spinal block (DSB) were
   used to study each patient's underlying pain mechanisms,
   and then subjects were randomly assigned to one of two different methods of acupuncture, meridian loci needling
   (MLN) and tender area needling (TAN). [See A74 below
   for report of life change data.]

A74 Toomey, Timothy C.; Ghia, Jawahar N.; Mao, Willie; and
Gregg, John M.: Acupuncture and chronic pain mechanisms:
The moderating effects of affect, personality, and stress on
response to treatment. Pain 3:137-145, 1977.
This companion article to A73 above reports data collected
from administration of the Schedule of Recent Experience
RC73p 356and the Seriousness of Illness Rating Scale as well as from
the following instruments: the MMPI, the Zung Depression
Inventory, Spielberger's State-Trait Anxiety Inventory,
Rotter's Internal-External Locus of Control Scales, the
Global Pain Estimate, and a Performance Profile designed
for this study.

GENERAL ILLNESS:
Reviews and Theoretical Discussions
(A75-A118)

A75 Andrews, Gavin, and Tennant, Christopher: Being upset and
becoming ill: An appraisal of the relation between life events
and physical illness. Medical Journal of Australia 1:324-327,
1978.
This review and analysis of the literature on the relation of
"psychological stress" to illness onset gives special attention to the consequences of major disasters, the effects of
cumulative life event stress, and the consequences of conjugal bereavement.

A76 Birley, J. L. T.: Stress and disease. Journal of Psycho-
somatic Research 16:235-240, 1972.
The author briefly surveys research fields related to "Life
Events and Psychosomatic Disorder," the theme of the 15th
RC52.J6 annual conference of the Society for Psychosomatic Research.
The study was presented at that conference in London,
England, on October 1, 1971.

A77 Cassel, John: Psychosocial processes and "stress": Theoretical formulation. International Journal of Health Services 4:
471-482, 1974.
The author attributes failures to document the role of psychosocial processes in disease etiology to inadequacies in
the theoretical framework of epidemiologic studies. He
presents an alternative interpretation of "stress theory,"

using Nuckolls's study of life change and psychosocial assets in pregnant women [see A340] as a pivotal point in his argument.

A78 Cobb, Sidney: A model for life events and their consequences. In Stressful Life Events: Their Nature and Effects. Barbara Snell Dohrenwend and Bruce P. Dohrenwend (Eds.), pp. 151-156. New York: Wiley, 1974.

The author discusses the three preceding chapters by Theorell (A292), Hudgens (A192), and Paykel (A169) and proposes a "metatheoretical model" as a basis for further theorizing. His construct takes into account many variables in personal characteristics and social situations and their relation to the life event-illness model.

A79 Coleman, James C.: Life stress and maladaptive behavior. American Journal of Occupational Therapy 27(4):169-180, 1973.

This review of the literature on "stress" gives special emphasis to techniques for measuring different kinds of stress (muscle tension, autonomic changes, life change events),

to coping patterns, precipitants of disease, and the effects of rapid social change on patterns and incidence of maladaptive behavior.

A80 Crisp, Arthur H.: Psychosomatic research today: A clinician's overview. International Journal of Psychiatry in Medicine 6:159-166, 1975.

The author discusses the need for short-term prospective clinical studies to complement long-term survey studies of personality, life events, and disease.

A81 Eastwood, M. R.: Epidemiological studies in psychosomatic medicine. International Journal of Psychiatry in Medicine 6: 123-132, 1975.

The author discusses use of the epidemiological triad of host, agent, and environment as a model for research into psychosomatic disorders; reviews efforts to overcome methodological and sampling difficulties of such research; and proposes "vulnerability to illness" and "clustering of illness" as the research areas that pose the greatest challenge for future epidemiological research.

A82 Frank, Jerome D.: Psychotherapy of bodily disease: An overview. Psychotherapy and Psychosomatics 26:192-202, 1975.

Clinical and experimental studies of the relationship between psychological states (including the readjustment required by life events) and diseases are reviewed. Special consideration is given to the psychotherapist's role in diagnosis, prevention, and treatment of such conditions.

A83   Gottschalk, Louis A.: Psychosomatic medicine today: An overview. Psychosomatics 19:89-93, 1978.
The author reviews the current status of research in specificity theory, life changes, peptic ulcers, and neuropsychopharmacology, and discusses their relevance to the practice of psychosomatic medicine.

A84   Greene, William A.: Hematology and the derivation of psychosomatic concepts. Archives of Internal Medicine 135:1338-1343, 1975.
The author presents a historical review of leukemia and lymphoma research at the University of Rochester under the direction of Dr. Lawrence Young. The development of new psychosomatic concepts at Rochester is then related to later developments, including the life change research of Holmes and Rahe.

RIIA725

A85   Gunderson, E. K. Eric: Introduction. In Life Stress and Illness. E. K. Eric Gunderson and Richard H. Rahe (Eds.), pp. 3-7. Springfield, Illinois: Charles C Thomas, 1974.
The editor provides a brief description of the symposium that generated this volume of research reports and an outline of the topics of the contributors.

RC49.G85

A86   Hinkle, Lawrence E., Jr.: The concept of "stress" in the biological and social sciences. International Journal of Psychiatry in Medicine 5:335-357, 1974.
The author traces the historical development of the concept of "stress" and its application to biological and social systems as an explanation for the apparent nonspecificity of disease reactions. He reviews evidence subsequently accumulated and concludes that the "stress concept" is no longer useful and, in fact, even hampers present research efforts.

A87   Holmes, Thomas H.: Life situations, emotions, and disease. Psychosomatics 19:747-754, 1978.
This article is an adaptation of the lecture presented at the third Weiss-English Symposium at Temple University in Philadelphia on October 29, 1977. The author reviews historically the research questions and methods undertaken in the Holmes laboratory over the course of 30 years.

A88 Holmes, Thomas H., and Masuda, Minoru: Psychosomatic syndrome: When mother-in-law or other disasters visit, a person can develop a bad, bad cold. Or worse. Psychology Today 5:71-72, 1972 (April).

BFIP835

The authors briefly review the development of the Schedule of Recent Experience, the Social Readjustment Rating Scale, and the Seriousness of Illness Rating Scale; their use in research on life change and illness; and their potential use in the prevention of illness.

A89 Holmes, T. Stephenson, and Holmes, Thomas H.: Risk of illness. Continuing Education for the Family Physician 3:48-51, 1975.

The authors present a brief history of the development of the Schedule of Recent Experience as an instrument to measure risk of illness. An illustrative case history is presented along with suggestions for applying the SRE to the clinical practice of family medicine.

A90 Hurst, Michael W.; Jenkins, C. David; and Rose, Robert M.: The relation of psychological stress to onset of medical illness. Annual Review of Medicine: Selected Topics in the Clinical Sciences 27:301-312, 1976.

Two models of "psychological stress" are discussed: one model defines it in terms of emotional responses and the other in terms of the occurrence of stimulus situations which require adjustment. The authors review the literature relating psychological stress to the onset of cardiovascular and neoplastic diseases, discussing the relationship of each model of psychological stress to heart disease and cancer. Suggestions are offered for future research design and clinical applications.

A91 Ierodiakonou, C. S.; Kokantzis, N.; and Fekas, L.: Stressful factors in Greek life leading to illness. In Life Stress and Illness. E. K. Eric Gunderson and Richard H. Rahe (Eds.), pp. 189-194. Springfield, Illinois: Charles C Thomas, 1974.

RC49. G85

This summary paper reviews research done by several teams. These are reports of the timing and disruption of crucial life situations which are associated with illness occurrence: going away to college, getting married or having sexual relations, having children at a later age.

A92 Kagan, Aubrey: Psychosocial factors in disease: Hypotheses

RC49. G85

and future research. In Life Stress and Illness. E. K. Eric

Gunderson and Richard H. Rahe (Eds.), pp. 41-57. Springfield, Illinois: Charles C Thomas, 1974.
> The author discusses problems, strategies, techniques,
> and directions of needed future research into psychosocial
> factors in disease.

A93   Kagan, Aubrey R., and Levi, Lennart: Health and environment—psychosocial stimuli: A review. Social Science and
Medicine 8:225-241, 1974.

PℇR

> The authors present a model of psychosocial factors and
> disease by describing six subsystems (psychosocial stimuli,
> psychobiological program, mechanisms, precursors of
> disease, disease, and interacting variables) and by review-
> ing the literature concerning relationships among the six.
> The authors discuss the implications of the current state of
> knowledge for health planners.

A94   Kimball, Chase Patterson: Conceptual developments in psychosomatic medicine: 1939-1969. Annals of Internal Medicine 73:
307-316, 1970.
> The author reviews theoretical developments and shifts in
> psychosomatic medicine over 30 years, tracing the work
> and influence of Cannon, Dunbar, Alexander, Wolff, Mason,
> Miller, Engel and the Rochester school, and many other
> researchers. He compares the earlier linear model of
> causality to the more recent cyclical model.

A95   Leigh, Hoyle, and Reiser, Morton F.: Major trends in psychosomatic medicine: The psychiatrist's evolving role in medicine. Annals of Internal Medicine 87:233-239, 1977.

RIIA84

> The authors discuss changes in the concept of "psychomatic
> illness" that have shifted the emphasis away from psycho-
> dynamic investigations to psychophysiologic and psycho-
> social research that is aimed at a holistic understanding of
> the biologic, psychologic, and social systems of both medi-
> cal and psychiatric patients. The importance of life events
> research in this shift is discussed. The changing role of
> consultation-liaison psychiatry in the general hospital is
> emphasized.

A96   Levi, Lennart: Psychosocial stress and disease: A conceptual
model. In Life Stress and Illness. E. K. Eric Gunderson and
Richard H. Rahe (Eds.), pp. 8-33. Springfield, Illinois:
RC40.G85 Charles C Thomas, 1974. [For a comment on Levi's presentation, see W. T. Singleton's remarks on pp. 34-40.]

Surveying the present knowledge of the relationships between psychosocial stimuli and disease, the author presents a model for psychosocially mediated disease. Detailed consideration is given to the following: physiological mechanisms, interaction variables, precursors of
disease and disease itself, an analysis of the design of
psychosomatic research and of the "stress concept" of
Selye.

A97   Levi, Lennart: Stress, distress and psychosocial stimuli.
Occupational Mental Health 3(3):2-10, 1973.
This review article begins with a discussion of Selye's
definition of stress and includes the life change research
of Holmes, Rahe, and Theorell.

A98   Levi, Lennart: A synopsis of ecology and psychiatry: Some
theoretical psychosomatic considerations, review of some
studies and discussion of preventive aspects. Report No. 30,
Laboratory for Clinical Stress Research. Stockholm:
Karolinska Institutet, 1972. [Available from the Laboratory
for Clinical Stress Research, Box 60205, S-104 01 Stockholm, Sweden.]
The role of extrinsic, psychosocial stimuli in the causation of disease is the realm of study which unites ecology
and psychiatry. The author presents theory, data from
recent studies, and viewpoints on prevention of illness.

A99   Lipowski, Z. J.: New perspectives in psychosomatic medicine. Canadian Psychiatric Association Journal 15:515-525,
1970.
This is the first in a series of three reviews of advances
in psychosomatic medicine and research. The author
discusses theoretical frameworks, methodological im-
provements, and clinical applications of current research.
Life events research is included in the discussion of the
multifactorial approach to the study of health and disease.
(See also A100 and A101.)

A100   Lipowski, Z. J.: Psychosomatic medicine in a changing
society: Some current trends in theory and research.
Comprehensive Psychiatry 14:203-215, 1973.
This is the second of three reviews by the author. (See
A99 and A101.)

A101   Lipowski, Z. J.: Psychosomatic medicine in the seventies:
An overview. <u>American Journal of Psychiatry</u> 134:233-244,
1977.
RC321A52   This is the third and most recent review of advances in
psychosomatic medicine and research by the author. (See
A99 and A100.)

A102   Luborsky, Lester; Docherty, John P.; and Penick, Sydnor:
Onset conditions for psychosomatic symptoms: A comparative review of immediate observation with restrospective
research. <u>Psychosomatic Medicine</u> 35:187-204, 1973.
This is a detailed review of 53 research studies of onset
conditions, including two life change studies. The authors
compare psychological antecedents of symptoms reported
in 23 "immediate-context" studies and in 30 "broad-
context" (mainly retrospective) studies. Methods are
suggested for the study of mediation of psychological antecedents and symptoms.

A103   Mason, John W.: A historical view of the stress field.
Part I. <u>Journal of Human Stress</u> 1(1):6-12, 1975.
The author traces the development of "stress theory" and
research both before and after Selye's formulations. In
analyzing the grounds for the present-day controversy and
confusion over both concepts and terminology, he gives
special emphasis to the importance of the "nonspecificity
concept." Recent studies are reviewed and guidelines for
future research methods and directions are proposed.

A104   Mason, John W.: A historical view of the stress field.
Part II. <u>Journal of Human Stress</u> 1(2):22-36, 1975.
This is the second half of the discussion described in A103.
(See also A114 for a reply by Hans Selye.)

A105   Mechanic, David: Discussion of research programs on relations between stressful life events and episodes of physical
illness. In <u>Stressful Life Events: Their Nature and Effects</u>.
Barbara Snell Dohrenwend and Bruce P. Dohrenwend (Eds.),
pp. 87-97. New York: Wiley, 1974.
BF575.S75   The author comments on three preceding chapters in this
C64 1973   volume by Hinkle (A18), Holmes and Masuda (A19), and
Rahe (H111) and discusses alternative models of illness,
the conceptions of life events and their impact, and illness behavior.

A106   Minter, Richard E., and Kimball, Chase Patterson: Life
        events and illness onset: A review. Psychosomatics 19:
        334-339, 1978.
            This review of the literature emphasizes the need to es-
        tablish clear documentation of illness onset by controlling
        sick role and illness behavior variables.

A107   Modlin, Herbert C.: Does job stress alone cause health
        problems? Occupational Health and Safety 47(5):38-39, 1978.
            The author reviews briefly the basic concepts of life
        events research and their applicability to job-related
        problems.

RC963.A372

A108   Petrich, John, and Holmes, Thomas H.: Life change and
        onset of illness. The Medical Clinics of North America:
        Symposium on Psychiatry and Internal Medicine 61:825-838,
        1977.
            The authors describe the measurement of life changes
        using the Schedule of Recent Experience and the Social
        Readjustment Rating Scale, and then they review studies
        of the relationship of life change to the onset of illness
        (cardiac disease, minor illness, diabetes mellitus,
        duodenal ulcer, tuberculosis, fractures, athletic injuries,
        traffic injuries, depression, suicide, and alcoholism).
        The development of the Seriousness of Illness Rating
        Scale and its use in relation to life change magnitudes is
        also reviewed. Clinical applications of life change re-
        search findings are illustrated.

RC60M4

A109   Rabkin, Judith G., and Struening, Elmer L.: Life events,
        stress, and illness. Science 194:1013-1030, 1976.
            The authors selectively review and critique the research
        on the relationship of life events, stress, and the onset of
        illness. Particular attention is given to analysis of re-
        search trends, conceptual and methodological approaches,
        and the study of mediating variables.

A110   Rahe, Richard H., and Arthur, Ransom J.: Life change and
        illness studies: Past history and future directions. Journal
        of Human Stress 4(1):3-15, 1978.
            After reviewing early retrospective studies and later
        prospective studies, the authors present a model for the
        life change-illness relationship which illustrates the key
        role of intervening variables. They propose the further
        investigation of such intervening variables as the most
        fruitful direction for future research.

A111 Rees, W. Linford: Stress, distress and disease. <u>British Journal of Psychiatry</u> <u>128</u>:3-18, 1976.

 This discussion of theoretical concepts and research findings was presented as the Presidential Address at the annual meeting of the Royal College of Psychiatrists held in London on July 9, 1975.

A112 Schmale, Arthur H.: Giving up as a final common pathway to changes in health. <u>Advances in Psychosomatic Medicine</u> <u>8</u>:20-40, 1972.

 In a section of his presentation called "Studies which Support the Concept of Giving Up as a Final Common Pathway to Changes in Health," the author discusses life change research, particularly the Social Readjustment Rating Scale.

A113 Schmale, Arthur H., Jr.: Importance of life setting for disease onset. <u>Modern Treatment</u> <u>6</u>:643-655, 1969.

 The author reviews the literature relating factors in life setting to changes in health (including use of the Schedule of Recent Experience to study life change and illness patterns). Emphasis is placed on the utility and applicability of such information in the nonpsychiatric physician's treatment methods.

A114 Selye, Hans: Confusion and controversy in the stress field. <u>Journal of Human Stress</u> <u>1</u>(2):37-44, 1975.

 The author replies in detail to Mason's analysis of present controversy and confusion in the "stress field" (see A103 and A104).

A115 Smith, C. Kent; Cullison, Sam W.; Polis, Emily; and Holmes, Thomas H.: Life change and illness onset: Importance of concepts for family physicians. <u>Journal of Family Practice</u> <u>7</u>:975-981, 1978.

 This review of the literature, directed to practitioners in family medicine, illustrates the clinical implications of life changes research with two case histories.

A116 Steele, G. P.: Editorial: Life event research and its clinical implications. <u>Medical Journal of Australia</u> <u>1</u>:312-313, 1978.

 After discussing some of the contradictory evidence and claims of life event research, the author proposes reaffirmation of multifactorial approaches by clinicians to study the complexities of the individual patient's situation.

A117   Thurlow, H. John: General susceptibility to illness: A
selective review. <u>Canadian Medical Association Journal</u> <u>97</u>:
1397–1404, 1967.

>The author discusses the notion of a "general susceptibil
>ity to illness" by reviewing research into the distribution
>of illness, the clustering of illnesses, illness and the
>"giving-up" reaction, and illness and the "sick-role ten
>dency."

A118   Wilkins, Walter L.: Social stress and illness in industrial
society. In <u>Life Stress and Illness</u>. E. K. Eric Gunderson
and Richard H. Rahe (Eds.), pp. 242–254. Springfield,
Illinois: Charles C Thomas, 1974.

>The author reviews and discusses theoretical issues
>raised by contributors to this volume of research reports
>and by others, and he posits several conceptual models.

SPECIFIC ILLNESS:
Infectious and Parasitic Diseases
(A119–A122)

A119   Hawkins, Norman G.; Davies, Roberts; and Holmes, Thomas
H.: Evidence of psychosocial factors in the development of
pulmonary tuberculosis. <u>The American Review of Tuberculosis and Pulmonary Diseases</u> <u>75</u>:768–780, 1957.

>Subjects: 20 employees of a sanatorium who became ill
>with tuberculosis, individually matched to 20 fellow em
>ployees who did not develop the disease.
>Method: Each subject completed the original version of
>the Schedule of Recent Experience (annual frequency and
>distribution of life events for a 10-year period) and the
>Cornell Medical Index.

A120   Holmes, Thomas H.; Hawkins, Norman G.; Bowerman,
Charles E.; Clarke, Edmund R., Jr.; and Joffe, Joy R.:
Psychosocial and psychophysiologic studies of tuberculosis.
<u>Psychosomatic Medicine</u> <u>19</u>:134–143, 1957.

>Subjects: A representative sample of 215 patients.
>Method: This report includes several different studies:
>interviewing 100 consecutive sanatorium admissions to
>gather data on general characteristics of the tuberculosis
>population; ecologic studies of tuberculosis using census
>tract data to study incidence of disease by economic resi
>dential areas; a psychosocial study of 33 children hospital-

ized for tuberculosis; and a study of psychophysiologic relationships (17-ketosteroid excretion). The life change study collected data (using the original Schedule of Recent Experience and interview) on life event occurrences for the 12 years prior to hospitalization of 215 patients, and then plotted the temporal relationships of life crisis to on-set of disease.

A121   Katcher, Aaron Honori; Brightman, Vernon; Luborsky, Lester; and Ship, Irwin: Prediction of recurrent herpes labialis and systemic illness from psychological measure-ments. Journal of Dental Research 52:49-58, 1973.
Subjects: 49 first-year nursing students.
Method: An initial interview with each subject was held to collect personal and medical history and to conduct physi-cal examinations. Subjects completed a battery of ques-tionnaires: the Cornell Medical Index, the Johns Hopkins Symptom Index, the Clyde Mood Scale, a newly designed social assets scale [C101], and a modified Schedule of Recent Experience (past 2 years). Each subsequent month subjects turned in a calendar/diary of health-related events, and when reporting RHL lesions the subjects also provided specimens for antibody titration and virus isola-tion. This paper reports the first year's findings in this 3-year study.

A122   Wilder, Russell M.; Hubble, Jayne; and Kennedy, Carroll E.: Life change and infectious mononucleosis. Journal of the American College Health Association 20(2):115-119, 1971.
Subjects: 54 college students hospitalized with infectious mononucleosis, 9 college students with acute bronchitis, and 400 college students attending a variety of classes.
Method: All subjects completed the Life Change Index, a 51-item questionnaire modeled on the Schedule of Recent Experience and adapted to the experiences of college stu-dents.

SPECIFIC ILLNESS:
Neoplasms
(A123-A138)

A123   Greene, William A.: The psychosocial setting of the develop-ment of leukemia and lymphoma. Annals of the New York Academy of Sciences 125:794-801, 1966.

Subjects: Three series of patients with leukemia or lymphoma, all at least 20 years old: 16 men, 32 women, 61 men.

Method: Each patient was interviewed for details about his or her psychological and social experiences with particular emphasis on the setting in which the manifest leukemia or lymphoma developed.

A124　Greene, William A., and Swisher, Scott N.: Psychological and somatic variables associated with the development and course of monozygotic twins discordant for leukemia. Annals of the New York Academy of Sciences 164:394-408, 1969.

Subjects: 3 sets of monozygotic twins discordant for leukemia (all were males and all were teenagers when the disease developed).

Method: Extensive interviews were conducted with each twin and one or both parents. Data were collected regarding gestational circumstances, past illness experience, personality development, and social characteristics, including family relationships. Medical records and high school counselors' records were used to confirm interview information.

A125　Greer, Steven, and Morris, Tina: Psychological attributes of women who develop breast cancer: A controlled study. Journal of Psychosomatic Research 19:147-153, 1975.

Subjects: 160 women consecutively admitted to hospital for breast tumor biopsy.

Method: The day before the operation (without knowledge of any provisional diagnoses), interviews and testing were conducted with each subject. Questionnaires included the Hamilton Rating Scale for Depression, the Eysenck Personality Inventory, and the Caine and Foulds Hostility and Direction of Hostility Questionnaire. The interview included inquiries about the occurrence of any events the subject considered stressful during the 5 years preceding the appearance of the breast lump. Separate interviews with husbands or close relatives were used to verify all data. Results are based on statistical comparisons of the 69 patients found to have breast cancer and the remaining 91 patients with benign breast disease. [See also A126.]

A126　Greer, Steven, and Morris, Tina: The study of psychological factors in breast cancer: Problems of method. Social Science and Medicine 12A:129-134, 1978.

The authors review the literature and discuss in detail the problems of method they find there. They describe their own controlled study (see A125) and discuss its findings and limitations. They conclude with recommendations for more stringent methods.

A127   Grissom, Julie J.; Weiner, Barbara J.; and Weiner, Elliot A.: Psychological correlates of cancer. Journal of Consulting and Clinical Psychology 43:113, 1975.
        Subjects: 30 male patients with lung cancer, 30 male patients with emphysema, and 30 male well controls.
        Method: Each subject completed the Recent Life Changes Questionnaire and the Tennessee Self-Concept Scale.

A128   Haney, C. Allen: Illness behavior and psychosocial corre-lates of cancer. Social Science and Medicine 11:223-228, 1977.
        After reviewing the literature on psychosocial precursors of cancer, the author proposes "illness behavior" as the intervening variable which might account for the research findings that associate life events and cancer. Life events may influence the individual's awareness of his own func-tioning and symptoms and thus trigger the help-seeking behavior which leads to eventual diagnosis and treatment for cancer.

A129   Hurlburt, Kathryn Elizabeth: Life change events as they re-late to the onset of breast tumors in women (Doctoral dis-sertation, University of Oregon, 1974). Dissertation Ab-stracts International 35:7651-A, 1975.
        Subjects: 84 women with breast tumors (undiagnosed as cancerous or benign at time of study).
        Method: Each subject completed the Schedule of Recent Experience for the 3 years preceding referral to the can-cer clinic for examination and diagnosis of breast tumor.

A130   Kissen, David M.: Psychosocial factors, personality and lung cancer. British Journal of Medical Psychology 40:29-43, 1967.
        Subjects: 218 male patients with lung cancer and 148 male control patients (hospitalized with other chest diseases), aged 55-64.
        Method: All subjects were interviewed by a researcher who did not know the patient's diagnosis. Subjects were interviewed about childhood and adult experiences, friends

and family relationships, occupational attitudes and satisfaction, and specific adverse experiences (life events such
as financial troubles, sexual difficulties, bereavements,
etc.). Each subject was also tested using the Short
Maudsley Personality Inventory (neuroticism scale). [See
also A131.]

A131   Kissen, David M.; Brown, R. I. F.; and Kissen, Margaret:
        A further report on personality and psychosocial factors in
        lung cancer. Annals of the New York Academy of Sciences
        164:535-545, 1969.
            Subjects: 550 male lung cancer and control patients.
            Method: Preliminary results are presented from further
            samples of patients drawn from the same hospital wards
            as reported in a 1967 study (see A130). The method of
            the earlier study was modified in several ways. The
            Eysenck Personality Inventory superseded the Short
            Maudsley Personality Inventory; data were gathered on
            smoking habits; a new 11-item scale, the Awareness of
            Autonomic Activity, was administered; and the interviews
            for psychosocial variables were analyzed not only for data
            on the occurrence of adverse situations but also for dif-
            ferences in the way subjects reported them.

A132   Muslin, Hyman L.; Gyarfas, Kalman; and Pieper, William J.:
        Separation experience and cancer of the breast. Annals of
        the New York Academy of Sciences 125:802-806, 1966.
            Subjects: 165 women admitted to hospital for breast
            biopsy.
            Method: All subjects completed a questionnaire about
            early (first 9 years of life) and recent (3 years preceding
            diagnosis of lesion) separation experiences. A subsample
            of matched pairs (one benign case and one malignant case
            with similar backgrounds) was interviewed about their
            separation experiences.

A133   Paloucek, Frank P., and Graham, John B.: The influence
        of psycho-social factors on the prognosis in cancer of the
        cervix. Annals of the New York Academy of Sciences 125:
        814-816, 1966.
            Subjects: 135 women with diagnosed cases of primary in-
            vasive cancer of the cervix, 14 women with uterine can-
            cer, and 4 women with cancer of the ovary.
            Method: Subjects were interviewed for data concerning
            various psychosocial factors: childhood experiences,

marital satisfaction, sexual history, patient's view of
prognosis, precipitating factors ("debilitating" life events
prior to manifestation of tumor). Cervical cancer patients
were followed for 5-year survival rate after treatment.

A134   Pech, Karel: Psychological factors in cancer. International
Mental Health Newsletter 16(2):1, 12, 1974.
The author briefly presents a hypothetical model to account for the observed phenomenon of drastic changes in
an individual's life preceding the onset of cancer. The
hypothesis is illustrated with representative clusters of
drastic changes (e.g., widowhood, divorce and new marriage, radical changes in social and climatic environment).

A135   Schmale, Arthur, and Iker, Howard: The psychological setting of uterine cervical cancer. Annals of the New York
Academy of Sciences 125:807-813, 1966.
Subjects: 51 essentially healthy women awaiting cone
biopsy after referral because of a positive Pap smear.
Method: Subjects were administered a battery of psychological tests (including three subscales of the MMPI) and
were interviewed about their responses to life events in
the 6 months prior to the first positive Pap smear. Predictions were made and recorded at the end of the interview: cancer was predicted for those women who reported
responding with feelings of hopelessness to a recent life
event, while predictions of no cancer were made for
women who did not report such feelings. Predictions
were then checked against subsequent histological findings.

A136   Schonfield, Jacob: Psychological and life-experience differences between Israeli women with benign and cancerous
breast lesions. Journal of Psychosomatic Research 19:229-
234, 1975.
Subjects: 112 Israeli women awaiting breast biopsy for a
suspicious tumor.
Method: On the day before biopsy each subject was administered Hebrew versions of three subscales of the
MMPI (Lie, Morale Loss, Well-being), the IPAT scales
of overt and covert anxiety, and the Schedule of Recent
Experience. Data were analyzed by grouping patients
according to birthplace (Europe, America, Middle East)
and diagnosis (cancerous or benign).

A137   Snell, Laura, and Graham, Saxon: Social trauma as related to cancer of the breast. <u>British Journal of Cancer</u> <u>25</u>:721-734, 1971.

        <u>Subjects</u>: 352 women with breast cancer and 670 controls with other types of cancer and nonneoplastic diseases.
        <u>Method</u>: Each subject was interviewed about the occurrence of deaths, separations, divorces, unemployment, and illnesses within her immediate family and those of other relatives. She was also asked about her own illnesses, sleep habits, work experience, periods of fatigue, financial troubles, and episodes of emotional distress.

A138   Walters, Candace Ann: The association between life changes and cervical cytology. Unpublished master's thesis, University of Washington, 1977.

        <u>Subjects</u>: 25 women awaiting their Pap smear or cervical biopsy procedure.
        <u>Method</u>: Each subject completed a personal history questionnaire and the Schedule of Recent Experience. When laboratory results were known, the subjects were divided into three groups for analysis and comparison: those with normal cervical cytology (N=14), abnormal cervical cytology (N=7), and the metaplastic cervical group (N=4).

SPECIFIC ILLNESS:
Endocrine, Nutritional, and Metabolic Diseases
and Immunity Disorders
(A139–A143)

A139   Grant, Igor; Kyle, G. C.; Teichman, A.; and Mendels, J.: Recent life events and diabetes in adults. <u>Psychosomatic Medicine</u> <u>36</u>:121-128, 1974.

        <u>Subjects</u>: 37 adult diabetic patients.
        <u>Method</u>: At each visit to their physicians during a period of 8-18 months, subjects completed a modified Schedule of Recent Experience for the interval since their previous visit; after completing the life events questionnaire, subjects received physical examinations. At the end of the study, an objective rater used the medical records to assess changes in the subject's physical condition from one visit to the next. Correlations were then calculated between life events scores (Total Life Events <u>vs</u>. Undesirable Life Events) and changes in diabetic condition.

A140 Hong, Kang-E Michael, and Holmes, Thomas H.: Transient diabetes mellitus associated with culture change. Archives of General Psychiatry 29:683-687, 1973.

> Subjects: 31-year-old male Korean physician who came to the United States for medical training.
> Method: This is a case history reporting the onset, course, and disappearance of diabetic symptoms in a 3-year period, at the end of which the patient had adapted to his new culture. The Schedule of Recent Experience was administered to measure the magnitude of life change from the 2 years preceding migration through 3 years following onset of disease.

RC321A66

A141 Katz, Jack L., and Weiner, Herbert: Psychosomatic considerations in hyperuricemia and gout. Psychosomatic Medicine 34:165-182, 1972.

> The authors review the literature and present several possible models for the role of psychosocial factors in the etiology, pathogenesis, and course of gout.

A142 Metzger, Genevieve V.: A follow up study of the diabetic regimen and life events of fifteen diabetic subjects in control and fifteen diabetic subjects out of control. Unpublished master's thesis, University of Oregon Medical School, 1972.

> Subjects: 30 diabetic subjects who had attended a clinic for classes in how to control their disease and its effects.
> Method: During home interviews subjects were asked for information about their medical history, diabetic routine, utilization of information learned in classes, and their own and their family's attitudes toward the disease. A modified Schedule of Recent Experience was administered to each subject.

A143 Stein, Stefan P., and Charles, Edward: Emotional factors in juvenile diabetes mellitus: A study of early life experience of adolescent diabetics. American Journal of Psychiatry 128: 700-704, 1971.

> Subjects: 38 adolescent diabetic patients and 30 nondiabetic, chronically ill controls (drawn from a clinic treating heritable blood diseases).

RC321A52

> Method: The medical records and histories of each subject were used to document subject's age, sex, time of disease onset, and incidence of major life events (deaths in family, separations, divorces, severe illnesses, and a number of kinds of family disturbances).

SPECIFIC ILLNESS:
Mental Disorders—General Psychiatric
(A144-A180)

A144   Andrews, Gavin, and Tennant, Christopher: Editorial: Life
event stress and psychiatric illness. Psychological Medicine 8:545-549, 1978.
       The authors present an analytical review of the major re-
search findings on life events and psychiatric illness by
the most prominent research teams (e.g., Brown and
associates, Paykel and associates, Jacobs, Myers, et
al.). Problems in past research are discussed and considerations for future research are offered.

A145   Aponte, Joseph F., and Miller, Francis T.: Stress-related
social events and psychological impairment. Journal of
Clinical Psychology 28:455-458, 1972.
       Subjects: 50 recently admitted psychiatric inpatients.
Method: Each subject was interviewed within 14 days of
admission to the hospital wards. A modified Schedule of
Recent Experience (divided into 4 intervals during the
past 3 years and a fifth section of "more than three years
ago") was read to each subject and responses were recorded by the interviewer. Measures of "psychological
impairment" included number of times previously committed, length of past and present hospitalizations, and
number and weighting of exhibited symptoms.

A146   Beaumont, P. J. V.; Abraham, Suzanne F.; Argall, W. J.;
George, G. C. W.; and Glaun, Daphne E.: The onset of
anorexia nervosa. Australian and New Zealand Journal of
Psychiatry 12:145-149, 1978.
       The authors report a retrospective study and a controlled
prospective study, respectively:
Subjects: 34 patients with anorexia nervosa.
Method: Case notes and medical records were studied to
    document experiential (life events) and psychological
    factors of possible importance to the psychogenesis of
    anorexia nervosa.
Subjects: 20 incoming clinic patients with anorexia nervosa.
Method: Both the patient and her family were interviewed
    by a team composed of a psychiatrist, a psychologist,
    and a dietician, who later pooled notes to compile a de-
    tailed clinical history of the disease. The difficulty of
    determining the onset of anorexia nervosa and the

consequent ineffectiveness of life change questionnaires is discussed.

A147   Beisser, Arnold R., and Glasser, Norbert: The precipitating
        stress leading to psychiatric hospitalization. Comprehensive
        Psychiatry 9:50-61, 1968.
        Subjects: 200 first-admission cases in a state mental
        hospital.
        Method: Working with the files of a state mental hospital,
        the investigators abstracted the following information
        about each case: patient's sex, marital status, and type
        of admission (voluntary or involuntary commitment), and
        the "external precipitating stress leading to hospitaliza-
        tion" as stated in the file by the psychiatric examiner.

A148   Blum, Jeffrey D.: On changes in psychiatric diagnosis over
        time. American Psychologist 33:1017-1031, 1978.
        Subjects: All male psychiatric inpatients (N=2,134) dis-
        charged in 1954, 1964, and 1974 from one hospital.
        Method: First a survey was made of the entire population:
        the age and primary diagnosis of each of the 2,134 dis-
        charged patients were collected. Then a detailed study
        was made of 794 patients randomly selected from the sur-
        vey population. The medical record of each of those pa-
        tients was studied to collect data on 13 variables in the
        patient's personal history (including life events in the 2
        years prior to admission) and the patient's diagnosis and
        course of treatment before discharge.

A149   Brown, George W.: Life-events and psychiatric illness:
        Some thoughts on methodology and causality. Journal of
        Psychosomatic Research 16:311-320, 1972.
RC52.J6 The author summarizes the main points developed in two
        earlier papers written with his colleagues at Bedford Col-
        lege and the Institute of Psychiatry (see A150 and A151)
        on the problems in measurement and the nature of the
        causal link in studies of life events and psychiatric illness.

A150   Brown, G. W.; Harris, T. O.; and Peto, J.: Life events
        and psychiatric disorders. Part 2: Nature of causal link.
        Psychological Medicine 3:159-176, 1973.
        Using their Camberwell (London) studies of depressive and
        schizophrenic disorders to illustrate their presentation,
        the authors describe methods for measuring the degree and
        nature of the causal effect of life events in psychiatric

disorders. Their method distinguishes between a "formative effect" and a "triggering effect" of life events in the onset of depressive and schizophrenic disorders. (See A151 for Part 1 of this report.)

A151   Brown, G. W.; Sklair, F.; Harris, T. O.; and Birley, J. L. T.: Life-events and psychiatric disorders. Part 1: Some methodological issues. Psychological Medicine 3:74-87, 1973.

Using their Camberwell (London) studies of schizophrenia (50 patients, 325 general population) and depression (114 patients, 200 general population) as illustrations, the authors discuss problems in the design of studies and the analysis of data. Three possible sources of error are discussed: (1) the definition and categorization of events; (2) the independence or dependence of life events and subsequent disorders; and (3) dating of life events and measurement and dating of illness onset. The Camberwell methods and findings are compared to those of Hudgens and associates in St. Louis studies (see A165, A193, H100). The authors suggest ways to control error and bias in studies of life events and psychiatric disorders. (See A150 for Part 2 of this report.)

A152   Clum, George A.: Personality traits and environmental variables as independent predictors of posthospitalization outcome. Journal of Consulting and Clinical Psychology 46:839-843, 1978.

Subjects: 79 psychiatric inpatients.
Method: At time of hospitalization and again one year later at a follow-up evaluation, patient and his or her significant other completed the following instruments to collect data about the patient: a biographic inventory, the "Life Change Inventory" (a modified Recent Life Changes Questionnaire) for past year, a measure of expectations for patient's improvement, and the Katz Adjustment Scale.

BFI.J575

A153   Clum, George A.: Role of stress in the prognosis of mental illness. Journal of Consulting and Clinical Psychology 44:54-60, 1976.

Subjects: 196 consecutively admitted psychiatric inpatients.
Method: At hospitalization and again one year later, each patient completed the "Life Change Inventory" (a modified Recent Life Changes Questionnaire) and the Katz Adjust-

BFI.J575

ment Scale. The patient's "significant other" also completed the research instruments at patient's hospitalization and one year later.

A154   Cohler, Bertram J.; Grunebaum, Henry U.; Weiss, Justin L.;
        Gallant, David H.; and Abernathy, Virginia: Social relations,
        stress, and psychiatric hospitalization among mothers of
        young children. Social Psychiatry 9:7-12, 1974.
            Subjects: 42 formerly hospitalized mothers and 42 matched
            well controls.
            Method: Each woman was interviewed. The occurrence
            of 11 categories of stressor events was tabulated for each
            subject and for members of her family. Social role per-
            formance was assessed for each subject in terms of social
            maladjustment (MMPI scale), social affiliation (Social
            Role Performance Instrument subscale), and social net-
            work (frequency and intensity of contacts).

A155   Cohler, Bertram J.; Grunebaum, Henry U.; Weiss, Justin L.;
        Hartman, Carol R.; and Gallant, David H.: Perceived life-
        stress and psychopathology among mothers of young children.
        American Journal of Orthopsychiatry 45:58-73, 1975.
            Subjects: 47 recently hospitalized married women with
            young children and 48 never-hospitalized well women
            (matched controls).
            Method: Each subject was individually administered the
RA790A1A5   MMPI, and each was interviewed regarding the occurrence
            of 11 categories of life events for herself, her husband and
            children, and her extended family. In addition, each for-
            mer patient was seen by two project psychiatrists who de-
            termined her diagnosis and assessed her prognosis for
            recovery; at the end of the project, the degree of overall
            change shown by mentally ill mothers was evaluated.

A156   Colligan, Michael J., and Smith, Michael J.: A methodologi-
        cal approach for evaluating outbreaks of mass psychogenic
        illness in industry. Journal of Occupational Medicine 20:
        401-402, 1978.
            The authors report their progress in the development of a
            questionnaire to assess the state and trait characteristics
            that make affected workers vulnerable to mass psycho-
            genic illness and to determine the transmission mecha-
            nisms by which symptoms and beliefs are spread in the
            workplace. The section of the questionnaire devoted to
            assessing the worker's state characteristics includes a
            modified Schedule of Recent Experience.

A157   Cooper, Brian, and Sylph, Judith: Life events and the onset
        of neurotic illness: An investigation in general practice.
        Psychological Medicine 3:421-435, 1973.
>   Subjects: 53 care-seeking patients with neurotic illness of
            clearly defined onset within the past 3 months, and 34
            matched controls who also consulted their doctors but
            were free from psychiatric disturbance in the previous
            3 months.
            Method: Goldberg's standardized clinical interview was
            administered to both groups of patients to determine their
            psychiatric status, and then each patient was interviewed
            at home concerning recent life events experienced in the
            past 3 months. Brown and Birley's life event interview
            method was used, and data were analyzed using Brown
            and Birley's classification of events by class (independent
            vs. possibly independent), by severity of threat, and by
            timing and effect.

A158   Dressler, David M.; Donovan, James M.; and Geller, Ruth A.:
        Life stress and emotional crisis: The idiosyncratic interpre-
        tation of life events. Comprehensive Psychiatry 17:549-558,
        1976.
            Subjects: 40 patients hospitalized on an emergency treat-
            ment unit of a mental health center.
            Method: Each subject was interviewed in detail about his
            or her life situation, and a semistructured questionnaire
            was administered to gather details of events which pre-
            ceded and precipitated hospitalization.

A159   Fratani, Romano Roy: An assessment of the Lüscher Color
        Test on psychiatric and nonpsychiatric cases (Doctoral dis-
        sertation, United States International University, 1975).
        Dissertation Abstracts International 36:2466-B, 1975.
            Subjects: 20 male and 22 female psychiatric inpatients
            and 20 male and 21 female nonpsychiatric hospitalized
            patients.
            Method: To determine whether color stimuli preference
            and responses can indicate group differences, the psy-
            chiatric and nonpsychiatric subjects were administered
            the Lüscher Color Test. To evaluate the Lüscher Color
            Test's ability to assess personality and to measure "stress,"
            both groups also completed the Cornell Medical Index and
            the Schedule of Recent Experience.

A160   Giel, R.; Ten Horn, G. H. M. M.; Ormel, J.; Schudel,
W. J.; and Wiersma, D.: Mental illness, neuroticism and
life events in a Dutch village sample: A follow-up. Psychological Medicine 8:235-243, 1978.
> Subjects: 32 Dutch subjects identified as having psychi-
> atric disorders and a matched group of well controls.
> Method: In 1969 a community survey was conducted in a
> Dutch village and a random sample of the population was
> screened for mental illness; 32 subjects identified then as
> clear psychiatric cases were reevaluated in 1975 and com-
> pared to a matched group of well controls. In the follow-
> up study each subject and control participated in a psy-
> chiatric interview (30 minutes), completed a self-report
> questionnaire covering neuroticism and psychosomatic
> complaints, and provided life event information for the
> past year. The life event interview followed the Brown
> and Birley method, and data were analyzed using the
> Brown and Birley classifications of event independence,
> severity of threat, and timing and effect.

A161   Grant, Igor; Sweetwood, Hervey L.; Yager, Joel; and Gerst,
Marvin S.: Patterns in the relationship of life events and
psychiatric symptoms over time. Journal of Psychosomatic
Research 22:183-191, 1978.
> Subjects: 89 male psychiatric outpatients and 107 hospital
> and university employees.
> Method: All subjects completed a modified Schedule of
> Recent Experience and a Symptom Checklist (SCL) every
> 2 months for 18 months.

A162   Healey, E. Shevy: The onset of chronic insomnia and the
role of life-stress events (Doctoral dissertation, The Ohio
State University, 1976). Dissertation Abstracts International
37:6326-B, 1977.
> Subjects: 31 chronic insomniacs and 31 matched good-
> sleepers.
> Method: All subjects completed a health history, a sleep
> questionnaire, and several personality and psychological
> tests (including the Adjective Check List, Rotter's
> Internal-External Locus of Control Scale, and a Life Sat-
> isfaction Scale). A modified Schedule of Recent Experi-
> ence was administered by interview (covering 5 years and
> beginning 2 years before onset of insomnia).

A163   Howard, Carolyn Ruth: A comparison of the life changes in
        the lives of a state hospital patient group and of a nonpatient
        group (Doctoral dissertation, West Virginia University,
        1976). Dissertation Abstracts International 37:6329-B, 1977.
            Subjects: 110 state mental hospital inpatients and 44 non-
            patients from the same geographical region.
            Method: The Schedule of Recent Experience and a social
            support index were administered to all subjects.

A164   Lahniers, C. Edward, and White, Kim: Changes in environ-
        mental life events and their relationship to psychiatric hos-
        pital admissions. Journal of Nervous and Mental Disease
        163:154-158, 1976.
            Subjects: 116 psychiatric inpatients (44 first admission,
            72 readmission) representing three diagnostic groups
            (schizophrenia, depressive neurosis, alcohol addictions).
            Method: A modified Schedule of Recent Experience (for
            past year) was administered by interview to each patient,
            and data were analyzed to determine the relationship of
            life events to sex, diagnostic classification, and to first
            vs. successive admission to inpatient psychiatric care.

A165   Morrison, James R.; Hudgens, Richard W.; and Barchha,
        Ramnik G.: Life events and psychiatric illness: A study of
        100 patients and 100 controls. British Journal of Psychiatry
        114:423-432, 1968.
            Subjects: 100 hospitalized psychiatric patients and 100
            matched general hospital patients with no history of psy-
            chiatric illness.
            Method: A structured interview was used to collect data
            on present illness; medical, social, and psychiatric his-
            tory; mental status; and recent as well as remote ocur-
            rence of specified life events.

A166   Murphy, George E.; Robins, Eli; Kuhn, Nobuko Obayashi;
        and Christensen, Roger F.: Stress, sickness and psychiatric
        disorder in a "normal" population: A study of 101 young
        women. Journal of Nervous and Mental Disease 134:228-
        236, 1962.
            Subjects: 101 women interviewed shortly after normal
            delivery of a full-term pregnancy.
            Method: Each subject was interviewed to determine
            presence of psychiatric illness. The 26 women who were
            determined to be psychiatrically ill and the remaining
            well group were compared on the basis of "potentially

stressful experiences" (number, kind, and patterns) and the seeking of medical attention in the year prior to interview.

A167   Murthy, R. Srinivasa: Methodological problems in the study of life stress and psychiatric illness: A review. Indian Journal of Psychology 50:1-10, 1975.

BF I I39

The problems of method discussed include the following: dating the onset of illness, definition of life events and estimation of their impact, selection of homogeneous patient samples and appropriate controls, and reliability of recall. The author also compares three life event research instruments: the Schedule of Recent Experience, the Life Event Scale, and the interview method.

A168   Paykel, E. S.: Contribution of life events to causation of psychiatric illness. Psychological Medicine 8:245-253, 1978. In this review and discussion of life events and psychiatric illness research, the author argues that the epidemiological concept of "relative risk" can be usefully applied as a measure of association in retrospective controlled studies. He proposes multifactorial causation as the appropriate model for this kind of research.

A169   Paykel, Eugene S.: Life stress and psychiatric disorder: Applications of the clinical approach. In Stressful Life Events: Their Nature and Effects. Barbara Snell Dohrenwend and Bruce P. Dohrenwend (Eds.), pp. 135-149. New York: Wiley, 1974.

BF575.S
75C64
1973

This chapter summarizes the research of Paykel and his colleagues into the relationship of life events to clinical psychiatric disorders; the data come primarily from the New Haven studies. Included are comparisons between depressives and general population controls; follow-up studies; studies in the perceptions and qualities of life events (degree of upset, exits vs. entrances, desirable vs. undesirable, controllable vs. uncontrollable); studies of life events and suicide attempts; life events and schizophrenia studies; and studies of neurotic syndromes.

A170   Pilowsky, I.: Psychiatric aspects of stress. Ergonomics 16:691-698, 1973. In the context of life change and illness research, the author discusses the way in which studies of individuals in stressful situations have contributed to the understanding of the role of ego functions in adaptation.

A171   Raskin, Marjorie; Rondestvedt, Joanne W.; and Johnson,
George: Anxiety in young adults: A prognostic study.
Journal of Nervous and Mental Disease 154:229-237, 1972.
   Subjects: 50 young adults beginning treatment for states
of anxiety.
   Method: The subjects were followed for 2-3 years to determine which of a number of social and psychological
variables were significantly related to recovery (remis-
sion of anxiety). One of the variables was "precipitating
stress," defined as the recent (in the 6 months preceding
treatment) or imminent occurrence of a life change event.

RC321.J83

A172   Robins, Lee N.: Psychiatric epidemiology. Archives of
General Psychiatry 35:697-702, 1978.
   The author discusses recent advances in the field of psychiatric epidemiology, including studies of life events and
psychiatric disorders, and discusses their applicability
to prevention of illness, intervention, and social policy.
She calls for prospective studies of significant life crises
(e.g., marriage, divorce, death of parents of middle-
aged subjects, major economic changes in a community)
as the next step in the study of who gets sick and why.

RC321A66

A173   Sack, William; Cohen, Stanley; and Grout, Christine: One
year's survey of child psychiatry consultations in a pediatric
hospital. Journal of the American Academy of Child Psychiatry 16:716-727, 1977.
   Subjects: 98 hospitalized children seen in psychiatric
consultations.
   Method: The medical records of the 98 patients were reviewed to determine family background characteristics of
children who received psychiatric consultation and to evaluate their utilization of the liaison service. A follow-up
study collected data concerning 2-year outcome and adjustment and health care utilization after hospitalization.
Families were evaluated and studied as "disordered"
(based on the occurrence of any of 11 "family disorder
events" in the year prior to child's hospitalization) or
"nondisordered" families.

A174   Schless, A. P., and Mendels, J.: Life stress and psychopathology. Psychiatry Digest 28(3):25, 29-31, 34-35, 1977.
   The authors review the research findings which clearly
associate life events and psychopathology and they discuss
important methodologic problems.

A175 Schless, Arthur P.; Teichman, Alicia; Mendels, J.; and
DiGiacomo, Joseph N.: The role of stress as a precipitating factor of psychiatric illness. British Journal of Psychiatry 130:19-22, 1977.

Subjects: 56 psychiatric inpatients, 56 medical and surgical inpatients, and a comparison "normal" population
independently studied by J. K. Myers (New Haven data).
RC 321B856X Method: The psychiatric and nonpsychiatric patients were
administered a modified Schedule of Recent Experience by
interview (for the year preceding hospitalization). The
life event experience of the two groups was compared to
that of the "normal" community sample of 938 studied by
Myers in New Haven [see C22].

A176 Seligman, Roslyn; Gleser, Goldine; Rauh, Joseph; and
Harris, Leonard: The effect of earlier parental loss in
adolescence. Archives of General Psychiatry 31:475-479,
1974.

Subjects: 85 adolescents referred for psychiatric evaluation from the adolescent medical services of a hospital.
RC321A66 Method: The occurrence of earlier parental loss in the
hospital population was documented by referral to their
medical records. Comparison samples were drawn from
two local junior high schools (N=179) and from two medical adolescent clinics (N=186), and a questionnaire concerning "losses" was administered to the two control
groups.

A177 Smith, William G.: Critical life-events and prevention
strategies in mental health. Archives of General Psychiatry 25:103-109, 1971.

Subjects: 880 mental hospital patients admitted consecutively in a 2-year period, and 2,414 survey respondents
in a stratified random sample of the entire population of
a state.
RC321A66 Method: All patients were interviewed about the occurrence in the 12 months preceding admission of 37 critical
life-events designated "potential risk-markers" for mental disturbance requiring hospitalization. In the survey
of the general population, data were gathered concerning
the occurrence of 19 of the original 37 events in the 12
months prior to interview. Life event frequencies of
patient and general population samples were compared.
When five of the 19 life events proved to be positive risk-
markers, a second phase of study was undertaken with a

second patient sample to determine the temporal relationship between occurrence of risk-marker and onset of disorder.

A178   Smith-Meyer, H.; Valen, H. A.; Flekkoy, K.; Floistad, I.; Haseth, K.; and Astrup, C.: Psychophysiological studies of a geographically defined population. Activitas Nervosa Superior 18:145-156, 1976.

> Subjects: 22 neurotic patients, 12 psychotic patients, and 16 normal control subjects drawn from a 30-year follow-up study of psychiatric morbidity in a Danish fishing village.
> Method: Subjects were administered a battery of psychophysiological tests and cognitive measures. A modified Social Readjustment Rating Questionnaire was administered to obtain patient groups' and normals' subjective evaluation of life change magnitudes.

A179   Swart, Edward Carl: Differential life change in psychiatric patient and control groups: A retrospective study (Doctoral dissertation, Wayne State University, 1976). Dissertation Abstracts International 37:2531-B, 1976.

> Subjects: 3 diagnostic groups (patients with schizophrenia, neurosis, or personality disorder) and 1 control group.
> Method: All subjects completed the Schedule of Recent Experience (for past year). The MMPI standard and content scales for females were used in the analysis of sex differences.

A180   Weissman, Myrna M., and Klerman, Gerald L.: Epidemiology of mental disorders: Emerging trends in the United States. Archives of General Psychiatry 35:705-712, 1978.

> The authors discuss recent advances in the field of psychiatric epidemiology and present a "Model for Epidemiology of Mental Disorders" that includes "life stress" as an independent variable.

SPECIFIC ILLNESS:
Mental Disorders—Depression
(A181–A216)

A181   Alarcon, Renato, and Covi, Lino: The precipitating event in depression: Some methodological considerations. Journal of Nervous and Mental Disease 155:379-391, 1972.

The authors review the literature and discuss problems that obscure or confuse the research findings: selection of representative patient samples and control groups, methods of reporting and defining life events, and statistical methods.

A182   Bebbington, Paul E.: The epidemiology of depressive disorder. Culture, Medicine and Psychiatry 2:297-341, 1978. This analytical review includes a section devoted to five problem areas in the life events approach to the study of depression: (1) retrospective method, (2) independence of events, (3) representative samples, (4) specificity of life events, and (5) quantification of data.

A183   Briscoe, C. William, and Smith, James B.: Depression in bereavement and divorce. Relationship to primary depressive illness: A study of 128 subjects. Archives of General Psychiatry 32:439-443, 1975.
RC 321 A66   Subjects: 43 recently divorced subjects, 22 recently bereaved subjects, and 88 hospitalized subjects, all with the same psychiatric diagnosis of primary affective disease ("unipolar depressed").
Method: The 88 hospitalized subjects were first screened to make certain none had experienced any of 9 specified precipitating life events. Then all subjects were interviewed and compared for the following factors: age, sex, history of previous episodes of depression, incidence of psychiatric illness in first-degree relatives, and differences in depressive symptoms.

A184   Brown, George W.: Life-events and the onset of depressive and schizophrenic conditions. In Life Stress and Illness. E. K. Eric Gunderson and Richard H. Rahe (Eds.), pp. 164-188. Springfield, Illinois: Charles C Thomas, 1974.
RC49. G85   The author describes the Camberwell (London) studies of depression and schizophrenia reported previously (see A220, A221, A150, A151), giving special attention to the way life events were selected for inclusion in the interviews, how life events were rated, and how they were evaluated. This paper concludes with a discussion of both the practical implications and the theoretical significance of the findings in the Camberwell studies.

A185   Brown, George W.; Bhrolchain, Maire Ni; and Harris, Tirril: Social class and psychiatric disturbance among
HM1S73   women in an urban population. Sociology 9:225-254, 1975.

Subjects: Two samples of women, aged 18-65, living in the Camberwell (South London) area: 220 women drawn from a random sample of the Camberwell community, and 114 female patients in treatment for primary depression (onset within a year of interview).

Method: All subjects were interviewed by trained interviewers following an established format. Two semistructured instruments were used as parts of the interview: the Present State Examination (for psychiatric disturbance within the past 12 months) and the Brown and Birley life-events interview and rating method.

A186 Brown, George W.; Bhrolchain, Maire Ni; and Harris, Tirril: A study of depression in women: A reply to Keith Hope's critical note. Sociology 11:527-531, 1977.

The authors give detailed responses to questions raised about their Camberwell study (A185) by Keith Hope (see A191).

A187 Brown, George W., and Harris, Tirril: Social origins of depression: A reply. Psychological Medicine 8:577-588, 1978.

The authors respond to Tennant and Bebbington's critique (A212) of their work. They refer some of the questions raised by Tennant and Bebbington to their book, Social Origins of Depression, while using other questions as the occasion for a discussion of the complexities of statistical analysis and interpretation of data.

A188 Brown, George W.; Harris, Tirril; and Copeland, John R.: Depression and loss. British Journal of Psychiatry 130: 1-18, 1977.

Subjects: 114 women being treated for depression by psychiatrists and 76 women found to be suffering from depression in a sample of 458 women living in the Camberwell area of London.

Method: Subjects were interviewed about recent losses (in the 2 years prior to onset of depression) and past losses (any time before the previous 2 years) of parents, sibling, husbands, and children. The nature of the loss as well as the timing of the loss was studied in relation to illness onset and severity of depressive symptoms.

A189 Cadoret, Remi J.; Winokur, George; Dorzab, Joe; and Baker, Max: Depressive disease: Life events and onset of illness. Archives of General Psychiatry 26:133-136, 1972.

Subjects: 100 inpatients with unipolar depressive illness.
Method: Data were gathered by interview about five types
of precipitating events: (1) loss of parents by death, divorce, or separation before age 16; (2) death of family
member or friend in the 12 months prior to hospitalization; (3) threatened personal losses; (4) recent physical
illness (previous 6 months); and (5) personal loss preceding onset of depressive symptoms. Losses by subjects
with earlier-onset disease (before age 40) were compared
to those by subjects with later-onset disease (after age 40),
and 51 well controls (matched for age and sex) were compared to the patient group reporting personal loss preceding onset of depressive symptoms.

A190   Hall, Kathleen S.; Dunner, David L.; Zeller, Gary; and
        Fieve, Ronald R.: Bipolar illness: A prospective study of
        life events. Comprehensive Psychiatry 18:497-502, 1977.
        Subjects: 38 bipolar manic-depressive patients who were
        being treated chronically with lithium carbonate.
        Method: The subjects were studied prospectively for 10
        months by collecting life event data at each physician visit
        and comparing the life event experience of the four out-
        come groups (21 remained euthymic, 6 became hypomanic
        or manic, 8 became depressed, and 3 became hypomanic
        and depressed). Subjects completed an 86-item life event
        questionnaire for the interval between visits and then were
        interviewed about the reported events: degree of "stress"
        the event created (5-point scale), desirability of the event
        (4-point scale), and required readjustment of daily rou-
        tine (4-point scale). In addition, subjects were asked to
        report which, if any, events they anticipated experiencing
        before their next visit.

A191   Hope, Keith: Critical note: Comments on a study of depres-
        sion in women. Sociology 10:321-323, 1976.
        The author raises six questions about procedure and
HMI573 method used by Brown and associates in their Camberwell
        study (see A185). The questions concern sampling pro-
        cedure, assignment of social class, and class differences
        in perception and exposure to misfortunes and threatening
        events. (See A186 for Brown et al. reply to Keith Hope.)

A192   Hudgens, Richard W.: Personal catastrophe and depression:
        A consideration of the subject with respect to medically ill
        adolescents, and a requiem for retrospective life-event

studies. In <u>Stressful Life Events: Their Nature and Effects</u>. Barbara Snell Dohrenwend and Bruce P. Dohrenwend (Eds.), pp. 119-134. New York: Wiley, 1974.

<u>Subjects</u>: 101 adolescents hospitalized on medical and surgical wards for nonpsychiatric disorders.

<u>Method</u>: Each patient and a relative were extensively interviewed for psychiatric, medical, social, scholastic, and family histories. Medical records and school records were also consulted. The 22 subjects who were found to have current or past depressive syndrome were compared to the 78 psychiatrically well subjects for the nature, timing, and duration of life-event "stress" and its relation to the onset of depressive syndrome.

A193   Hudgens, Richard W.; Morrison, James R.; and Barchha, Ramnik G.: Life events and onset of primary affective disorders. <u>Archives of General Psychiatry</u> <u>16</u>:134-135, 1967.

<u>Subjects</u>: 40 hospitalized patients with primary affective disorders (34 depression, 6 mania) and 40 matched controls from the medical and surgical hospital wards who had no history of psychiatric illness.

<u>Method</u>: Each subject was interviewed extensively and medical records were also examined to obtain detailed medical, social, and psychiatric histories, including the occurrence of life events in the remote and recent past. Temporal relationships of life events and illness onset were studied.

A194   Johnson, G. F. S., and Leeman, M. M.: Onset of illness in bipolar manic-depressives and their affectively ill first-degree relatives. <u>Biological Psychiatry</u> <u>12</u>:733-741, 1977.

<u>Subjects</u>: 35 patients and their available first-degree relatives.

<u>Method</u>: Subjects and their relatives were interviewed for family history and illness data. One variable studied was "type of stress," including life events, reported as precipitating initial episode of illness in subjects and their relatives.

A195   Johnson, Norma Jean Wohlgamuth: Life events and depression (Doctoral dissertation, Rutgers University, 1977). <u>Dissertation Abstracts International</u> 38:2864-B, 1977.

<u>Subjects</u>: A "large research sample" of recently hospitalized depressed women and well controls.

Method: Each subject was administered a modified
Schedule of Recent Experience (for the 2 months preceding hospitalization or interview). Subjects' life events
and measures of depression-related affects and behaviors
were compared. Case histories of two clinically depressed
subjects are also presented, and the findings of the case
study method are related to the findings of the larger research study.

A196   Klerman, Gerald L., and Paykel, Eugene S.: Depressive
pattern, social background, and hospitalization. Journal of
Nervous and Mental Disease 150:466-478, 1970.
Subjects: 57 depressed patients from three psychiatric
inpatient facilities (a general hospital psychiatric ward,
a mental health center, and a state mental hospital).
Method: Each subject was interviewed by a research
psychiatrist soon after admission for data on history and
clinical symptomatology. After clinical improvement or
recovery, 47 of the original subjects were again interviewed; a modified Schedule of Recent Experience was
administered by interview (for the 6 months preceding
symptomatic onset of current depressive episode) and
subjects completed the Maudsley Personality Inventory.

A197   Leff, Melitta J.; Roatch, John F.; and Bunney, William
E., Jr.: Environmental factors preceding the onset of
severe depressions. Psychiatry 33:293-311, 1970.
Subjects: 13 patients with "endogenous" and 27 patients
with "nonendogenous" types of depression.
Method: Patients and their families were interviewed for
environmental and behavioral events occurring prior to
the onset of severe depression. Types of events studied
ranged from life change events such as moving, bereavement, and physical illness, to "stressful" events such as
"failure of children to meet parents' goals," "damage to
social status," and "made to face denied reality."

A198   Okuma, Teruo, and Shimoyama, Naoko: Course of endogenous manic-depressive psychosis, precipitating factors and
premorbid personality—a statistical study. Folia Psychiatrica et Neurologica Japonica 26:19-33, 1972.
Subjects: 134 patients with endogenous manic-depressive
psychosis who had had more than 3 manic or depressive
episodes in their history.

Method: Subjects were interviewed, a personality inventory was administered, and medical records were reviewed. Subjects were compared to determine age at onset of disease, length of symptom-free interval, hereditary factors, premorbid personality, and precipitating factors of illness episodes (defined as "any psychic or physical events which occurred or lasted within 3 months preceding the episode and which were judged by the authors to have been stressful to the patients").

A199   Parsons, Oscar A.: Life events, stress and depression. Biological Psychology Bulletin 4:143-151, 1975.

The author briefly reviews the retrospective and prospective studies of the relationship of life events to the onset of illness, describing methods and tools such as the life chart, the Schedule of Recent Experience, and the Social Readjustment Rating Scale.

A200   Patrick, V.; Dunner, D. L.; and Fieve, R. R.: Life events and primary affective illness. Acta Psychiatrica Scandinavica 58:48-55, 1978.

Subjects: 183 patients with primary affective disorder who were attending a research lithium clinic.
Method: Subjects completed a life events questionnaire to document possibly relevant precipitants in the 3 months prior to illness onset. The list of events was derived from a study of the medical records of more than 200 former clinic patients, and it included all life events covered by the Schedule of Recent Experience and by Paykel's life events questionnaire. Medical records, research records, and direct interviews were used to collect family histories of affective disorder in parents and siblings.

A201   Paykel, E. S.: Classification of depressed patients: A cluster analysis derived grouping. British Journal of Psychiatry 118:275-288, 1971.

Subjects: 165 depressed patients from a variety of treatment settings.
Method: The same procedure described in A207 was followed: Each subject was interviewed and rated for clinical symptoms, previous history, recent life events, and premorbid neuroticism. A special cluster analysis was performed on the ratings to classify individuals into 4 groups.

A202   Paykel, Eugene S.: Correlates of a depressive typology.
Archives of General Psychiatry 27:203-210, 1972.
    Subjects: 165 depressed patients.
    Method: This study presents further analysis of the 4-
RC321A66   group typology derived in A201 above. In this work, additional correlates were examined to test the validity of
the typology.

A203   Paykel, Eugene S.: Life events and acute depression. In
Separation and Depression, John Paul Scott and Edward C.
Senay (Eds.), pp. 215-236. Publication No. 94. Washington, D.C.: American Association for the Advancement of
Science, 1973.
RC537. S46   The author reviews selected studies, particularly controlled studies of separations and depressions. He discusses evidence on the topics of specificity of stress and
the qualities of life events, perceptions of life events by
"normals" and depressives, the nature of endogenous depression, and elements which modify the relationship of
life events to depression.

A204   Paykel, Eugene S.: Life stress, depression and attempted
suicide. Journal of Human Stress 2(3):3-12, 1976.
The author summarizes a series of controlled studies
carried out with colleagues at Yale University concerning
the relationship of life events to depression and suicide
attempts. (For original reports of studies summarized
here see A205, A208, B102, H23, A211, A196, A224,
and C38.)

A205   Paykel, Eugene S.: Recent life events and clinical depression. In Life Stress and Illness. E. K. Eric Gunderson and
Richard H. Rahe (Eds.), pp. 134-163. Springfield, Illinois:
Charles C Thomas, 1974.
    The author summarizes research carried out with col-
RC49.G85   leagues at Yale University between 1967 and 1971. The
discussion covers a wide range of topics: methodological
issues, comparisons between depressives and general
population controls, categories of life events, specificity,
follow-up studies, magnitude of effect in life event studies,
scaling of life events, perceptions of stress, endogenous
depressions, and life event and symptom patterns.

A206   Paykel, E. S.; Klerman, G. L.; and Prusoff, B. A.: Prognosis of depression and the endogenous-neurotic distinction. Psychological Medicine 4:57-64, 1974.
    Subjects: 190 depressed patients.
    Method: These subjects, drawn from the original survey of depressed patients reported in A207, were reinterviewed 10 months after admission to the survey. Predictor variables were derived from the original data of the survey study and included a Recent Life Events score. [See also A201, A202.]

A207   Paykel, Eugene S.; Klerman, Gerald L.; and Prusoff, Brigitte A.: Treatment setting and clinical depression. Archives of General Psychiatry 22:11-21, 1970.
    Subjects: 220 depressed patients from four kinds of treatment settings (100 from outpatient clinics, 30 from a day hospital, 25 briefly hospitalized at an emergency treatment service, and 65 hospital inpatients).
    Method: A clinical interview based on the Hamilton Rating Scale for Depression was conducted by a research psychiatrist soon after admission to obtain patient's history and clinical symptomatology. After clinical improvement or recovery, 185 patients were again interviewed. Self-report instruments were administered at that time and ratings were made on the following factors: sociodemographic characteristics; recent life events (Paykel et al.'s 60-item Recent Life Events interview for the past 6 months, with scores based on life event weightings derived from the Holmes and Rahe Social Readjustment Rating Scale); premorbid adjustment (Maudsley Personality Inventory); psychiatric history; and history of present illness and clinical symptoms.

RC321A66

A208   Paykel, Eugene S.; Myers, Jerome K.; Dienelt, Marcia N.; Klerman, Gerald L.; Lindenthal, Jacob J.; and Pepper, Max P.: Life events and depression: A controlled study. Archives of General Psychiatry 21:753-760, 1969.
    Subjects: 185 depressed patients from a variety of inpatient and outpatient treatment settings and 185 matched well controls drawn from a New Haven community survey.
    Method: All subjects were interviewed for life event experience, using a list of life events based on items in the Social Readjustment Rating Scale. Patients were asked about events in the 6 months prior to onset of depression; controls were asked about events in the 12 months prior

RC321A66

to interview. Analysis of data includes frequency of individual events and categorization of events (desirable vs. undesirable, exits vs. entrances of the social field, area of activity).

A209   Paykel, Eugene S.; Prusoff, Brigitte; and Klerman, Gerald L.: The endogenous-neurotic continuum in depression: Rater independence and factor distributions. Journal of Psychiatric Research 8:73-90, 1971.

    Subjects: 220 depressed patients.

RC321.J838 Method: The same procedures described in A207 were followed. Data were analyzed for correlations of life event scores, neuroticism, and independently rated clinical symptoms in terms of the endogenous-neurotic distinction.

A210   Paykel, Eugene S.; Prusoff, Brigitte A.; Klerman, Gerald L.; Haskell, David; and DiMascio, Alberto: Clinical response to amitriptyline among depressed women. Journal of Nervous and Mental Disease 156:149-165, 1973.

    Subjects: 85 female depressed patients.

RC321.J83 Method: The patients were treated for four weeks with amitriptyline, and predictive analyses of outcome were performed using two models—typological and regressional—based on the same 29 predictor variables. [For descriptions of four-group typology, cluster analysis derivation, and multiple variables including recent life event experience, see A201, A202, and A207.]

A211   Paykel, E. S., and Tanner, J.: Life events, depressive relapse and maintenance treatment. Psychological Medicine 6:481-485, 1976.

    Subjects: 30 recovered depressed women undergoing clinical relapse and 30 matched patients who did not relapse.

    Method: In a controlled trial of maintenance treatment with amitriptyline and psychotherapy, subjects in different treatment subgroups were interviewed at 2, 4, and 8 months for their monthly life event experience in the interval between interviews. When a subject relapsed, she was interviewed again to document life events in the period between last interview and relapse. Data were collected by a semistructured 60-item life event interview.

A212 Tennant, Christopher, and Bebbington, Paul: The social causation of depression: A critique of the work of Brown and his colleagues. Psychological Medicine 8:565-575, 1978.
The authors critique the Camberwell (London) studies of Brown and colleagues (A185 and A188), with particular emphasis placed on methodology, delineation of variables, statistical methods, and mode of argument. (See A187 for a reply by Brown and Harris.)

A213 Thomson, Kay C., and Hendrie, Hugh C.: Environmental stress in primary depressive illness. Archives of General Psychiatry 26:130-132, 1972.
Subjects: 74 patients with primary depressive disorders, and 2 control groups (21 patients with early polyarthritis and 37 hospital staff members and their friends) matched for age and sex.
Method: All patients were interviewed to determine onset of illness, and patients were asked to complete the Schedule of Recent Experience for the year prior to illness onset. The staff control group completed the Schedule of Recent Experience for the previous year. Half the depressed patients and the staff control group also completed a "self-rating stress scale" (5-point scale ranging from "much less" to "much more stress than usual"). A family history rating was assigned to each patient based on interview data concerning illness in relatives. The depressed patients were studied in 3 groups: negative vs. positive family history; endogenous vs. reactive depression groups; and bipolar vs. unipolar group.

RC321A66

A214 Tonks, Clive M.; Paykel, Eugene S.; and Klerman, Gerald L.: Clinical depressions among Negroes. American Journal of Psychiatry 127:329-335, 1970.
Subjects: 31 black and 187 white depressed patients.
Method: Each subject was interviewed and rated for history and clinical symptomatology using a modification of the Hamilton Rating Scale for Depression. A semistructured interview for recent life events (6 months prior to illness onset) was conducted and a Total Recent Life Events Score was calculated using item values from the Social Readjustment Rating Scale. Subjects also completed the Maudsley Personality Inventory. A psychiatrist judged each patient's severity of illness on a 7-point scale, and the Hollingshead Two-Factor Index of social class was also used to compare the two groups and to select a matched

RC321A52

subsample of 31 blacks and 31 whites who were then compared on the basis of 38 variables.

A215   Weissman, Myrna M., and Klerman, Gerald L.: Sex differences and the epidemiology of depression. Archives of General Psychiatry 34:98-111, 1977.

RC321A66

The authors review the research reports of different rates of depression between the sexes in the United States and around the world, and they then analyze the possible explanations for such findings. Two topics included in the discussion are the higher frequencies of life events in women's lives and women's perceptions of life events.

A216   Weissman, Myrna M.; Prusoff, Brigitte A.; and Klerman, Gerald L.: Personality and the prediction of long-term outcome of depression. American Journal of Psychiatry 135: 797-800, 1978.

Subjects: 150 women who had undergone treatment on an outpatient basis for acute depression.

Method: At follow-up interviews 8, 20, and 48 months after the occurrence of an acute episode, data were col-

RC321A52

lected to assign patients to one of three outcome groups: asymptomatic, moderate, and chronic. A number of pretreatment variables were analyzed for their ability to predict long-term outcome: age, race, social class, marital status, religion, number of previous depressions, number of suicide attempts, early deaths of or separations from significant others during childhood, neurotic traits as a child, life events in the 6 months prior to acute episode (measured by Paykel's Recent Life Events Scale), severity of pretreatment symptoms, and personality (Maudsley Personality Inventory, neuroticism and extroversion scales).

SPECIFIC ILLNESS:
Mental Disorders—Schizophrenia
(A217-A232)

A217   Bagley, Christopher: The social aetiology of schizophrenia in immigrant groups. International Journal of Social Psychiatry 17:292-304, 1971.

Subjects: 27 West Indian schizophrenics, 27 West Indians in the community who had never had a psychiatric consultation, and 27 English-born schizophrenics: all males and

all drawn from an epidemiologic survey of mental illness
in ethnic minorities in the Camberwell district of London.
Method: Each subject was interviewed by a research psychiatrist for data concerning three possible factors in
West Indians' schizophrenia: (1) life crises, measured
using the Brown and Birley life events interview method;
(2) chronic environmental hazards (overcrowding, poverty,
working conditions, etc.); and (3) stresses of "goal-
striving" in the face of limited opportunities.

A218   Beck, James C.: Social influences on the prognosis of
schizophrenia. Schizophrenia Bulletin 4:86-101, 1978.
This selective review of the literature includes discussion
of the influence of life events on the course and prognosis
of schizophrenia.

A219   Beck, James C., and Worthen, Kathy: Precipitating stress,
crisis theory, and hospitalization in schizophrenia and depression. Archives of General Psychiatry 26:213-219, 1972.
Subjects: 50 consecutively admitted psychiatric ward inpatients (15 with schizophrenia, 21 with depression, 14
with other disorders).

RC321A66

Method: In addition to data collected in the usual clinical
interview with the patient, life event experience data were
collected in 4 subsequent research interviews (48 hours
after admission, at discharge, and then at 6 weeks and at
3 months after hospitalization). Lists of the 50 reported
life event situations preceding hospitalization were given
to 100 nonpsychiatric outpatients who rated the events on
a 5-point scale ("not at all upsetting" to "the most upsetting thing if it happened to mc"). Social characteristics
of patients and hazardousness of precipitant situation were
studied within and between diagnostic groups.

A220   Birley, J. L. T., and Brown, G. W.: Crises and life changes
preceding the onset or relapse of acute schizophrenia: Clinical aspects. British Journal of Psychiatry 116:327-333, 1970.
Subjects: 50 hospitalized schizophrenic patients who had

RC321 B856X

experienced an acute onset or relapse within 3 months of
admission.
Method: This companion article to A221 presents data on
the clinical aspects of the Brown and Birley schizophrenia
study. The life events data (12 weeks prior to onset or relapse) obtained from interviewing patients or their relatives are studied in relation to type and timing of onset,

diagnostic category, symptomatology, and medication reduction or stoppage.

A221 Brown, George W., and Birley, J. L. T.: Crises and life changes and the onset of schizophrenia. Journal of Health and Social Behavior 9:203-214, 1968.

Subjects: 50 patients with an acute onset of schizophrenia and a general population comparison group of 325 employed adults.

Method: Patients and their relatives were interviewed separately about the occurrence of life events in their family in the 13 weeks prior to the onset of schizophrenic symptoms; the comparison group from the general population was given the same interview concerning events in the preceding 3 months. A detailed description of the Brown and Birley life events interview method is presented, including selection and dating of life events and the distinctions made between "independent" and "possibly independent" life events. [See A220 for the companion report on clinical aspects of this study.]

R11.J687

A222 Dencker, S. J.; Frankenberg, K.; Malm, U.; and Zell, B.: A controlled one-year study of pipotiazine palmitate and fluphenazine decanoate in chronic schizophrenic syndromes: Evaluation of results at 6 and 12 months' trial. Acta Psychiatrica Scandinavica 241(Supplement):101-118, 1973.

Subjects: 67 schizophrenic patients who needed maintenance therapy with neuroleptics.

Method: To evaluate the dosage, effects, and side effects of the two drugs, monthly monitoring was conducted for 12 months. In addition to laboratory examinations at the end of each 6 months of the trial, patients were assessed and rated on the following: background data, global rating, symptoms, extrapyramidal side-effects, social function, and life events (Schedule of Recent Experience).

RC331.A248X

A223 Jacobs, Selby, and Myers, Jerome: Recent life events and acute schizophrenic psychosis: A controlled study. Journal of Nervous and Mental Disease 162:75-87, 1976.

Subjects: 62 first-admission schizophrenic patients and 62 matched "normal" adults from a community health survey.

Method: All subjects were interviewed about the occurrence of life events in the year prior to onset of illness (time of interview for control group). The 58-item life

RC321.J83

event list was based on schedules developed by Holmes and Rahe, Antonovsky and Kats, and Paykel and Myers. Data were analyzed for differences between schizophrenics and normals in the overall reporting of life events and for differences in the kinds of reported life events (area of social activity, desirability, entrances or exits from social field, etc.).

A224 Jacobs, S. C.; Prusoff, B. A.; and Paykel, E. S.: Recent life events in schizophrenia and depression. Psychological Medicine 4:444-453, 1974.

Subjects: 50 first-admission schizophrenic patients and 50 matched depressive patients.

Method: All subjects were interviewed for the occurrence of life events in the 6 months prior to onset of illness. The 59-item list of life events was based on schedules developed by Holmes and Rahe, Antonovsky and Kats, and modifications by Paykel and Myers. Data were analyzed for differences between schizophrenics and depressives in number, type, severity, and pattern of recent life events, including categorization of events by social area, desirability, and control.

A225 Langsley, Donald G.; Pittman, Frank S.; and Swank, Glenn E.: Family crises in schizophrenics and other mental patients. Journal of Nervous and Mental Disease 149:270-276, 1969.

Subjects: 50 schizophrenic patients and their families and 50 nonschizophrenic mental patients and their families.

Method: Half of the subjects in each patient group were admitted to the hospital for treatment, while the remaining half in each patient group was treated by family crisis therapy on an outpatient basis. Baseline (admission to treatment) and follow-up (6 months after termination of treatment) data were collected using a newly developed instrument. It measures the intensity and frequency of troubles within a family (a schedule of 30 "hazardous events" given scores based on similar life events in the Social Readjustment Rating Scale) and the manner in which each problem is resolved.

A226 Leff, J. P.; Hirsch, S. R.; Gaind, R.; Rohde, P. D.; and Stevens, B. C.: Life events and maintenance therapy in
schizophrenic relapse. British Journal of Psychiatry 123: 659-660, 1973.

Subjects: 39 acute and 77 chronic schizophrenia patients
in two placebo-controlled clinical trials.
Method: Patients were randomly assigned to drug or
placebo treatment. Each patient was administered the
Brown and Birley life events interview at the end of the
trial period if the subject remained well, or at time of
relapse. Data were analyzed by comparing well vs. relapsed and drug vs. placebo patient groups in terms of
number, kind, and timing of reported life events.

A227 Malm, Ulf: Discussion on assessment of psychiatric and
social state. British Journal of Clinical Pharmacology 3
(Supplement):391-393, 1976.
In discussing an article by Dr. J. P. Leff, the author
proposes use of a modified Schedule of Recent Experience
to assess a schizophrenic patient's "ability to encounter
change and to initiate actions in real life." Methods to
assess changes over time are needed to complement the
existing, reliable assessment methods for psychopathology.

A228 McCabe, Michael S.: Reactive psychoses and schizophrenia
with good prognosis. Archives of General Psychiatry 33:
571-576, 1976.
Subjects: 40 consecutively admitted patients diagnosed in
RC321A66 Aarhus, Denmark, as having reactive psychoses, and 28
consecutively admitted patients diagnosed in St. Louis,
Missouri, as having schizophrenia with good prognosis.
Method: Each patient was interviewed systematically for
social, medical, and psychiatric history data (including
precipitating life events), and each was evaluated with the
Present State Examination (PSE). A clinical comparison
of patients from the two studies is made in terms of differences in diagnostic criteria and duration of index episode, premorbid functioning, precipitating events, hallu-
cinations, delusions, and other disturbances, affective
symptoms, and first-rank symptoms of schizophrenia.

A229 Schwartz, Carol C., and Myers, Jerome K.: Life events and
schizophrenia. I. Comparison of schizophrenics with a community sample. Archives of General Psychiatry 34:1238-
1241, 1977.
RC321A66 Subjects: 132 formerly hospitalized schizophrenics living
in the community and 132 matched, nonpatient subjects
also living in the community.

Method: Each former patient was interviewed 2 to 3 years after discharge from the hospital; the control group was drawn from the 1967 New Haven field study of Myers et al. [see C22]. Psychiatric impairment was measured by the Gurin Mental Status Index. A list of 64 life events, drawn from the work of Holmes and Rahe and of Antonovsky and Kats, was constructed and subjects were queried about their occurrence in the 6 months prior to interview. Life events were categorized in four ways: by area of social activity, as exits or entrances in the social field, by desirability, and as controlled or uncontrolled events. [See A230 for Part II of this study.]

A230 Schwartz, Carol C., and Myers, Jerome K.: Life events and schizophrenia. II. Impact of life events on symptom configuration. Archives of General Psychiatry 34:1242-1245, 1977.

Subjects: 132 formerly hospitalized schizophrenics living in the community.

Method: Data collected by interviews described in Part I (A229) are used to study the importance of life events in determining psychiatric impairment in relation to other predictor variables (9 treatment variables, 8 natural history variables, and 8 sociodemographic variables). Life events are rated in terms of number, psychological control dimension, and qualitative nature. Symptom dimensions were measured using data from the Gurin Mental Status Index, the Psychiatric Evaluation Form, and the New Haven Schizophrenia Index.

A231 Steinberg, Harry R., and Durell, Jack: A stressful social situation as a precipitant of schizophrenic symptoms: An epidemiological study. British Journal of Psychiatry 114: 1097-1105, 1968.

Subjects: Every uncommissioned soldier in the U.S. Army who was hospitalized for schizophrenia during the period 1956-1960.

Method: Medical and service records were reviewed to determine rates of hospitalization for schizophrenia according to length-of-service categories (early months of service vs. second year of service). Two subsamples of patients' records were studied to determine whether the finding of increased rates of onset in early months of service was the result of early detection of chronic cases or a genuine increase.

A232 Zubin, Joseph, and Spring, Bonnie: Vulnerability—a new
view of schizophrenia. Journal of Abnormal Psychology 86:
103-126, 1977.
      After reviewing six etiological approaches to psycho-
pathology, the authors propose "vulnerability" as the
common denominator and discuss methods for finding
"markers" of vulnerability. The theoretical presentation includes sections devoted to the relationship of premorbid coping ability and life events to vulnerability and
adaptation.

RC321.J7

SPECIFIC ILLNESS:
Mental Disorders—Alcoholism and Drug Addiction
(A233-A254)

A233 Andersen, Marcia Susan DeCann: Life change and illness in
two drug treatment modalities (Doctoral dissertation, University of Michigan, 1978). Dissertation Abstracts International 39:2742-B, 1978.
      Subjects: 47 drug-dependent clients, 28 of whom were
outpatients in methadone clinics and 23 of whom were in
residential therapeutic communities.
      Method: All subjects completed a modified Schedule of
Recent Experience and the Recent Life Changes Questionnaire (for the past 2 years). Illness reports were obtained for the same 2-year period (number of illnesses,
type, time of onset, and perceived severity), and medical
records were reviewed to obtain data on the percentage of
urine samples found to contain illicit drugs.

A234 Bell, D. S.: The precipitants of amphetamine addiction.
British Journal of Psychiatry 119:171-177, 1971.
      Subjects: 34 amphetamine addicts.
      Method: Subjects were interviewed for a history of the
life events preceding onset of addiction.

BC321B
856X

A235 Bell, Roger A.; Keeley, Kim A.; Clements, Ray D.; Warheit, George J.; and Holzer, Charles E., III: Alcoholism,
life events, and psychiatric impairment. Annals of the New
York Academy of Sciences 273:467-480, 1976.
      Subjects: 122 recently admitted patients in a detoxifica-
tion unit and a "normative" sample of 2,029 respondents
to a community survey.

Method: Detoxification patients were interviewed with a
215-item schedule to obtain data concerning demographic
variables, social history, family and interpersonal relationships, alcohol behavior history, mental health, and
social well-being. The Health Opinion Survey (HOS) measured psychiatric impairment, and a "Stressful Life
Events Inventory" documented numbers and kinds of experienced life events. Respondents in the community survey were interviewed with a 403-item schedule which collected comparable data.

A236   Bell, Roger A.; Warheit, George J.; Bell, Richard A.; and
Sanders, Grover: An analytic comparison of persons arrested
for driving while intoxicated and alcohol detoxification patients.
Alcoholism: Clinical and Experimental Research 2:241-248,
1978.
Subjects: 247 detoxification unit patients and 118 drivers
arrested for driving while intoxicated and now attending
DWI school.
Method: All subjects were administered a structured interview for the following data: sociodemographic characteristics; drinking attitudes and behaviors; functioning and
social consequences; life crisis events (number in past
year, number in lifetime, and kinds of events); the Leighton Health Opinion Survey (mental health score); self-
report health history; and perceptions of self and relations
to others.

A237   Blum, J., and Levine, J.: Maturity, depression, and life
events in middle-aged alcoholics. Addictive Behaviors 1:
37-45, 1975.
Subjects: 28 middle-aged hospitalized alcoholics.
Method: Subjects were administered the following instru-
ments: the Rudie and McGaughran Essential-Reactive
Alcoholism Scale, the Phillips-Ziegler Social Competence
Index, the Beck Depression Inventory and the Zung Self-
Rating Depression Scale (each given twice, for "before
hospitalization" and "now"), and the Schedule of Recent
Experience (for the 2 years prior to testing).

A238   Dembo, Richard, and LaGrand, Louis E.: A research model
for a comprehensive, health service oriented understanding
of drug use. Journal of Drug Issues 8:355-371, 1978.
The authors review the literature and then present an outline for a research model. One section of the proposed

model includes the assessment of the relationship of life changes to use of drugs.

A239   Dudley, Donald L.; Mules, Janet E.; Roszell, Douglas K.; Glickfeld, Gail; and Hague, William H.: Frequency and magnitude distribution of life change in heroin and alcohol addicts. International Journal of the Addictions 11:977-987, 1976.
> Subjects: 50 male heroin addicts and 66 male alcohol addicts.
> Method: This companion article to A240 reports and analyzes in greater detail the Schedule of Recent Experience data collected in the first study.

A240   Dudley, Donald L.; Roszell, Douglas K.; Mules, Janet E.; and Hague, William H.: Heroin vs alcohol addiction—quantifiable psychosocial similarities and differences. Journal of Psychosomatic Research 18:327-335, 1974.
> Subjects: 50 male heroin addicts and 66 male alcohol addicts.
> Method: All subjects completed three instruments: the Schedule of Recent Experience (to measure life change during previous 3 years), the Social Readjustment Rating Questionnaire (to measure perception of life change event magnitude), and the Seriousness of Illness Rating Questionnaire (to measure perception of seriousness of illness). Results are also compared to "normative values" originally obtained by Holmes, Rahe, Wyler, and Masuda in developing the SRRQ and SIRQ instruments. [See also A239.]

RC52.J6

A241   Duncan, David F.: Life stress as a precursor to adolescent drug dependence. International Journal of the Addictions 12: 1047-1056, 1977.
> Subjects: 31 drug-dependent adolescents.
> Method: Each subject was interviewed for admission to a halfway house for adolescent drug abusers and was asked for a history of his or her drug use. Each subject then completed Coddington's Schedule of Recent Experience for junior and senior high school students (for events in the year prior to first use of illicit drugs). Coddington's "normative" data are compared to drug abusers' life change data.

A242   Duncan, David F.: Stress and adolescent drug dependence: A brief report. IRCS Medical Science: Psychology and Psychiatry; Social and Occupational Medicine 4:381, 1976.

Subjects: 31 drug-dependent adolescents.
Method: This is a preliminary report of results obtained
using Coddington's Schedule of Recent Experience for adolescents. A more detailed report and analysis of data
appears in A241.

A243   Goldstein, Leonide; Temple, Robert J.; and Pollack, Irwin W.:
EEG and clinical assessment of subjects with drug abuse problems. Research Communications in Psychology, Psychiatry
and Behavior 1:193-210, 1976.
Subjects: 19 subjects with drug abuse problems.
Method: Subjects were administered a clinical interview,
urine samples were analyzed, and clinical and quantitative
EEG recordings were obtained. The evaluation instruments administered included the SCL-90 (symptom checklist), Gurin Mental Status Index, Hamilton Rating Scale
for Depression, the MMPI, and the Schedule of Recent
Experience. Clinical findings classified by four symptom
groups (anxiety, depression, paranoia, and symptom-
free) were compared to quantitative data, particularly
correlations to EEG data.

A244   Hoffman, Helmut, and Noem, Avis A.: Social background
variables, referral sources and life events of male and female alcoholics. Psychological Reports 37:1087-1092, 1975.
Subjects: 650 males and 74 female alcoholics in rural
state hospitals.
Method: Subjects were interviewed using a social history
inventory that included queries about "stressful life events"
which preceded a period of drinking.

A245   Hore, Brian D.: Life events and alcoholic relapse. British
Journal of Addiction 66:83-88, 1971.
Subjects: 28 alcoholics.
Method: Subjects were prospectively studied for up to 6
months. At regular intervals relapse data and life events
data were collected by clinical interview and through use
of the Brown and Birley interview method.

A246   Lawson, Thomas R., and Winstead, Daniel K.: Toward a
theory of drug use. British Journal of Addiction 73:149-154,
1978.
The authors present a model of drug use and a formula to
quantify the factors that lead to drug use: Factor A
(amount of internal stress: personality) plus Factor B

HV5800 B7

(amount of external stress: environment) equals Level of
Discomfort (where Level of Discomfort determines category of drug use or abuse). The authors propose use of
the MMPI to quantify Factor A and the Schedule of Recent
Experience to quantify Factor B.

A247   Leavy, Richard Lawrence: Stressful life events and in-
        creases in alcohol consumption among male problem drink-
        ers (Doctoral dissertation, University of Massachusetts,
        1976). Dissertation Abstracts International 37:4689-B, 1977.
        Subjects: 38 male problem drinkers in a hospital alcohol
        treatment unit.
        Method: Subjects were interviewed to obtain longitudinal
        self-report data on the amount of alcohol consumed and the
        major life events in their adult lives (using a life events
        inventory based on the Schedule of Recent Experience).

A248   Morrissey, Elizabeth R., and Schuckit, Marc A.: Stressful
        life events and alcohol problems among women seen at a de-
        toxication center. Journal of Studies on Alcohol 39:1559-
        1576, 1978.
        Subjects: 293 females newly admitted to a detoxification
        center.
        Method: Subjects were administered a structured inter-
        view for psychiatric history, demographic characteris-
        tics, educational and familial histories, alcohol and drug
        use and related life problems, gynecological history, anti-
        social and arrest history, and family history of psychiatric
        disorders. Each woman was asked her age at the first oc-
        currence of selected life events, her age when specified
        alcohol-related difficulties first occurred, and her subjec-
        tive estimate of her age at the onset of problem drinking.

A249   Mules, Janet E.; Hague, William H.; and Dudley, Donald L.:
        Life change, its perception and alcohol addiction. Journal of
        Studies on Alcohol 38:487-493, 1977.
        Subjects: 68 confirmed male alcoholics.
        Method: Subjects completed the Schedule of Recent Ex-
        perience (to measure life change) and the Social Readjust-
        ment Rating Questionnaire (to measure perception of life
        change event magnitudes). Manson's ALCADD test was
        administered to obtain alcohol addiction scores. Data are
        compared to Holmes and Rahe's "normative" SRRQ data.

A250   Prusoff, Brigitte; Thompson, W. Douglas; Sholomskas, Diane; and Riordan, Charles: Psychosocial stressors and depression among former heroin-dependent patients maintained on methadone. Journal of Nervous and Mental Disease 165:57-63, 1977.

Subjects: 106 former heroin addicts on a methadone maintenance treatment program.

Method: A structured interview was conducted with each subject to obtain sociodemographic, psychiatric, and drug use history data. The clinical rater who conducted interviews used the Raskin Depression Scale to assess clinical depression, and Paykel's 61-item Recent Life Events semistructured interview was used to collect life change data for the previous six months.

A251   Roszell, D. K.; Mules, J. E.; Glickfeld, G.; and Dudley, D. L.: Life change, disease, perception and heroin addiction. Drug and Alcohol Dependence 1:57-69, 1975.

Subjects: 50 male heroin addicts, all patients in a hospital Drug Dependency Unit.

Method: All subjects completed the Schedule of Recent Experience (to measure life change in the past 3 years), the Social Readjustment Rating Questionnaire (to measure perception of life change events), and the Seriousness of Illness Rating Questionnaire (to measure perception of the seriousness of illnesses). Data were compared to "normative" population findings.

A252   Tonowski, Richard Frank: Depressed alcoholic women: Personality characteristics and life events (Doctoral dissertation, Rutgers University, 1978). Dissertation Abstracts International 39:1001-B, 1978.

Subjects: 78 nonalcoholic depressive inpatients, 31 alcoholic depressive inpatients, and 83 nonpatient controls— all females and between the ages of 18 and 65.

Method: All subjects completed three self-report inventories: the Rutgers Inventory of Dysphorias (recent depressive symptoms), the Rutgers Depression-Prone Inventory (selected personality characteristics of depressives), and a modified Schedule of Recent Experience (life change events). Psychiatric staff members rated the two patient groups using the Wittenborn Psychiatric Rating Scale.

A253 Weissman, Myrna M.; Slobetz, Frank; Prusoff, Brigitte; Mezritz, Marjorie; and Howard, Pat: Clinical depression among narcotic addicts maintained on methadone in the community. American Journal of Psychiatry 133:1434-1438, 1976.

> Subjects: 106 outpatients of a methadone maintenance clinic.
>
> Method: Subjects were interviewed for sociodemographic characteristics, drug history, and family and patient psychiatric history. The Raskin Depression Scale and the Hamilton Rating Scale for Depression were used to evaluate clinical status (34 patients were determined to be depressed, 72 were not). Subjects completed the self-report Hopkins Symptom Checklist. The Social Adjustment Scale was used to assess social functioning in the past 2 months, and a semistructured 61-item life events interview was administered (for past 6 months).

RC321A52

A254 Westermeyer, Joseph: Opium smoking in Laos: A survey of 40 addicts. American Journal of Psychiatry 131:165-169, 1974.

RC321A52

> Subjects: 40 opium addicts in Laos.
>
> Method: Subjects were interviewed for a detailed social and family history of the year prior to onset of addiction, including open-ended questions about precipitating events.

SPECIFIC ILLNESS:
Nervous System and Sense Organs
(A255-A257)

A255 Cohen, Samuel I., and Hajioff, J.: Life events and the onset of acute closed-angle glaucoma. Journal of Psychosomatic Research 16:335-341, 1972.

RC52.J6

> Subjects: 52 patients with acute closed-angle glaucoma and 52 matched controls from other ophthalmic wards.
>
> Method: Glaucoma patients were interviewed within a week of the onset of their acute attack; matched controls were given the same interview upon selection for the study. A full history of physical illness and accidents was obtained, and special emphasis was given to major changes in life situation in the preceding 3 months, anniversaries of major bereavements within 3 months, and early bereavement.

A256 Crary, William G. , and Wexler, Murray: Meniere's disease:
A psychosomatic disorder? Psychological Reports 41:603-
645, 1977.
Subjects: A large sample of patients with Meniere's disease, and control groups of (a) patients with Meniere's
disease who chose not to participate in the long-term study
and (b) controls with otological problems other than
Meniere's disease (both vertiginous and nonvertiginous).
Method: All subjects were administered the following
standard or specially constructed tests: General questionnaire (sociodemographic data); Scaled Dizziness Questionnaire (vertigo, tinnitus, nausea, and related symptoms); the MMPI; Taylor Manifest Anxiety Scale and Spielberger's State Anxiety Scale; a psychosomatic symptom
checklist for subjects and for their blood relatives; a self-
esteem scale and a personal beliefs test; and the Recent
Life Changes Questionnaire (for the 2 years prior to onset
of Meniere's disease symptoms or current otological disorder). The Meniere's disease subjects and the non-
Meniere's disease controls were followed during the course
of the research program and retested at the end of the
study.

A257 Mei-Tal, Varda; Meyerowitz, Sanford; and Engel, George L.:
The role of psychological process in a somatic disorder:
Multiple sclerosis. I. The emotional setting of illness onset and exacerbation. Psychosomatic Medicine 32:67-86,
1970.
Subjects: 17 United States patients with diagnosed multiple
sclerosis and 15 Israeli patients with diagnosed multiple
sclerosis.
Method: Subjects were extensively interviewed, medical
records and attending physicians were consulted, and,
when possible, family members were also interviewed.
Data collection was focused on the details of the life setting in which illness occurred: occurrence, nature, timing, and significance of life events before onset or exacerbation of illness; psychological stress experienced
in conjunction with those events; lifelong and situational
coping patterns; family relationships; and patient attitudes, personality, and functioning. Illustrative case
histories are included in the discussion.

SPECIFIC ILLNESS:
Circulatory System—Coronary Heart Disease
(A258-A299)

A258   Bianchi, Geoffrey; Fergusson, David; and Walshe, James:
        Psychiatric antecedents of myocardial infarction. Medical
        Journal of Australia 1:297-301, 1978.
            Subjects: 40 survivors of myocardial infarction and 40
            matched controls.
            Method: All subjects were administered a semistructured
            interview to obtain data on preinfarct or preinterview (con-
            trols) variables: symptoms of anxiety and depression,
            personality traits, recognized risk factors (smoking, etc.),
            and life events (modified Schedule of Recent Experience).
            Close informants provided corroborating information on
            all subjects.

A259   Bruhn, John G., and Wolf, Stewart: Update on Roseto, PA.:
        Testing a prediction. Psychosomatic Medicine 40:86, 1978.
        (Abstract)
            Subjects: The communities of Roseto and Bangor, Penn-
            sylvania.
            Method: Data on deaths from myocardial infarction from
            1955-1975 were collected for the two communities to test
            the prediction that Roseto's "relative immunity to death
            from myocardial infarction" would diminish as the sup-
            portive social structure based on "Old World values" of
            the Italian-American community eroded in later genera-
            tions and as Roseto came to resemble its neighboring
            city, Bangor. [See also A5 for life change and illness in
            Roseto.]

A260   Byrne, D. G.: Personality, stress and coronary heart dis-
        ease. Medical Journal of Australia 2:469-470, 1978.
            The author briefly reviews the literature describing the
            influence of psychosocial factors on not only the onset of
            primary episodes but also recurrent episodes and the
            course of recovery from myocardial infarction.

A261   Connolly, Joseph: Life events before myocardial infarction.
        Journal of Human Stress 2(4):3-17, 1976.
            Subjects: 91 myocardial infarction patients and 91
            matched, well comparison subjects.

Method: Subjects were interviewed following the Brown and Birley life events interview method (for the 3-month period preceding myocardial infarction or interview).

A262 De Faire, Ulf: Life change patterns prior to death in ischaemic heart disease. A study of death-discordant twins. Journal of Psychosomatic Research 19:273-278, 1975.

Subjects: 27 male pairs of Swedish twins (9 monozygotic, 18 dizygotic) death-discordant with respect to ischaemic heart disease (myocardial infarction and/or sudden death). Method: The surviving twin of each pair and a close informant of the deceased twin completed a Swedish translation of a modified Schedule of Recent Experience for the 4-year period preceding death discordance (data collected in 6-month segments). The Swedish Social Readjustment Rating Scale developed by Theorell and used to score the Swedish Schedule of Recent Experience is reproduced in Table 1.

RC52.J6

A263 De Faire, Ulf, and Theorell, Tores: Life changes and myocardial infarction: Epidemiological and clinical considerations. Preventive Medicine 6:302-311, 1977.

The authors review recent studies of life change and myocardial infarction and then discuss the relevance and applicability of life change measurement to epidemiological and clinical study. Suggestions to improve research design include using a prospective method, determining subjects' habitual level of life change, using subjective ratings of life events, and recording other risk factors and psychological variables as well as life change data.

RA421P684

A264 De Faire, Ulf, and Theorell, Tores: Life changes and myocardial infarction: How useful are life change measurements? Scandinavian Journal of Social Medicine 4(3):115-122, 1976.

The authors discuss modifications in life change measurement that will improve studies of its relation to myocardial infarction. [See A263.]

A265 Dimsdale, Joel E.: Emotional causes of sudden death. American Journal of Psychiatry 134:1361-1366, 1977.

The author reviews studies relating emotional setting to cardiovascular responses that can lead to sudden death. One section of the discussion is devoted to life change research done by Rahe and colleagues in Helsinki (see A287).

RC321A52

A266   Doehrman, Steven R.: Psycho-social aspects of recovery
        from coronary heart disease: A review. Social Science and
        Medicine 11:199-218, 1977.
             This extensive and analytical review covers the litera-
        ture published since 1970. The author divides the pub-
        lished reports into three categories ("advocacy articles,"
        "clinical papers," and "empirical reports"), evaluates
        the quality of their contributions, and outlines future re-
        search needs and directions.

PER

A267   Edwards, Margaret K.: Life crisis and myocardial infarc-
        tion. Unpublished master's thesis, University of Washing-
        ton, 1971.
             Subjects: 75 participants in an exercise rehabilitation
        program for cardiac and pulmonary patients (44 with
        diagnosed myocardial infarction and 31 without a diag-
        nosed myocardial infarction).
             Method: Subjects completed the Schedule of Recent Ex-
        perience (for the preceding 3 years).

A268   Ell, Kathleen Obier: Stressful life events and onset, sever-
        ity, and recovery from myocardial infarction (Doctoral dis-
        sertation, University of California, Los Angeles, 1978).
        Dissertation Abstracts International 39:2219B-2220B, 1978.
             Subjects: 63 patients with a first myocardial infarction.
             Method: Subjects were patients consecutively admitted to
        a public hospital CCU; all completed the Recent Life
        Changes Questionnaire (for past 2 years), and the severity
        of their infarctions was measured by Killip classification
        I-IV. A follow-up sample of 28 patients with characteris-
        tics similar to the initial sample completed the Recent
        Life Changes Questionnaire to provide life change data
        for the 6 months prior to illness and the 3 months post-
        infarct. Level of recovery at 3 months postinfarct was
        measured by the American Health Association classifica-
        tions I-IV.

A269   Eliot, Robert S.: Stress and cardiovascular disease. Euro-
        pean Journal of Cardiology 5:97-104, 1977.
             The author presents an overview of present knowledge,
        with particular emphasis on the following: risk factors,
        myocardial pathophysiology, sudden death, predictive
        environmental factors, and modification of risk factors.

A270   Engelsmann, Frank: The psychologist's role in psychosomatics. Psychosomatics 18(5):47-52, 1977.

The author reviews the development and current status of
concepts in psychosomatic medicine such as specificity
theory. His discussion includes life change research as
an example of one of the nonspecific models for illness,
and he compares life change studies of myocardial infarction survivors with personality-specific studies of Type A
subjects. Particular attention is given to the psychologist's active role in diagnosis, psychological testing, and
therapy for psychophysiological disorders.

A271   Glass, David C.: Stress, behavior patterns, and coronary
disease. American Scientist 65:177-187, 1977.

Subjects: 45 patients in the coronary care unit of the
Houston Veterans Administration Hospital, 77 hospitalized
control subjects (from the general-medical and surgical
wards), and 50 healthy nonhospitalized controls (building-
maintenance employees).

Method: All subjects were administered two instruments:
the Jenkins Activity Survey (Type A behavior) and a modified Schedule of Recent Experience. Selected life events
were analyzed as "losses" (uncontrollable events, help-
lessness-inducing events) or simply "negative" events
("stressful" but not necessarily uncontrollable or help-
lessness-inducing).

A272   Greene, William A.; Speegle, E. K.; Bayer, L.; Littlefield,
N.; Davis, H.; and Cromwell, R. L.: Psychosocial variables
and heart attacks. II. Well-being $1\frac{1}{2}$ years after acute coronary events. Psychosomatic Medicine 38:63-64, 1976.
(Abstract)

Subjects: 272 patients below age 66 admitted to two CCUs
with myocardial infarction (76%) or coronary insufficiency
(24%).

Method: Subjects were followed at 4-month intervals after
discharge from hospital. Data collected at time of hospitalization and at each follow-up interview were similar:
demographic data, symptoms, moods, family setting,
social changes and life events, home satisfaction, 6-hour
ECG. A Well-Being score was derived from moods and
symptom data; baseline and follow-up correlations of well-
being and psychosocial variables were examined.

A273   Hiland, David Neil: Type A behavior, anxiety, job-satisfaction and life stress as risk factors in myocardial infarction (Doctoral dissertation, University of South Florida, 1978). Dissertation Abstracts International 39:3516-B, 1979.

     Subjects: 40 male patients who had sustained at least one documented myocardial infarction, and 40 matched non-coronary control subjects.

Z5053.D57

     Method: Subjects completed the Jenkins Activity Survey (Type A behavior), the State-Trait Anxiety Inventory, the Job-Descriptive Index, and a modified Schedule of Recent Experience (for 10 years).

A274   Jenkins, C. David: Psychologic and social precursors of coronary disease [in two parts]. New England Journal of Medicine 284:244-255 [Part 1], 307-317 [Part 2], 1971.

     This is a detailed review of journal articles published from 1965 to 1969 (162 references). The review is divided into the following sections: recent review papers, sociologic indexes, social mobility and status incongruity, anxiety and neuroticism, life dissatisfactions, stress, coronary-prone behavior pattern, and other personality traits.

A275   Jenkins, C. David: Recent evidence supporting psychologic and social risk factors for coronary disease [in two parts]. New England Journal of Medicine 294:987-994 [Part 1], 1033-1038 [Part 2], 1976.

     This review covers serial publications from 1970 through the beginning of 1975. This detailed review of the literature (88 references) follows the same organizational format as its predecessor (see A274 above) with a few additions: a section on "other reactive characteristics" follows the "anxiety and neuroticism" section, "life problems" are added to the "life dissatisfactions" section, and the "stress" section is here expanded to "stress and life change." [The review of life change research appears in part two of the review on pp. 1033-1034.]

A276   Lehman, Edward W.; Schulman, Jay; and Hinkle, Lawrence E., Jr.: Coronary deaths and organizational mobility: The 30-year experience of 1,160 men. Archives of Environmental Health 15:455-461, 1967.

MICRO
FILM

RC963A22

     Subjects: An age cohort of 1,160 men employed by the Bell Telephone System (median age of 30 on January 1, 1935).

Method: Using company occupational records to follow the cohort, the investigators compared the mobility experience (number of changes in 9 dimensions of work experience: promotion/demotion/lateral move, working conditions, responsibilities, job changes, work locations, etc.) of those men who died of coronary heart disease before age 60 (N=65) to the mobility experience of matched subjects who did not suffer from coronary heart disease. Each "coronary man" was matched to one man who also died but from another cause and to another man who was still living and on the company payroll on January 1, 1965.

A277 Levene, Donald L.: Letter to the editor: Psychological factors in the genesis of myocardial infarction. Canadian Medical Association Journal 111:499, 501, 1974.

Subjects: 15 patients with a first myocardial infarction.
Method: The subjects, who were consecutively admitted patients on a CCU, were interviewed during their hospitalization regarding the "quality of life preceding hospitalization": friends and family, home life and work life, situational changes (life events, conflicts, etc.), and health and mental health.

A278 Lundberg, Ulf; Theorell, Tores; and Lind, Evy: Life changes and myocardial infarction: Individual differences in life change scaling. Journal of Psychosomatic Research 19:27-32, 1975.

RC52.J6

Subjects: 56 Swedish survivors of myocardial infarction and 33 matched control subjects.
Method: All patients completed a life change events questionnaire, reporting any of 46 life events which occurred in the year prior to infarction; controls reported life changes for a corresponding period. Patients and controls were then randomly divided into two groups: 6 months later one patient-control group rated the 46 life events for degree of "adjustment" required by the event, while the other mixed-subject group rated them for "how upsetting" the events would be. Each subjective estimation was made on a scale of 1-100. Three types of life change rating scales were derived from the two kinds of subjective estimates: a life change rating mean scale for "the average person," separate mean scales for infarction patients and for control subjects, and individual scales for each subject.

A279   Mayou, Richard; Foster, Ann; and Williamson, Barbara:
Psychosocial adjustment in patients one year after myocardial infarction. Journal of Psychosomatic Research 22:447–
453, 1978.

> Subjects: 100 patients with a first myocardial infarction.
> Method: Subjects and their spouses were interviewed
> three times (during hospitalization, then 2 months and 1
> year after discharge) and were rated for levels of activity
> at work and in leisure time, family and social life, diffi-
> culties and life events (Brown and Birley interview method),
> changes in activities and in satisfaction, and appropriate-
> ness and quality of adjustment.

RC52.J6

A280   Ossenkop, Kathleen Ann: Reported life changes and their
relationship to recovery following myocardial infarction.
Unpublished master's thesis, University of Washington, 1973.

> Subjects: 16 patients with myocardial infarction and their
> spouses.
> Method: All subjects completed the Schedule of Recent
> Experience for the 3 years preceding patient's illness.
> Life change data were then studied in relation to level of
> recovery 2 months postmyocardial infarction. Recovery
> was measured by a modified Family Task Performance
> form, a modified Leisure Activities form, and the Health
> Opinion Survey (symptoms of "stress").

A281   Rahe, Richard H.: Stress and strain in coronary heart disease. Journal of the South Carolina Medical Association 72
(Supplement):7–14, 1976.

> The author reviews the historical development of the terms
> "stress" and "strain," describes the development and ap-
> plication of the Recent Life Changes Questionnaire (RLCQ)
> and the Work, Striving, Time and Life Satisfaction Ques-
> tionnaire, and discusses some of the results of studies
> using the two instruments to investigate coronary heart
> disease. The two questionnaires are included in the text.

A282   Rahe, Richard H.; Arajarvi, Heikki; Arajarvi, Seija; Punsar,
Sven; and Karvonen, Martti J.: Recent life changes and coro-
nary heart disease in East versus West Finland. Journal of
Psychomatic Research 20:431–437, 1976.

> Subjects: 592 male East Finns and 695 West Finns, all
> participants in a 10-year follow-up study of coronary
> heart disease in two age cohorts.

RC52 .J6

Method: At the time of their scheduled 10-year exam for coronary heart disease, all subjects also completed the Recent Life Changes Questionnaire (past 2 years). The development of coronary heart disease in the two age cohorts (born 1909 and 1919) since the study began was documented, and the two regional subject groups were compared for life change experience, physiological risk factors, and coronary heart disease.

A283   Rahe, Richard H.; Bennett, Linda; Romo, Matti; Siltanen, Pentti; and Arthur, Ransom J.: Subjects' recent life changes and coronary heart disease in Finland. American Journal of Psychiatry 130:1222-1226, 1973.

RC321A52

Subjects: 279 survivors of myocardial infarction and 226 victims of sudden coronary death, all drawn from the Helsinki Ischaemic Heart Disease Register.
Method: Survivors of myocardial infarction and spouses of deceased subjects provided life change data for the 2 years preceding infarct or death to nurse-interviewers using the Finnish translation of the Schedule of Recent Experience (divided into 6-month units). Subjects were assigned to subgroups based on presence or absence of illness before index episode, and then the degree of increase (marked, moderate, none) in life change before infarct or death was examined.

A284   Rahe, Richard H., and Lind, Evy: Psychosocial factors and sudden cardiac death: A pilot study. Journal of Psychosomatic Research 15:19-24, 1971.

RC52.J6

Subjects: 39 Swedish male cases of sudden cardiac death.
Method: Close informants completed the Swedish translation of the Schedule of Recent Experience for subjects' experience during the 3 years prior to death. Subjects were assigned to subgroups based on presence or absence of coronary heart disease symptoms prior to their sudden deaths.

A285   Rahe, Richard H., and Paasikivi, Juhani: Psychosocial factors and myocardial infarction: II. An outpatient study in Sweden. Journal of Psychosomatic Research 15:33-39, 1971.

RC52.J6

Subjects: 30 Swedish outpatients who had experienced an initial myocardial infarction from 1 to 4 years prior to the study.
Method: In late 1968 all subjects completed the Swedish translation of the Schedule of Recent Experience for the

previous 4 years (1965, 1966, 1967, 1968). Individual
Life Change Unit (LCU) totals were calculated for all year-
quarters (3 months) before and since infarction. Mean
year-quarter LCU totals were calculated for each patient
group (13 with infarctions in 1965, 8 in 1966, 9 in 1967)
to examine patterns of life change build up and decrease
in relation to infarction. [See A299 for Part I of this
study.]

A286   Rahe, Richard H., and Romo, Matti: Recent life changes
and the onset of myocardial infarction and coronary death in
Helsinki. In Life Stress and Illness. E. K. Eric Gunderson
and Richard H. Rahe (Eds.), pp. 105-120. Springfield, Illinois: Charles C Thomas, 1974.

RC49. G85   Subjects: 279 survivors of a documented myocardial infarction and 226 victims of sudden coronary death, all
drawn from the Helsinki Ischaemic Heart Disease Register.
Method: Survivors of myocardial infarction and spouses of
coronary death victims provided information about the 2
years preceding infarct or death to nurse-interviewers
using the Finnish translation of the Schedule of Recent
Experience. The Finnish Life Change Unit (LCU) weights
used to score the Finnish Schedule of Recent Experience
are listed.

A287   Rahe, Richard H.; Romo, Matti; Bennett, Linda; and Siltanen,
Pentti: Recent life changes, myocardial infarction, and
abrupt coronary death. Archives of Internal Medicine 133:
221-228, 1974.

Subjects: 279 survivors of myocardial infarction (including 61 females) and 226 cases of abrupt coronary death
(including 42 females), all drawn from the Helsinki
Ischaemic Heart Disease Register.

RIIA725   Method: Survivors of myocardial infarction and spouses
of deceased subjects provided life change data for the 2
years preceding infarct or death to nurse-interviewers
using the Finnish translation of the Schedule of Recent
Experience. Subjects were assigned to subgroups of "recently ill" vs. "no recent illness"; the coronary death
group was also subdivided into "sudden-death" and "de-
layed-death" groups. Two sections of this report are devoted to special topics: the life change patterns of the 103
female subjects, and comparison of life change reporting
by myocardial infarction survivors and reports by their
spouses.

A288 Rahe, Richard H.; Tuffli, Charles F., Jr.; Suchor, Raymond
J., Jr.; and Arthur, Ransom J.: Group therapy in the outpatient management of post-myocardial infarction patients.
International Journal of Psychiatry in Medicine 4:77-88, 1973.
  Subjects: 23 first-myocardial infarction patients in a
  group therapy program and 21 similar patients followed
  as controls (no intervention).
  Method: All subjects completed the Schedule of Recent
  Experience; case histories are presented to illustrate the
  build up of life changes preinfarct. Group therapy sessions were held every other week, and intervention subjects attended 4-6 sessions. This report describes patients' perceptions of the convalescence experience, their
  perceptions of life changes before and after infarct, and
  their attitudes toward resuming physical activity and returning to work.

A289 Siltanen, P.: Life changes and sudden coronary death. Advances in Cardiology 25:47-60, 1978.
  The author reviews the method and findings of the Helsinki
  studies of life change preceding myocardial infarction and
  sudden death (reported earlier in A287 and A283). He includes related findings from research in and outside of
  Finland. The Finnish Life Change Unit (LCU) weights
  used to score the Finnish version of the Schedule of Recent Experience are listed in a table.

A290 Spittle, Bruce, and James, Basil: Psychosocial factors and
myocardial infarction. Australian and New Zealand Journal
of Psychiatry 11:37-43, 1977.
  Subjects: 61 male survivors of a first myocardial infarction and a comparison group (controlled for age and social
  status) who had not had an infarction.
  Methods: Patients and controls completed two questionnaires (total of 370 questions) which included the following: the Edwards Personality Preference Schedule, the
  Anxiety and the Depression subscales of the MMPI, the
  Cochrane and Robertson Life Events Inventory, and a
  series of questions based on known risk factors for myocardial infarction.

A291 Stern, Melvin J.; Pascale, Linda; and Ackerman, Anne:
Life adjustment postmyocardial infarction: Determining
predictive variables. Archives of Internal Medicine 137:
1680-1685, 1977.

Subjects: 68 patients with diagnosed myocardial infarctions.

Methods: Subjects were followed for 1 year after the onset of their infarct to study their psychological state and rehabilitation progress. Interviews were held twice during hospitalization and again at 6 weeks, 3 months, 6 months, and 1 year postinfarct. During the interviews the Zung Self-Rating Depression Scale and the Taylor Manifest Anxiety Scale were administered; a new questionnaire was constructed to assess denial. During hospitalization, the following instruments were administered: Jenkins Activity Survey (Type A behavior); the Schedule of Recent Experience (past 6 months); Rotter's Internal-External Locus of Control Scale; and the Structured and Sided Interview to Assess Maladjustment (SSIAM). The Schedule of Recent Experience was readministered at 6-month and 1-year follow-up interviews; the SSIAM was administered at every follow-up interview.

A292   Theorell, Tores: Life events before and after the onset of a premature myocardial infarction. In Stressful Life Events: Their Nature and Effects. Barbara Snell Dohrenwend and Bruce P. Dohrenwend (Eds.), pp. 101-117. New York: Wiley, 1974.

BF575.S75
C641973

The author reviews his and his colleagues' studies with Swedish patients using a modified Schedule of Recent Experience. This review focuses on the following areas: life events and catecholamines; retrospective reports of life events during the whole life span and recent life events; scaling experiments and total Life Change Unit scores of premature myocardial infarction patients and control subjects; prospective studies, including the author's work in progress.

A293   Theorell, T.: Psychosocial factors and myocardial infarction—why and how? Advances in Cardiology 8:117-131, 1973.
The author summarizes his research with Swedish male myocardial infarction patients aimed at identifying individuals susceptible to myocardial infarction and the timing of susceptible periods. The author reviews studies of myocardial infarction patients' sociological characteristics, attitudes, life change experience prior to infarct, and covariations between catecholamines and life changes.

A294 Theorell, Tores: Psychosocial factors in relation to the onset of myocardial infarction and to some metabolic variables—
a pilot study. Unpublished medical thesis, Department of
Medicine, Seraphimer Hospital, Karolinska Institute, Stockholm, 1970.
    This study was the basis for research subsequently pur-
    sued and published in collaboration with colleagues in
    Stockholm (see A296 and A299).

A295 Theorell, T.; Lind, E.; and Floderus, B.: The relationship
of disturbing life-changes and emotions to the early development of myocardial infarction and other serious illnesses.
International Journal of Epidemiology 4:281-293, 1975.
    Subjects: 6,579 Swedish males, all members of the con-
    struction building workers trade union in Stockholm and
    between the ages of 41 and 61.
    Method: Subjects completed a postal questionnaire which
    included a modified Schedule of Recent Experience (for
    previous 12 months), a discord index (dissatisfaction with
    work, home, and social relationships), and an illness his-
    tory (for episodes of 30 or more consecutive days of sick
    leave in the past year). All subjects were followed for
    the subsequent 12-15 months for incidence of death (from
    all causes) and hospitalization for myocardial infarction.
    The sample's urban dwellers (N=3,289) were also fol-
    lowed for incidence of other serious illnesses (ulcer or
    gastritis, accidents, degenerative joint disease, neurosis,
    and all new illnesses which caused 30 or more days of
    sick leave).

A296 Theorell, Tores; Lind, Evy; Froberg, Jan; Karlsson, Claes-
Goran; and Levi, Lennart: A longitudinal study of 21 subjects with coronary heart disease: Life changes, catechola-
mine excretion and related biochemical reactions. Psychosomatic Medicine 34:505-516, 1972.
    Subjects: 21 male, well-rehabilitated survivors of myo-
    cardial infarction.
    Method: During a 2-4 month period, each subject followed
    strict dietary regulations before weekly clinic appoint-
    ments (always same day, same hour) to provide urine
    specimens and blood samples for laboratory analysis. At
    each visit subjects completed a modified Swedish version
    of the Schedule of Recent Experience for the interval be-
    tween appointments. Intersubject and intrasubject varia-
    tions and correlations of life change data (Life Change

Units/week) and selected physiologic measures (epinephrine and norepinephrine output, serum cholesterol, serum triglyceride, serum uric acid, and serum creatine) were evaluated.

A297   Theorell, Tores, and Rahe, Richard H.: Life change events, ballistocardiography and coronary death. Journal of Human Stress 1(3):18-24, 1975.

Subjects: 18 postmyocardial infarction patients who survived over a 6-year period and 18 myocardial infarction patients who died from their coronary disease before the 6-year follow-up.

Method: In this retrospective study, data were derived from a larger study conducted at the University of Oklahoma in which myocardial infarction patients were followed for 6 years. Life change data were gathered by reviewing medical records containing physicians' notes of interviews with patients at their regular follow-up examinations. The investigators calculated Life Change Unit (LCU) scores by completing the Schedule of Recent Experience for each subject. LCU scores for the 2 years preceding coronary death for deceased subjects were then compared to LCU scores for matched survivors for the corresponding 2-year period, divided into 6-month segments. The ballistocardiograms made during clinic visits were examined and compared to the LCU patterns for the same 2-year period for both deceased and surviving subjects.

A298   Theorell, Tores, and Rahe, Richard H.: Psychosocial characteristics of subjects with myocardial infarction in Stockholm. In Life Stress and Illness. E. K. Eric Gunderson and Richard H. Rahe (Eds.), pp. 90-104. Springfield, Illinois: Charles C Thomas, 1974.

RC49.G85   The authors summarize their Stockholm studies, both retrospective and prospective, of psychosocial factors related to myocardial infarction. The Swedish version of the Schedule of Recent Experience was used to document and to quantify life change of patients and controls in many of the studies.

A299   Theorell, Tores, and Rahe, Richard H.: Psychosocial factors and myocardial infarction: I. An inpatient study in RC52.J6   Sweden. Journal of Psychosomatic Research 15:25-31, 1971.

Subjects: 54 Swedish male survivors of myocardial infarction and a healthy comparison group of 14 of their
friends (matched for sex, age, education, occupation,
and social class) who had no previous history of coronary
heart disease.
Method: All subjects completed the Swedish version of
the Schedule of Recent Experience for each quarter of the
year in the 3-4 years prior to infarction (or contact, for
controls). Year-quarter (3-month) Life Change Unit
totals and patterns were compared for patients vs. comparison group and for patients with no previous coronary
heart disease histories vs. patients with recent illness
episodes. [See A285 for Part II of this study.]

SPECIFIC ILLNESS:
Circulatory System—Other Circulatory Diseases
(A300-A305)

A300   Dimsdale, Joel E.; Hackett, Thomas P.; Block, Peter C.;
        and Hutter, Adolph M.: Emotional correlates of Type A be-
        havior pattern. Psychosomatic Medicine 40:580-583, 1978.
            Subjects: 99 male and 10 female hospital patients await-
        ing cardiac catherization (presumptive coronary artery
        disease manifested by angina).
            Method: All subjects were administered the following in-
        struments: the Jenkins Activity Survey, Form B (Type A
        behavior pattern); the Hackett-Cassem semistructured in-
        terview for denial of cardiac illness; the Schedule of Re-
        cent Experience (for past 4 months); and the Profile of
        Mood States (to measure tension, depression, anger,
        vigor, fatigue, and confusion). The distribution and
        correlations of psychosocial variables were examined.

A301   Gianturco, D. T.; Breslin, M. S.; Heyman, A.; Gentry,
        W. D.; Jenkins, C. D.; and Kaplan, B.: Personality pat-
        terns and life stress in ischemic cerebrovascular disease.
        1. Psychiatric findings. Stroke 5:453-460, 1974.
            Subjects: 10 white males hospitalized with completed
        cerebral infarction, 16 white males hospitalized with
        transient cerebral ischemic attacks, and 14 white male
        control subjects hospitalized with acute nonvascular ill-
        nesses.
            Method: All subjects were interviewed for a detailed his-
        tory of cardiovascular and other illnesses. A semistruc-

tured psychiatric interview was also conducted to rate
each subject on 6 personality and behavioral factors:
"pressured pattern," object relating style, affect at onset of illness, patterns of coping with anger, circumstances evoking anger, and "nature of life stress preceding illness" (life events were noted and then later classified as either internal or external and by degree of severity).

A302 Gillum, Richard F., and Paffenbarger, Ralph S., Jr.:
Chronic disease in former college students. XVII. Sociocultural mobility as a precursor of coronary heart disease
and hypertension. American Journal of Epidemiology 108:
289-298, 1978.
Subjects: A cohort of 13,728 male former Harvard University students examined as entering students in 1939-
1950.
Method: All subjects were followed for coronary heart
disease deaths. The 8,852 subjects who returned follow-
up questionnaires in 1962, 1966, and 1972 reported doctor-
diagnosed incidence of nonfatal myocardial infarction,
angina pectoris, and essential hypertension. Four well
control subjects were selected for each case of fatal
coronary heart disease (98), nonfatal myocardial infarction (78), and angina pectoris (48); one well control subject was selected for each case of hypertension (319).
Subjects and controls were compared for intergenerational
mobility (differences from father's occupational status)
and intragenerational mobility (number of changes in line
of work and number of residential changes since college
but before illness onset).

A303 Jenkins, C. David: Behavioral risk factors in coronary ar-
tery disease. Annual Review of Medicine: Selected Topics
in the Clinical Sciences 29:543-562, 1978.
The author reviews the concept of "coronary-prone behavior pattern" developed by Rosenman, Friedman,
Jenkins, and others, and then applies eight evaluation
criteria to the existing research evidence on coronary-
prone behavior. After evaluating Type A behavior research,
he also reviews research into other psychosocial risk factors, including life change research.

A304 Moody, Philip M.: Effect of smoking and recent life changes
upon onset of diseases of the circulatory system. Public
Health Reports 93:443-445, 1978.

Subjects: 149 adults hospitalized with diagnosed diseases of the circulatory system.
Method: Subjects completed the Schedule of Recent Experience for the year prior to hospitalization (divided into 6-month segments). They also completed a questionnaire about their smoking status: smoker (N=80), former smoker (N=43), and nonsmoker (N=26).

A305   Penrose, R. J. J.: Life events before subarachnoid haemorrhage. Journal of Psychosomatic Research 16:329-333, 1972.

Subjects: 44 patients hospitalized for subarachnoid hemorrhage (first admission and confirmed by lumbar puncture).
Method: Subjects were divided into two groups: those with aneurysms (N=27) and those without aneurysms (N=17). Two or more close informants were interviewed about subject's life events in the 3 months preceding onset (Brown and Birley interview method), his or her physical activity immediately before the ictus, drug use, and previous psychiatric history. Life events data were compared to Brown and Birley's "normative" group of 325 control subjects.

SPECIFIC ILLNESS:
Respiratory System
(A306-A313)

A306   Boyce, W. Thomas; Jensen, Eric W.; Cassel, John C.; Collier, Albert M.; Smith, Allan; and Ramey, Craig T.: Influence of life events and family routines on childhood respiratory tract illness. Pediatrics 60:609-615, 1977.

Subjects: 58 children attending a day care-elementary school complex.

Method: Respiratory illness data were collected for one year: daily observations for illness were made, and biweekly nasopharyngeal cultures for pathogenic bacteria, mycoplasmas, and viruses were carried out. At the onset of clinical illness additional cultures were obtained. After illness data had been collected, an interview was conducted with the family of each child. Life change scores were calculated using Coddington's Schedule of Recent Experience for children, and an inventory devised for this study was used to score the strength of each family's routines.

A307 De Araujo, Gilberto; Van Arsdel, Paul P., Jr.; Holmes, Thomas H.; and Dudley, Donald L.: Life change, coping ability and chronic intrinsic asthma. Journal of Psychosomatic Research 17:359-363, 1973.

RC52.J6

> Subjects: 36 chronic asthmatic patients.
> Method: Subjects completed the Schedule of Recent Experience (for past 2 years) and were evaluated by an investigator using the Berle Index (measure of psychosocial assets). One year later the medical records of each subject were reviewed, and a mean daily steroid dose was calculated for the subject. Data were analyzed for relationships of life change (high vs. low Life Change Unit scores), psychosocial assets (high vs. low scores), and steroid dose (high vs. low mean daily amount).

A308 Dudley, Donald L.; Holmes, Thomas H.; Van Arsdel, Paul P., Jr.; and De Araujo, Gilberto: Quantification of psychosocial variables in intrinsic asthma: Relationship to physiologic variability. Psychotherapy and Psychosomatics 24: 129-131, 1974.

RC321A

2853

> Subjects: 36 chronic asthmatic patients.
> Method: All subjects completed the Schedule of Recent Experience, and the Berle Index was used to evaluate coping ability (psychosocial assets). Steroid dose was calculated for each patient and studied in relation to Berle Index and life change scores. In addition, 13 patients underwent psychiatric interviews designed to elicit discussion of events (past and present) associated with distressing emotion; the interviews were alternated with measurements of pulmonary ventilation. Emotionally induced physiologic change was examined in relation to life change and Berle Index scores.

A309 Greene, W. A.; Betts, R. F.; Ochitill, H. N.; Iker, H. P.; and Douglas, R. G.: Psychosocial factors and immunity; preliminary report. Psychosomatic Medicine 40:87, 1978. (Abstract)

> Subjects: 33 volunteer subjects (18 males, 15 females; ages 18-35).
> Method: Subjects were confined to a motel for 7 days. On Day 1 subjects completed Anderson's College Schedule of Recent Experience and the Profile of Mood States; signs and symptoms were rated. On Day 2 subjects were inoculated intranasally with influenza A/Victoria/75H3N2 virus. On Days 2-7, signs and symptoms were rated twice daily

and immune measures were made (e.g., nasal virus shed). Correlations of clinical and immune measures with mood and life change scores were examined.

A310 Jacobs, Phyllis Clark: Patterns of stress in patients with respiratory diseases. Unpublished master's thesis, Washington University, St. Louis, 1967.

Subjects: 17 hospitalized respiratory patients matched by age and sex to 17 undiagnosed patients returning to the Health Department for a second x-ray because initial small x-ray was suspicious.

Method: Subjects completed the Schedule of Recent Experience (for past 10 years) and the Macmillan Health Opinion Survey.

A311 Kurata, John H.; Glovsky, M. Michael; Newcomb, Robert L.; and Easton, James G.: A multifactorial study of patients with asthma. Part 1: Data collection and rapid feedback. Annals of Allergy 37:231-245, 1976.

Subjects: 49 asthma patients and 11 controls (nonallergic relatives of patients).

Method: This report describes the development of a computer-assisted research, treatment, and education program for patients with asthma. In addition to routine clinical and laboratory procedures and allergy histories, daily punched-card diaries of symptoms, medications, and exposures to irritants are kept by patients. These data are then analyzed in relation to weekly pollen counts (by geographical region only), monthly pulmonary function tests and scores on a modified Schedule of Recent Experience, and annual scores on the State-Trait Anxiety Inventory and Luborsky's Social Assets Scale. Monthly interviews are also held with each patient.

A312 Rowlett, David B., and Dudley, Donald L.: COPD: Psychosocial and psychophysiological issues. Psychosomatics 19: 273-279, 1978.

The authors describe the chronic nature of the disease process in asthma, chronic bronchitis, and emphysema and the distinctive emotional characteristics and psychophysiological changes associated with those conditions. Reducing the effects of life change and increasing the patient's psychosocial assets to cope with disease are discussed as key elements in the treatment of patients with chronic obstructive pulmonary disease.

A313　Wright, Diana Dryer; Kane, Robert L.; Olsen, Donna M.; and Smith, Thomas J.: The effects of selected psychosocial factors on the self-reporting of pulmonary symptoms. Journal of Chronic Diseases 30:195-206, 1977.

> Subjects: 1,110 smelter and mine workers.
> Method: Subjects were interviewed and questionnaires were administered to collect data on respiratory symptoms, attitudes (job satisfaction, hypochondriasis, etc.), life events (modified Schedule of Recent Experience for previous 4 years), work history (location, exposure to sulfur dioxide), and various sociodemographic factors. Subjects also performed pulmonary function tests measuring FEV_1 and FVC.

RB156.J6

SPECIFIC ILLNESS:
Digestive System
(A314-A325)

A314　Almy, Thomas P.: Therapeutic strategy in stress-related digestive disorders. Clinics in Gastroenterology 6:709-722, 1977.

> The author discusses the therapeutic relationship; diagnosis and prognosis (including use of the Schedule of Recent Experience as one of 4 indicators of prognosis for long-term improvement); first steps in treatment; goals and procedures in definitive treatment; psychiatric referrals; and the resources of behavioral psychiatry.

A315　Bock, O. A. A.: Alcohol, aspirin, depression, smoking, stress and the patient with a gastric ulcer. South Africa Medical Journal 50:293-297, 1976.

> Subjects: 194 consecutive patients with gastric ulceration seen in a South African hospital.
> Method: Subjects were interviewed concerning the presence of the following precipitating factors: smoking, drinking alcohol, use of salicylates, symptoms of depression, and "recent stress" ("out-of-the-ordinary physical, psychological or social upsets" such as car accident, job change with increased responsibility, death in the family).

A316　Fava, Giovanni A., and Pavan, Luigi: Large bowel disorders. I. Illness configuration and life events. Psychotherapy and Psychosomatics 27:93-99, 1977.

RC52.J6

Subjects: 60 consecutive patients with large bowel disorders (20 with ulcerative colitis, 20 with irritable bowel syndrome, and 20 with appendicitis).

Method: Two semistructured research interviews were conducted with each subject to collect data on the following: demographic variables, present medical illness, hospitalizations, medical and psychiatric symptoms, and life events in the 6 months preceding illness onset (using a modification of Paykel's method for distinguishing events as desirable and undesirable and as exits or entrances in the social field).

A317 Hislop, I. G.: Onset setting in inflammatory bowel disease. Medical Journal of Australia 1:981-984, 1974.

Subjects: 50 consecutive patients presenting with inflammatory bowel disease (35 with ulcerative colitis, 9 with granulomatous colitis, and 6 with regional enteritis) and 50 matched control subjects (hospital visitors not receiving medical treatment).

Method: All subjects were questioned about the frequency of 7 life events (family bereavement and terminal illness, marriage, divorce, pregnancy, childbirth, migration) in the preceding 12 months. Additional life events data were noted for patients, and the temporal relationship of life events to illness onset was examined.

A318 Marbach, Joseph J., and Lipton, James A.: Aspects of illness behavior in patients with facial pain. Journal of the American Dental Association 96:630-638, 1978.

Subjects: 170 consecutive patients referred to a TMJ (temporomandibular joint) facial pain clinic.

Method: A symptom and treatment history was obtained from each patient during the initial clinic visit; included in the symptom histories were questions about specific life events associated with the onset of pain. Clinic and radiographic examinations were also performed. Each patient was then interviewed for information on social and personal background of self, spouse, and parents.

A319 McKegney, F. Patrick; Gordon, Robert O.; and Levine, Stephen M.: A psychosomatic comparison of patients with ulcerative colitis and Crohn's disease. Psychosomatic Medicine 32:153-166, 1970.

Subjects: In Phase 1, 83 patients with ulcerative colitis and Crohn's disease; in Phase 2, 21 patients with ulcerative colitis and 19 patients with Crohn's disease.

Method: In Phase 1, a retrospective chart review was
conducted to survey over 50 demographic and psychosocial
characteristics (chronology of illnesses and other life
events; patient's personality and impression of the causes
of his or her disease; personal, family, and social history; and psychiatric history). In Phase 2, subjects were
interviewed following the protocol established in Phase 1.
In addition, a rating was assigned for severity of physical
disease (based on gastroenterologist's examination), and
patients completed the Cornell Medical Index as a measure
of the severity of emotional disturbance.

A320   Mendeloff, Albert I.; Monk, Mary; Siegel, Charles I.; and
        Lilienfeld, Abraham: Illness experience and life stresses in
        patients with irritable colon and with ulcerative colitis: An
        epidemiologic study of ulcerative colitis and regional enter-
        itis in Baltimore, 1960-1964. New England Journal of Medi-
        cine 282: 14-17, 1970.
        Subjects: 102 hospitalized patients with irritable colon,
        158 hospitalized patients with ulcerative colitis, and 735
        control subjects from the general population who were not
        hospitalized.
        Method: Structured interviews were conducted with all
        subjects to collect data on the following: demographic
        characteristics, religious and ethnic background, birth
        order, education, work experience, marital history,
        socioeconomic mobility, and possibly precipitating life
        events in the 6 months prior to onset of symptoms (or
        prior to interview, for controls).

A321   Piper, D. W.; Greig, Margaret; Shinners, Jane; Thomas,
        Joan; and Crawford, June: Chronic gastric ulcer and stress:
        A comparison of an ulcer population with a control population
        regarding stressful events over a lifetime. Digestion 18:
        303-309, 1978.
        Subjects: 50 Australian patients with gastric ulcer and 50
        control subjects (matched for age, sex, and social grade).
        Method: Subjects completed a questionnaire to indicate
        the occurrence of 31 life events (half of Paykel's list of
        62 events) at any time during the subject's life. Life
        events data were calculated three ways: by number of life
        events experienced, by "change" scores (Holmes and Rahe
        approach), and by "distress" scores (Paykel approach).
        Tennant and Andrews's life event scales [H29] were used
        to weight each event for change and distress values.

A322 Sessions, John T.; Raft, David; and Tate, Suzanne: The severity of Crohn's disease does not correlate with life stress, depression and anxiety. Gastroenterology 74:1144, 1978. (Abstract)

> Subjects: 47 patients with Crohn's disease.
> Method: The severity of each patient's disease was quantified using the Crohn's Disease Activity Index (CDAI). Subjects completed the Schedule of Recent Experience and the SCL-90 (Symptom Check List—anxiety and depression scales).

RC799A634

A323 Stevenson, David K.: Life change and the postoperative course of duodenal ulcer patients. Unpublished medical thesis, University of Washington, 1975. [An article based on this study was published subsequently by Stevenson and coauthors Donald C. Nabseth, Minoru Masuda, and Thomas H. Holmes in Journal of Human Stress 5(1):19-28, 1979.]

> Subjects: 42 male subjects with duodenal ulcer who had undergone either of two surgical procedures (hemigastrectomy or a drainage procedure) plus vagotomy.
> Method: In this retrospective study subjects completed a postal questionnaire containing the Schedule of Recent Experience (for the 4 years before and the 4 years after surgery). Medical records, discharge summaries, and records from a prospective study to evaluate surgical procedures in the treatment of duodenal ulcer were all reviewed; postoperative follow-up data were organized into 6-month periods. Subjects were assigned to postoperative clinical groups to reflect the amount, seriousness, and types of postoperative symptoms, and correlations with life change scores were examined.

A324 Susman, Paul Erwin: The relationship of ulcerative colitis and spastic colon to life change, ego strength and family disturbance (Doctoral dissertation, Northwestern University, 1976). Dissertation Abstracts International 37:3632-B, 1977.

> Subjects: 32 ulcerative colitis patients, 27 spastic colon patients, and two control groups (20 "routine medically healthy" individuals and 97 night school students).
> Method: Subjects completed "three objective psychological questionnaires" [unnamed in abstract] as measures of life change, ego functioning, and family disturbance. In addition, the two patient groups and one control group (N=20) participated in tape-recorded interviews concerning life change, family and patient interaction, parental dominance, and the expression of anger.

A325   Whybrow, Peter C.; Kane, Francis J.; and Lipton, Morris A.:
        Regional ileitis and psychiatric disorder. Psychosomatic
        Medicine 30:209-221, 1968.
            Subjects: 39 patients with proved regional ileitis.
            Method: In this retrospective study all available hospital
            records for each subject were reviewed. Data were col-
            lected in the following areas: major characteristics of
            the group, treatment by surgery and by steroids, preva-
            lence of psychiatric disorder, relationship between "life
            stress" and GI symptoms (precipitating events in illness
            onset and exacerbation}, psychiatric symptoms observed
            during hospitalization, and associated psychosomatic dis-
            ease. An illustrative case history is also presented.

                        SPECIFIC ILLNESS:
                        Genitourinary System
                          (A326-A331)

A326   Lodewegens, F. J.; Bos-van Run, I.; Groenman, N. H.;
        and Lappohn, R. E.: The effect of psychic factors on the
        spontaneous cure of secondary amenorrhoea: A comparison
        of cases with and without spontaneous cure. Journal of
        Psychosomatic Research 21:175-182, 1977.
            Subjects: 30 women with functional amenorrhoea of at
            least 6 months' duration.
            Method: In the prospective part of this study, each woman
RC52.J6   was interviewed by a consulting psychiatrist during her
            initial diagnostic inpatient examination, and two personal-
            ity inventories were administered: the ABV (Amsterdam
            Biographic Questionnaire), which produces neuroticism
            and extraversion scores, and the Dutch translation of the
            MMPI. At least 2 years later the subjects were reexam-
            ined to determine incidence of spontaneous cure (3 suc-
            cessive menstrual periods in the absence of medical
            therapy). At that time the retrospective part of the study
            was conducted: each woman completed the Schedule of
            Recent Experience for the preceding 2 years (divided into
            6-month segments).

A327   Malmquist, A.: A prospective study of patients in chronic
        hemodialysis. I. Method and characteristics of the patient
        group. Journal of Psychosomatic Research 17:333-337, 1973.
RC52.J6   Subjects: 23 Swedish patients admitted to the chronic
            hemodialysis program.

Method: This study was designed to test the validity of findings in an earlier follow-up study done with American patients (see A329). The same psychological and psychiatric testing and interviews for pretreatment variables were performed. Subjects were followed for 6-12 months during treatment. [See A328 for Part II of this study.]

A328   Malmquist, A.: A prospective study of patients in chronic hemodialysis. II. Predicting factors regarding rehabilitation. Journal of Psychosomatic Research 17:339-344, 1973.

Subjects: 23 Swedish patients admitted to the chronic hemodialysis program.

RC52.J6

Method: This paper reports the 6-month and 12-month outcome of patients on hemodialysis. Rehabilitation at 6 or 12 months is examined in relation to 150 pretreatment variables, including adaptability to life changes before and after onset of kidney symptoms. [See A327 for Part I of this study.]

A329   Malmquist, A.; Kopfstein, J. Held; Frank, E. T.; Picklesimer, K.; Clements, G.; Ginn, E.; and Cromwell, R. L.: Factors in psychiatric prediction of patients beginning hemodialysis: A follow-up of 13 patients. Journal of Psychosomatic Research 16:19-23, 1972.

Subjects: 13 American patients with chronic renal failure.

RC52.J6

Method: Subjects were patients selected by a medical team for admission to hemodialysis. After selection but before treatment began, subjects were tested and interviewed. Eight psychological tests were administered, and interview questions generated data on psychiatric and psychosocial variables (early relationships, family and social history, psychiatric and physical health histories, attitudes toward illness, adaptability to life changes before and after illness onset, etc.). Patients' adjustment to treatment was evaluated at 3 and 12 months after treatment had begun, and the relationship of pretreatment variables was examined. [See also A327 and A328.]

A330   Pond, D. A., and Maratos, Jason: Psychosocial interrelations of benign prostatic hypertrophy. Journal of Psychosomatic Research 21:201-206, 1977.

RC52.J6

Subjects: A total of 35 patients from two study groups (hospitalized patients with acute urinary retention plus patients admitted from a waiting list for prostatic surgery) and a control group (patients with carcinoma of the bladder).

Method: Several days after surgery, all subjects were
given a semistructured interview. They also completed
two questionnaires, the Middlesex Hospital Questionnaire
(for personality and symptoms of anxiety, depression,
etc.), and a modified Schedule of Recent Experience (covering the 2 years prior to hospitalization). Weight of re-
sected prostatic mass was used as an indicator of degree
of prostatic hypertrophy; correlations of gland size, personality, and life events were examined.

A331   Wilcoxon, Linda A.; Schrader, Susan L.; and Sherif,
Carolyn W.: Daily self-reports on activities, life events,
moods, and somatic changes during the menstrual cycle.
Psychosomatic Medicine 38:399-417, 1976.
    Subjects: 11 males, 11 females taking oral contracep-
    tives, and 11 females not taking oral contraceptives (all
    college students).
    Method: Subjects completed four questionnaires daily for
    35 consecutive days: the Pleasant Activities Schedule,
    the Menstrual Distress Questionnaire (to measure affec-
    tive, somatic, and behavior changes in the menstrual
    cycle, but instrument was given an indefinite name so
    subjects would not be alerted to its purpose), the Mood
    Adjective Checklist, and the Personal Stress Inventory
    (checklist of events and a 3-point scale to rate "degree of
    stressfulness" of each event experienced in the past 24
    hours). Male subjects were assigned a "pseudocycle,"
    and then the Males, Females-Pill, and Females-No Pill
    subject groups were compared across the three phases of
    the menstrual cycle.

SPECIFIC ILLNESS:
Pregnancy, Childbirth, and the Puerperium
(A332-A346)

A332   Dunn, Susan Irene: Life change magnitude, pregnancy, patterns of contraceptive use, and sexual activity in unmarried
females. Unpublished master's thesis, University of Washington, 1976.
    Subjects: 48 unmarried females, aged 18-27 (12 preg-
    nant, 36 not pregnant).
    Method: Subjects completed a two-part questionnaire.
    Part 1 contained Anderson's College Schedule of Recent
    Experience (for previous 2 years), and Part 2 contained

questions concerning demographic characteristics, contraceptive use, and sexual activity.

A333 Friederich, M. A., and Labrum, A. H.: The setting for pregnancy in women seen for elective abortion. Psychosomatic Medicine 37:89-90, 1975. (Abstract)

Subjects: 262 women who had an elective early abortion.
Method: Subjects were interviewed 4-8 weeks after the abortion. Data were obtained on the medical and psychological sequelae of the abortion and on the psychosocial setting (including life changes) at the time of conception.

A334 Gorsuch, Richard L., and Key, Martha K.: Abnormalities of pregnancy as a function of anxiety and life stress. Psychomatic Medicine 36:352-362, 1974.

Subjects: 111 pregnant women attending an obstetrics clinic serving primarily low-income patients.
Method: The State-Trait Anxiety Inventory was used to measure anxiety over time. At each subject's first clinic visit she was asked about prepregnancy anxiety and about anxiety since learning she was pregnant; at subsequent clinic visits she was asked about anxiety since last visit. A modified Schedule of Recent Experience was administered at each subject's first clinic visit to assess life change in the 2 years preceding pregnancy; after delivery, each woman completed the same life change instrument for the interval since her first clinic visit. Medical records were examined for data on any abnormalities of mother or infant.

A335 Jones, Arthur C.: Life change and psychological distress as predictors of pregnancy outcome. Psychosomatic Medicine 40:402-412, 1978.

Subjects: 122 pregnant women at a residential facility for indigent women.
Method: Several weeks before delivery, each subject was administered a battery of tests for possible predictors of labor complications: the Lykken Activity Preference Questionnaire, the Grimm Psychological Tension Battery, subject and investigator ratings of anxiety, the MMPI, and the Schedule of Recent Experience (2 years). An obstetric screening survey was used to assess medical and demographic high-risk factors. After delivery, medical records were examined for the presence or absence of six factors defined as labor complications.

A336   Kjaer, George Christian Dixen: Some psychosomatic aspects of pregnancy with particular reference to nausea and vomiting. Unpublished medical thesis, University of Washington, 1959.

        Subjects: 18 postpartum obstetric patients and 17 prenatal patients.

        Method: All subjects completed the Cornell Medical Index, the Schedule of Recent Experience (the early version developed by Hawkins and Holmes, covering 10 years and scored by simple counting of events), and a questionnaire concerning obstetric and gynecological history, symptoms during pregnancy, and attitudes toward pregnancy. An interview was also conducted to confirm and/or supplement data collected by questionnaire.

A337   Klinghoffer, Laura A.: Self-concept, stress and alcohol consumption during pregnancy. Unpublished master's thesis, University of Washington, 1978.

        Subjects: 17 pregnant women receiving prenatal care at a hospital family medical center.

        Method: Subjects completed the Schedule of Recent Experience and the "How I See Myself" Scale (self-concept). Data were collected by interview and questionnaire on the following factors: demographic characteristics; coffee, tea, cola, and alcohol consumption; smoking; medication and drug use; and knowledge of effects of alcohol consumption during pregnancy.

A338   Kruckemeyer, Margaret Irene: Psychosocial assets, life crisis and the incidence of miscarriage. Unpublished master's thesis, University of Washington, 1975.

        Subjects: 103 pregnant women receiving prenatal care at a military medical facility.

        Method: Subjects were in no later than the 14th week of gestation when they completed the Internal-External Support Systems (IESS) questionnaire. The IESS incorporates items from other instruments to measure the following: "self" support systems (ego strength, flexibility, hostility, self-esteem, etc.); psychosocial assets; external support systems (neighborliness scale); and life changes (Schedule of Recent Experience). Medical charts were reviewed after 20 weeks of gestation time had elapsed to document incidence of miscarriage (6 aborted by 20 weeks, 97 did not).

A339 Murphy, George E.; Kuhn, Nobuko Obayashi; Christensen, Roger F.; and Robins, Eli: "Life stress" in a normal population: A study of 101 women hospitalized for normal delivery. Journal of Nervous and Mental Disease 134:150-161, 1962.

RC321.J83

 Subjects: 101 postpartum women.
 Method: Subjects were interviewed about the occurrence of 27 life events in the 12 months prior to hospitalization for delivery.

A340 Nuckolls, Katherine B.; Cassel, John; and Kaplan, Berton H.: Psychosocial assets, life crisis and the prognosis of pregnancy. American Journal of Epidemiology 95:431-441, 1972.

 Subjects: 170 pregnant women.

RA421A37

 Method: Early in pregnancy each subject completed a new questionnaire, TAPPS (Total Adaptive Potential for Pregnancy Scale), designed to assess psychosocial assets. At 32 weeks the subjects completed the Schedule of Recent Experience (for the 2 years before and the 3 trimesters of pregnancy). Medical records were reviewed after each subject's delivery in order to designate the pregnancy as "normal" or "complicated."

A341 Peres, Katherine Eleanor: Emotional aspects of the pregnancy experience: Anxiety, life changes, and feminine identification (Doctoral dissertation, University of Florida, 1978). Dissertation Abstracts International 39:5081B-5082B, 1979.

Z5053.D57

 Subjects: 64 women in the first trimester of pregnancy.
 Method: Instruments [unnamed in abstract] were administered to measure state and trait anxiety, life changes, and somatic symptoms before and during pregnancy. The Bem Sex Role Inventory and the Attitudes Toward Women Scale were used to measure sexual identification and sex role preference.

A342 Schwartz, Jane Linker: A study of the relationship between maternal life change events and premature delivery. Unpublished master's thesis, University of Washington, 1973.

 Subjects: 25 mothers who delivered full-term (37-40 weeks) infants and 25 mothers who delivered premature (less than 37 weeks) infants.
 Method: Subjects were interviewed for demographic information, for histories of previous pregnancies, and for health associated with previous as well as present pregnancies. Subjects completed the Schedule of Recent

Experience (for the 2 years prior to and the 3 trimesters of pregnancy).

A343   Sugar, Max: At-risk factors for the adolescent mother and her infant. Journal of Youth and Adolescence 5:251-270, 1976. Subjects: 215 adolescent (age 14 and under) and 264 adult (20 years and over) mothers of premature or full-term infants.

HQ796.J625 Method: The author used the Social Readjustment Rating Scale to tabulate life event data of each mother during her pregnancy and then compared "Percent crises in pregnancies" of adolescent and adult mothers by infant's birth-weight.

A344   Swigar, Mary E.; Bowers, Malcolm B.; and Fleck, Stephen: Grieving and unplanned pregnancy. Psychiatry 39:72-80, 1976.

RC321 P93 Subjects: 7 women applying for abortion who experienced conception in very close temporal relationship to bereavement.

Method: Case histories are presented of women whose onset of pregnancy occurred within 2 months of the death (or of the knowledge of impending death from illness) of a close friend or loved one.

A345   Williams, Cindy Cook; Williams, Reg Arthur; Griswold, Manzer J.; and Holmes, Thomas H.: Pregnancy and life change. Journal of Psychosomatic Research 19:123-129, 1975.

RC52.J6 Subjects: 23 postpartum mothers who delivered prematurely and 23 who delivered at full-term gestation.

Method: Subjects completed the Schedule of Recent Experience (for pregnancy and 2 years prior to conception).

A346   Williams, Cynthia Ann: Life change units and length of gestation. Unpublished master's thesis, University of Washington, 1974.

This is the original study upon which the later publication, A345, was based.

SPECIFIC ILLNESS:
Skin and Subcutaneous Tissue
(A347-A351)

A347   Baughman, Richard, and Sobel, Raymond: Psoriasis, stress, and strain. Archives of Dermatology 103:599-605, 1971.

Subjects: 252 adults who had been hospitalized for psoriasis.

Method: Subjects completed a modified Schedule of Recent Experience (previous 5 years). A newly developed Psoriasis Severity Scale was used to calculate annual "severity" scores for the same 5-year period for each subject. A personality inventory was also administered.

A348 Brown, Dennis G.: Stress as a precipitant factor of eczema. Journal of Psychosomatic Research 16:321-327, 1972.

Subjects: 82 eczema patients and 123 control subjects (dental patients).

Method: Subjects completed questionnaires covering the following areas: incidence of potentially stressful life events (bereavement and separation experiences) in the past 12 months; incidence of "a severe shock, worry, or emotional upset" within 6 months of illness onset; childhood bereavement and separation experiences; past medical history (psychiatric illnesses, other skin disorders, other psychosomatic disorders); attitudes and emotional responses to difficulties. Questionnaire data were compared to responses and observations made during clinical interviews.

A349 Edwards, Allan E.; Shellow, William V. R.; Wright, Edwin T.; and Digman, Thomas F.: Pruritic skin disease, psychological stress, and the itch sensation. Archives of Dermatology 112:339-343, 1976.

Subjects: 18 men and 22 women.

Method: Subjects completed an illness history (to determine positive or negative history of a pruritic dermatosis) and a modified Schedule of Recent Experience (for the previous 90 days). Controlled levels of terminable itching were induced experimentally and subjects' perception of itching (threshold and intensity) was examined in relation to their positive or negative history of pruritic dermatosis and to their recent life change experience.

A350 Smith, Michael R.: Psychogenic factors in skin disease. Unpublished medical thesis, University of Washington, 1962.

Subjects: 105 dermatology clinic patients.

Method: In Part 1 of this study, baseline data regarding level of control and sebaceous gland activity were gathered by measuring sebum flow, skin temperature, urinary 17-ketosteroid level, and emotional status in a sample of

normal subjects; baseline data were then compared to data
for 4 dermatology patients. In Part 2 of this study, 105
subjects completed the Cornell Medical Index and the
Schedule of Recent Experience (the early version developed by Hawkins and Holmes, covering 10 years and
scored by simple counting of events).

A351   Ullman, Kenneth C.; Moore, Ralph W.; and Reidy, Mary:
Atopic eczema: A clinical psychiatric study. Journal of
Asthma Research 14:91-99, 1977.
    Subjects: 10 patients with atopic eczema and 9 normal
matched controls plus 1 nonmatched control subject.
    Method: Subjects completed a series of psychological
tests (MMPI, Draw-House-Tree-Person, and selected
TAT cards), and a clinical psychiatric interview was conducted with each subject. Interview data included the nature and timing of life events as precipitants of the onset
and exacerbation of eczema.

SPECIFIC ILLNESS:
Musculoskeletal System and Connective Tissues
(A352-A358)

A352   Heisel, J. Stephen: Life changes as etiologic factors in
juvenile rheumatoid arthritis. Journal of Psychosomatic
Research 16:411-420, 1972.
    Subjects: 34 patients with juvenile rheumatoid arthritis
and 68 well control subjects (two controls matched to
every patient).

RC52.J6   Method: Parents of subjects completed a modified version of Coddington's Schedule of Recent Experience for
children (for the 12 months preceding illness onset or interview). Medical records were examined to document
date and mode of illness onset for patients with juvenile
rheumatoid arthritis.

A353   Hendrie, H. C.; Paraskevas, F.; Baragar, F. D.; and
Adamson, J. D.: Stress, immunoglobulin levels and early
polyarthritis. Journal of Psychosomatic Research 15:337-
342, 1971.
RC52.J6   Subjects: 22 patients with early polyarthritis and two
control groups (37 hospital staff and friends and 74 patients with primary depression).

Method: Polyarthritic subjects were interviewed, the date of the onset of their joint symptoms was established, their immunoglobulin levels were measured, and they completed the Schedule of Recent Experience for the 3 years preceding onset of symptoms. The depressive control subjects completed the Schedule of Recent Experience for the year prior to the onset of their symptoms, and the staff control subjects completed the Schedule of Recent Experience for the past year.

A354   Lunghi, M. E.; Miller, P. McC.; and McQuillanl W. M.: Psychosocial factors in osteoarthritis of the hip. Journal of Psychosomatic Research 22:57-63, 1978.
Subjects: 18 outpatients with osteoarthritic hips.
Method: At the beginning of this 6-month study subjects were given a medical examination and x-rays were taken. The Eysenck Personality Inventory and the Zung Depression Scale were also administered, and subjects completed the Cochrane and Robertson Life Events Inventory. X-rays were taken again at 3 and at 6 months. The medical exam was repeated monthly, and at that time subjects completed the Life Events Inventory for the previous month. Between monthly examinations, subjects kept a weekly diary of 13 symptoms and two types (pleasant/unpleasant) of events experienced in the past week; the Affect Balance Scale (measure of psychological status) was administered with the weekly diaries. At the end of 6 months, subjects gave each Life Events Inventory item a score of 1-1000 for disruptiveness.

A355   Mooney, Vert; Cairns, Douglas; and Robertson, James: A system for evaluating and treating chronic back disability. Western Journal of Medicine 124:370-376, 1976.
The authors describe five methods used to evaluate cases of patients with prolonged pain disability at their Problem Back Treatment Center: patient pain drawings, pentothal pain studies, a modified Schedule of Recent Experience, the MMPI, and response to treatment challenge.

A356   Otto, Rosemarie, and Mackay, Ian R.: Psycho-social and emotional disturbance in systemic lupus erythematosus. Medical Journal of Australia 2:488-493, 1967.
Subjects: 20 female patients with systemic lupus erythematosus and 20 matched control subjects (patients who had a severe accidental hemorrhage in pregnancy).

RC52.J6

Method: The Eysenck Personality Inventory was administered, and all subjects were interviewed to obtain a life
history. Particular attention was given to childhood experiences and to the psychological and social stresses related to onset and exacerbation of illness.

A357 Pancheri, P.; Teodori, S.; and Aparo, U. L.: Psychological
aspects of rheumatoid arthritis vis-à-vis osteoarthrosis.
Scandinavian Journal of Rheumatology 7:42-48, 1978.
Subjects: 35 rheumatoid arthritis patients and 30 osteoarthrosis patients.
Method: The two arthritic groups were compared on the
basis of the following objective measures: the MMPI, the
State-Trait Anxiety Inventory, the M.H.P.A. (personality
traits evaluated and put into profile form), and ANAM (a
standardized anamnestic data record sheet that codifies
demographic characteristics, family and personal history
including life events preceding illness, and subject's
psychopathological history).

A358 Rimón, Ranan; Belmaker, Robert H.; and Ebstein, Richard:
Psychosomatic aspects of juvenile rheumatoid arthritis.
Scandinavian Journal of Rheumatology 6:1-10, 1977.
Subjects: 54 children hospitalized for juvenile rheumatoid
arthritis.
Method: Patients were observed during hospitalization
for psychiatric symptoms, rheumatological variables,
personality, and behavioral characteristics. Parents
were interviewed 1-3 times to collect data concerning
home atmosphere, family relationships, previous psychiatric disturbances, and major distressing life events preceding onset and exacerbation of juvenile rheumatoid
arthritis (e.g., parental divorce or separation, illness
and death in the family, important change in living conditions).

SPECIFIC ILLNESS:
Congenital Anomalies
(A359-A360)

A359 Dodge, J. A.: Psychosomatic aspects of infantile pyloric
stenosis. Journal of Psychosomatic Research 16:1-5, 1972.
Subjects: 394 children with infantile pyloric stenosis and
RC52.J6 two control groups (119 unselected school children and 62
children hospitalized for tonsillectomy).

Method: Mothers of subjects were interviewed concerning adverse social, domestic, or emotional circumstances during pregnancy, including 10 specified life events such as bereavement, family illness, marital disruption, housing and financial problems. In addition, 101 of the youngest pyloric stenosis patients were matched to 101 "normal" subjects, and their mothers' pregnancy experiences were compared.

A360   Revill, Susan I., and Dodge, J. A.: Psychological determinants of infantile pyloric stenosis. Archives of Disease in Childhood 53:66-68, 1978.

Subjects: 100 infants with infantile pyloric stenosis, 100 "normal" children whose mothers had not sought medical advice at any time concerning feeding problems, and 50 children with spina bifida.

Method: Mothers of all subjects completed the Cochrane and Robertson Life Events Inventory for the period of their pregnancy. They also completed the Eysenck Personality Inventory (Form A), the Multiple Affect Adjective Check List, and Linear Analogue Scales (to measure satisfaction and/or distress due to feeding infant).

RJ1A793X

SPECIFIC ILLNESS:
Certain Conditions Originating in the Perinatal Period
(A361-A362)

A361   Kirgis, Carol A.; Woolsey, Donna B.; and Sullivan, John J.: Predicting infant Apgar scores. Nursing Research 26:439-442, 1977.

Subjects: 51 newborn infants.

Method: Mothers of subjects were administered the Utah Test Appraising Health (UTAH) during the second or third trimester of pregnancy. UTAH is a 360-item instrument containing 16 scales to measure illness (past 10 years), life change (modified Schedule of Recent Experience for past year), and coping mechanisms (Health Predispositions Test) during pregnancy. After delivery medical records were reviewed to determine infant outcome as measured by the Apgar score 5 minutes after birth; length of labor and maternal health postdelivery were also documented.

RT1.N8

A362   Morgan, Susan A.; Buchanan, Diane; and Abram, Harry S.:
        Psychosocial aspects of hyaline membrane disease. Psycho-
        somatics 17:147-150, 1976.
            Subjects: 51 infants born with hyaline membrane disease
            and 35 infants born without hyaline membrane disease.
            Method: Both parents of the hyaline membrane disease
            infants and mothers of the control subjects were inter-
            viewed and asked to complete questionnaires concerning
            the following: family's social and psychological setting
            before and during pregnancy, psychosocial and physical
            problems during pregnancy, and impact of pregnancy and
            birth (or death) on the family structure. Life change data
            were extracted from interview and questionnaire responses,
            and the Social Readjustment Rating Scale was used to quan-
            tify life change scores for families before and during preg-
            nancy. The families with hyaline membrane disease
            births were followed at 6 months and at yearly intervals
            to study impact of hyaline membrane disease birth (and/or
            death) on family's structure and functioning.

SPECIFIC ILLNESS:
Symptoms, Signs, and Ill-Defined Conditions
(A363-A365)

A363   Cassidy, Catherine Angela: The relationship between ap-
        praisal of adjustment required by reported daily life events,
        physical symptoms and temperature range (Doctoral disser-
        tation, New York University, 1975). Dissertation Abstracts
        International 36:1654-B, 1975.
            Subjects: 40 female nursing students, aged 18-25.
            Method: Subjects kept a daily record of events and symp-
            toms experienced for a period of 14 days. In addition,
            they recorded their oral temperature at 2-hour intervals
            during wakefulness. At the end of 14 days of data collec-
            tion, each subject rated the amount of adjustment required
            by each event on the daily events checklist.

A364   Holmes, T. Stephenson, and Holmes, Thomas H.: Short-
        term intrusions into the life style routine. Journal of Psycho-
        somatic Research 14:121-132, 1970.
            Subjects: 55 individuals, aged 16-60, drawn as a sample
            of convenience.
            Method: The Schedule of Daily Experience (SDE), a modi-
            fication of the Schedule of Recent Experience, was devel-

oped to record life changes on a daily basis. Each subject completed the SDE daily for at least 2 (and up to 9) weeks, and at the same time kept a daily diary of health changes (signs, symptoms, inconveniences), giving possible reasons for symptoms and a brief description of general state of mind each day ("nervous," "elated," "moody," etc.).

A365   Peters, Jerome: The neurologist's use of rating scales, EEG, and tranquilizers in dealing with hysterical symptoms. Journal of Biological Psychology 18:40-42, 1976.
    Subjects: 20 neurology clinic outpatients, 10 with headaches and 10 with back pain unresponsive to treatment. Method: All subjects had pain unresponsive to traditional and standard methods of treatment, all had normal neurological and general physical examinations, and all had negative profiles for depression (Beck Depression Inventory and Hamilton Rating Scale for Depression). Three measures of anxiety were administered (Wolpe's "Willoughby Personality Schedule," "Fear Inventory," and "Bernreuter S-S Scale and Scoring Key"). A modified Schedule of Recent Experience was also administered to collect data on life events just prior to time of onset of pain. Subjects were followed for 1 year in the neurology clinic: after initial administration of three EEG tests (with saline, with chlordiazepoxide, and with chlorpromazine), subjects were treated with chlordiazepoxide for 6 months and with chlorpromazine for the next 6 months. Improvement under the two tranquilizers was compared.

SPECIFIC ILLNESS:
Injury and Poisoning
(A366–A370)

A366   Andreasen, N. J. C.; Noyes, Russel, Jr.; and Hartford, C.E.: Factors influencing adjustment of burn patients during hospitalization. Psychosomatic Medicine 34:517-525, 1972.
    Subjects: 32 patients in a hospital burn unit. Method: A psychiatric history was obtained from each patient shortly after admission, and a standardized social history was obtained from a close relative. In these histories special attention was directed to collecting data about premorbid personality and about the occurrence of

major life changes prior to injury. Daily progress notes
from medical charts were used to assess adjustment
("poor adjustment" was defined as developing severe depression or regression, violent or nearly unmanageable
behavior, delirium, or death).

A367   Erickson, Ruth Mae: Accidental poisoning in childhood and
life stress. Unpublished master's thesis, University of
Washington, 1976.
Subjects: 95 preschool children, aged 1-4, who had been
treated for a nonfatal ingestion of poison within the previous year.
Method: Parents or guardians of subjects completed a
postal questionnaire which included questions about the
poisoning incident and Coddington's Schedule of Recent
Experience for preschool children (with one event added,
"moving day"). Life change data for the poisoning subjects were compared to Coddington's "normative" data.

A368   Sibert, R.: Stress in families of children who have ingested
poisons. British Medical Journal 3:87-89, 1975.
Subjects: 105 young children admitted to hospital for accidental ingestion of poison and 105 control children matched
for age, sex, and family's socioeconomic status.
Method: One or both parents of subjects and controls were
interviewed, and their family settings were compared.
Special attention was directed to family history of childhood poisoning or accidents, occupation and health of parents, family's housing conditions, and to the occurrence
of specified life events in the recent past: family illness
or bereavement, pregnancy, change of residence, father
unemployed, one parent absent from home, and parental
seeking of treatment for depression or anxiety.

A369   Sobel, Raymond: The psychiatric implications of accidental
poisoning in childhood. Pediatric Clinics of North America
16:653-685, 1970.
Subjects: 367 children, ages 2-5, whose parents responded
to a survey of families living in a predominantly rural area
of New England.
Method: Parents of 115 children reported that an accidental poisoning incident had occurred to the index child; parents of 252 children reported no accident. Both groups of
families were studied and compared based on information
gathered during an initial home interview and at a follow-up

interview over a year later. The following instruments
were administered during interviews: the Family Life
Questionnaire (an extensive survey of parents' history,
marital relationship, psychopathology as well as child's
development and family relationships); a Hazard Survey
(inspection of home for types and accessibility of poisons);
the Childhood Symptom Rating Scale (a modification of
Prall's Symptom List to identify emotional disturbances
in children); a modified Schedule of Recent Experience
(parents' life changes in each of the preceding 8 years);
and the Van Allstyne Picture Vocabulary Intelligence Test
(administered to the child while parent being interviewed).

A370   Tollefson, DeEtte Joan: The relationship between the ocurrence of fractures and life crisis events. Unpublished master's thesis, University of Washington, 1972.
Subjects: 37 hospitalized adult patients with diagnosis of
fracture due to trauma.
Method: Subjects completed the Schedule of Recent Experience. The life crisis patterns constructed from their
life change data were compared to findings from other
studies using the Schedule of Recent Experience with dis-
similar subject groups.

LIFE CHANGE EVENTS
AND PERFORMANCE

PERFORMANCE:
Care-seeking
(B1 - B40)

B1   Andersen, Marcia DeCann, and Pleticha, Jane Marie: Emer-
      gency unit patients' perceptions of stressful life events.
      Nursing Research 23:378-383, 1974.
          Subjects: 52 emergency unit adult patients.
          Method: Subjects were administered a structured interview
      to collect data on demographic variables, life changes
      (modified Schedule of Recent Experience for previous 6
      months), and patient's estimation of severity of medical
      problem (mild/moderate/severe). Questionnaires were
      completed by attending physicians to document symptoms,
      diagnosis, and physician's perception of severity of patient's
      problem.

B2   Bieliauskas, Linas Augustine: Relationship of the Social Read-
      justment Rating Scale, 17-OHCS values, and MMPI K-Scale
      scores to aid-seeking in firefighters (Doctoral dissertation,
      Ohio University, 1976). Dissertation Abstracts International
      37:5823-B, 1977.
          Subjects: 40 firefighters who had sought professional med-
      ical or psychological aid in the past 6 months and 40 fire-
      fighters who had not sought aid.
          Method: Subjects completed a modified Schedule of Recent
      Experience, the MMPI Mini-Mult, and a questionnaire of
      potential covariate items. A 24-hour urine sample was

RTI.N8

analyzed for presence of 17-OHCS. Eight weeks later the MMPI was readministered and aid-seeking data were collected.

B3   Bieliauskas, Linas A., and Strugar, Debra A.: Sample size characteristics and scores on the Social Readjustment Rating Scale. Journal of Psychosomatic Research 20:201-205, 1976.

Subjects: Three groups of undergraduate psychology students: Group A = 253, Group B = 122, and Group C = 53.
Method: All subjects completed a modified Schedule of Recent Experience for college students (covering the past 6 months) and answered a single item asking them to indicate aid-seeking for physical or mental health in the past 6 months. Life Change Unit (LCU) scores were calculated for each subject in two ways (as the sum of single weighted items and as the sum of weighted items multiplied by frequency of occurrence) and examined in relation to aid-seeking. In addition to comparing differences among the three group sizes, investigators administered the modified Schedule of Recent Experience to a fourth group of 23 other undergraduate students at two different times in order to test reliability of LCU scores.

B4   Bieliauskas, Linas A., and Webb, James T.: The Social Readjustment Rating Scale: Validity in a college population. Journal of Psychosomatic Research 18:115-123, 1974.

Subjects: 116 female and 137 male college students.
Method: All subjects completed a questionnaire of 20 demographic variables including nature and frequency of aid-seeking in the past 6 months (hospitalizations and consultations for physical and mental health). Two modified versions of the Schedule of Recent Experience were completed by each subject: Form A for the general adult population and Form B for college students. Two scoring methods were used to calculate life change scores on both Forms (summing single weighted items and summing weighted items multiplied by frequency of occurrence). Correlations between life change and aid-seeking were examined for both Form A and Form B.

B5   Brown, B. Bradford: Social and psychological correlates of help-seeking behavior among urban adults. American Journal of Community Psychology 6:425-439, 1978.

Subjects: 606 urban adults who had encountered 1 or more of 16 specified life changes within a 4-year period.

Method: Subjects were interviewed about the occurrence of 16 life events and 10 role-related strains, their perceived distress and evaluation of events, and their help-seeking behavior. Those who had sought help (from formal or informal support systems) were compared to those who had not sought help on the basis of interview responses concerning demographic background, personal resources (coping strategies, self-esteem, mastery), social networks, and psychological barriers to help-seeking. [See B22 for description of larger study of this population.]

B6   Casey, Robert L.; Thoresen, A. Robert; and Smith, Frederick J.: The use of the Schedule of Recent Experience Questionnaire in an institutional health care setting. Journal of Psychosomatic Research 14:149-154, 1970.

Subjects: 206 young male trainees at a large military installation.

RC52.J6   Method: Subjects completed the Schedule of Recent Experience (for the 12 months prior to active duty) a few days before the beginning of basic training. Seven weeks later medical records of all subjects were reviewed for illness occurrence and health care utilization (frequency and levels of health care attained).

B7   Cleghorn, J. M., and Streiner, B. J.: Prediction of illness behavior from measures of life change and verbalized depressive themes. Psychosomatic Medicine 33:474-475, 1971. (Abstract)

Subjects: 29 student nurses.

Method: Subjects were interviewed for health history data, and six instruments were administered: a new instrument for measuring depressive themes in speech samples, the Schedule of Recent Experience, a modified Beck Depression Inventory, the MMPI Depression and Ego Strength scales, a Social Adjustment Scale, and the Gottschalk-Gleser Anxiety and Hostility scales. At 6-, 9-, and 12-month intervals, subjects were reinterviewed for illness data (illnesses experienced, symptom episodes, menstrual changes, and accidents). Clinic records were reviewed to determine attendance for documented illnesses.

B8   Corney, Robert T., and Roback, Howard B.: Life stress and psychiatric clinic referral. Southern Medical Journal 69:183-184, 1976.

Subjects: 179 new patients at an adult psychiatric outpatient clinic.

Method: Intake evaluation reports for all subjects were reviewed to determine which life events motivated patients to seek psychiatric help. The Social Readjustment Rating Scale was used to compare types and magnitudes of precipitating events.

B9   Dekker, Daniel J., and Webb, James T.: Relationships of the Social Readjustment Rating Scale to psychiatric patient status, anxiety and social desirability. Journal of Psychosomatic Research 18:125-130, 1974.

Subjects: 40 recently admitted psychiatric inpatients and 40 recently admitted psychiatric outpatients at mental health centers, and 40 "normal" subjects matched for age and social class with patients.

Method: All subjects completed three instruments: a modified Schedule of Recent Experience (for 6 months prior to admission/contact), the MMPI (At and So-R scales), and a demographic information form. Data were analyzed for differences among patients (inpatient vs. outpatient) and between patients and normals.

B10   DuBord, Robert J.: An evaluation of the College Schedule of Recent Experience. Unpublished master's thesis, North Dakota State University, 1972.

Subjects: 196 college students divided into the following groups: 46 who had not sought medical or mental health treatment in the past 3 months, 34 who had not sought medical treatment in the past 3 months, 99 seeking treatment at the college health center, and 17 seeking treatment at the counseling center.

Method: All subjects completed Anderson's College Schedule of Recent Experience (for past year).

B11   Fabrega, Horacio: Perceived illness and its treatment: A naturalistic study in social medicine. British Journal of Preventive and Social Medicine 31:213-219, 1977.

Subjects: 174 Mexican families living in a city.

Method: The families represented all three dominant ethnic groups: Ladinos (people of direct Spanish descent), Mestizos (people of mixed Spanish and Indian descent), and Indigenas (people of Indian descent). The female head of household was interviewed 6 times during one year and asked to report the following: specific family hardships and life events in the past two months and illness in the family in the past two weeks. For each reported illness, data were collected on severity; length of episode; emotional, physiological, and behavioral symptoms; and treatment-seeking (folk practitioner, physician, pharmacy).

B12   Farrington, Keith, and Linsky, Arnold S.: The scheduling of personal crises: Seasonal changes in the pace of social activities and help-seeking at mental health clinics. Paper presented at the meeting of the Society for the Study of Social Problems, New York, August, 1976. [The authors are from the University of New Hampshire.]

Subjects: The entire population of the State of New Hampshire.

Method: The Index of Changes in Social Activities (ICSA), an instrument to measure life change on a macroscopic level, was developed by modifying the Schedule of Recent Experience for application to an entire social system. The frequency of 25 life events was multiplied by the number of persons affected by the event and then by the event's Life Change Unit value (taken from the Social Readjustment Rating Scale). The ICSA scores for the entire state of New Hampshire were calculated for each of 15 consecutive months and then studied in relation to monthly admission rates at all community mental health clinics in the state for the same 15 months.

B13   Hebert, David J.: Life changes and seriousness of illness in female college students. Psychological Reports 43:1297-1298, 1978.

Subjects: 106 female college students who had consulted a physician for a physical illness within the past year.

Method: Subjects completed the Jacobs, Spilken, and Norman Life Change Inventory [B16] for the past year. They also indicated the illness for which they had sought treatment on a checklist version of Wyler's Seriousness of Illness Rating Scale. The number of life changes was studied in relation to seriousness of illness for which treatment was sought.

B14   Holmes, Thomas H.; Masuda, Minoru; and Kogan, W.: Life change magnitude and health care seeking behavior. Psychomatic Medicine 40:86, 1978. (Abstract)

Subjects: About 1,000 patients who had visited a rural family practice clinic, used the services of a prepaid health care facility, or been hospitalized.

Method: Subjects completed the Schedule of Recent Experience. The relationship of life change magnitude to health care seeking behavior was compared to the relationship of life change magnitude to time of illness onset or exacerbation.

B15   Ingham, J. G., and Miller, P. McC.: The determinants of illness declaration. Journal of Psychosomatic Research 20:309-316, 1976.

Subjects: 172 patients consulting a physician for a new illness and 172 control subjects who had not consulted in the past three months.

Method: All patients were waiting to see the doctor when asked to complete a checklist of symptoms (4 psychological and 5 physical) they intended to mention to the doctor; later during a home visit they completed two self-rating symptom scales (pair comparison and visual analogue scales). Control subjects provided symptom reports and ratings during a home interview. A subsample of 34 consulters and 34 controls was also interviewed about threatening life events in the previous three months (Brown and Birley interview method).

B16   Jacobs, Martin A.; Spilken, Aron; and Norman, Martin: Relationship of life change, maladaptive aggression, and upper respiratory infection in male college students. Psychosomatic Medicine 31:31-44, 1969.

Subjects: 29 male college students who sought treatment for sore throat and 29 who were free of sore throat symptoms for a year.

Method: After selection for the study, all subjects were examined to confirm initial diagnosis of upper respiratory infection or freedom from symptoms. All subjects completed the following instruments: the Life Change Inventory (to measure life change in the past year); the Boston University Personality Inventory (to measure adaptation styles: active, defiant vs. passive, compliant); the Adolescent Conflict Test (to measure coping styles); the Manifest Affect Rating Scale (self-rating measure of unpleasant affect). The Life Change Inventory (LCI) is an instrument in which subjects indicate the dates of occurrence in the past year of 47 life events. Life events are classified in three categories: personal failure or role crisis (19 events); loss of or changes in important relationships (18); and increases in personal achievements and responsibilities (10).

B17   Jacobs, Martin A.; Spilken, Aron Z.; Norman, Martin M.;
      and Anderson, Luleén S.: Life stress and respiratory illness.
      Psychosomatic Medicine 32:233-242, 1970.
          Subjects: 106 male college students who sought treatment
          (26 with hay fever, 14 with asthma, 50 with upper respira-
          tory infections, and 16 with anxiety or depression) and 73
          male college students who had not consulted a physician in
          the past year.
          Method: All subjects completed the Life Change Inventory
          (for past year), the Manifest Affect Rating Scale, and the
          Boston University Personality Inventory. This study re-
          ports findings on the relationship of life change and levels
          of manifest distress to degree of symptomatic incapacita-
          tion (with "neurotic" as highest degree and "hay fever" as
          least incapacitated) in aid-seeking and well subjects. [See
          B18 for companion report of measures of adaptation pat-
          terns and family background.]

B18   Jacobs, Martin A.; Spilken, Aron Z.; Norman, Martin M.;
      and Anderson, Luleén S.: Patterns of maladaption and respi-
      ratory illness. Journal of Psychosomatic Research 15:63-72,
      1971.
          Subjects: 106 male college students who sought treatment
          and 73 who had not consulted a physician in the past year.
RC52.J6 Method: This is the companion article to the study reported
          in B17. In addition to the measures of life change and
          manifest distress reported earlier, subjects also com-
          pleted three measures of coping styles to determine
          whether subjects were "intropunitive" (compliant) or
          "extropunitive" (defiant). One questionnaire (the Boston
          University Personality Inventory) and two projective tech-
          niques (the Family-Interaction Test—Crisis Resolution
          Series and the Adolescent Conflict Test) were administered.

B19   Keith, Pat M.: A comparison of factors associated with past
      use, projected use and perceived community need for health
      and social services. Sociological Abstracts 25(4):77SO7444
      (SSSP 1977 0898), 1977.
          Subjects: 62 men and 107 women aged 65 or over.
HM1.S67   Method: All subjects were interviewed for demographic
          and political variables, life change data, past use of health
          and social services, anticipated use of such services, and
          perception of needed services in their community.

B20 Lieberman, Morton A., and Bond, Gary R.: The problem of being a woman: A survey of 1,700 women in consciousness-raising groups. Journal of Applied Behavioral Science 12:363-379, 1976.

> Subjects: 1,669 women in consciousness-raising groups and four comparison groups of 219 women entering personal growth center groups, 57 women starting psychotherapy, 49 women entering sensitivity groups, and a "normative" group of 126 women.
>
> Method: Subjects completed a 26-page questionnaire which included the following: a section on demographic information, a modified version of Paykel's life event instrument, a modified Hopkins Symptom Check List, a self-rating measure of "motives for joining" (help-seeking, interest in women's issues, political activation, social needs, sexual awareness, curiosity), and a checklist of group processes found to be significant and helpful.

B21 Lieberman, Morton A., and Gardner, Jill R.: Institutional alternatives to psychotherapy. Archives of General Psychiatry 33:157-162, 1976.

> Subjects: 426 adults planning to participate in growth centers, 108 adults planning to attend National Training Laboratories programs, and 89 adult applicants at private psychiatric clinics.
>
> Method: All data were collected before subjects began participation in the different facilities. Subjects completed a questionnaire which included demographic questions, Paykel's 61-item life events questionnaire, a 35-item checklist of psychiatric symptoms, and questions concerning the following: how subject chose the specific institution; motivations for coming and expectations; attitudes toward and images of specific processes, leaders, authority; images of psychotherapy and previous experience in psychotherapy.

B22 Lieberman, Morton A., and Glidewell, John C.: Overview: Special issue on the helping process. American Journal of Community Psychology 6:405-411, 1978.

> The authors describe the organization and procedures of a joint effort by two research teams who coordinated their studies of a probability sample of adults in the Chicago area. The sample contained over 2,000 subjects who were interviewed in 1972 and over 1,000 who were interviewed again in 1976-77 for the following: 9 "nonnormative"

(disruptive, crisis) events, 8 "normative" events, role problems and role strains, perceived distress and evaluation of events, help-seeking behavior, measures of personal resources (coping strategies, mastery, and level of self-esteem). (See also B5 and B23.)

B23 Lieberman, Morton A., and Mullan, Joseph T.: Does help help? The adaptive consequences of obtaining help from professionals and social networks. American Journal of Community Psychology 6:499-517, 1978.

Subjects: A large probability sample of more than 2,000 adults in the Chicago area.

Method: Those subjects (N=1,106) who had experienced one of seven life events (3 transitions, 4 crises) between interviews at Time 1 (1972) and Time 2 (1976-77) were divided into "help-seeking behavior" categories: sought professional help, sought help only from social network, sought no help. The three groups were compared on 9 measures of adaptation: symptoms of anxiety and depression; strains in marital, occupational, and economic roles; and "perceived stress" in marital, occupational, economic, and parental roles. [See B22 for description of Chicago study's history and procedures.]

B24 Manuck, Stephen B.; Hinrichsen, James J.; and Ross, Elizabeth O.: Life-stress, locus of control, and treatment-seeking. Psychological Reports 37:589-590, 1975.

Subjects: 98 undergraduate students.

Method: At the beginning of the study 129 undergraduates completed the Jacobs, Spilken, and Norman Life Change Inventory (Category A), Rotter's Internal-External Locus of Control questionnaire, and Spielberger's State-Trait Anxiety Inventory. Six months later 98 subjects were available for follow-up and were interviewed by telephone for illness-related treatment-seeking during the previous 6 months. [See C74 for the first report on 129 subjects.]

B25 Matias, Ronald George: The relationship between client's reported stressful life events and judged severity of presenting problems at a university counseling service (Doctoral dissertation, University of Iowa, 1977). Dissertation Abstracts International 38:3128B-3129B, 1978.

Subjects: 96 clients using the university counseling service.

Method: Subjects completed a newly designed 95-item life event inventory (including whether the event was anticipated and the amount of perceived upset experienced with each event). Intake counselors rated severity of psychopathology of each subject using the Hopkins Psychiatric Rating Scale.

B26 McNeil, Jo, and Bergner, Lawrence: Use of mobile unit to provide health care for preschoolers in rural King County, Washington. Public Health Reports 90:344-348, 1975.
The authors describe the procedures and problems in the establishment of a mobile health unit to provide health screening and treatment for preschool children. They analyze first-year utilization and outcome data, noting the presence in half of the families served of life changes (e.g., residential change, job change) that "might be associated with an increased risk of illness or accident."

B27 Mechanic, David: Stress, illness, and illness behavior. Journal of Human Stress 2(2):2-6, 1976.
The author describes conceptual difficulties in the definition and measurement of life events and their relationship to health status. He emphasizes problems in distinguishing illness from illness behavior and illustrates distortions that can arise when medical records are used as a measure of physical health instead of as an indicator of illness behavior.

B28 Mickley, Sally L.: Life change and health care seeking behavior of patients utilizing an out-patient clinic. Unpublished master's thesis, University of Washington, 1975.
Subjects: 56 patients seeking health care at a clinic for active and retired military personnel and their dependents.
Method: All subjects completed the Schedule of Recent Experience and a questionnaire concerning demographic factors and health care seeking behavior (derived from Zola's 5 nonphysiological patterns of triggers: interpersonal crisis, social interference, presence of sanctioning, perceived threat, nature and quality of symptoms).

B29 Miller, P. McC.; Ingham, J. G.; and Davidson, S.: Life events, symptoms and social support. Journal of Psychosomatic Research 20:515-522, 1976.
Subjects: 34 people who had consulted their doctor in the past 7 days and 34 people who had not recently consulted (matched for age and sex).
Method: All subjects were interviewed at home to obtain the following: self-ratings on 5 physical symptoms

(headache, backache, palpitations, dizziness, breathlessness) and 4 psychological symptoms (anxiety, depression, tiredness, irritability) experienced in the past month; degree of social support (existence, availability, and reciprocity of confidant and number of acquaintances and friends); and life events in the past three months (modified Brown and Birley interview method). Life events were analyzed as "threatening" or "nonthreatening" events.

B30 Mueller, Daniel P.; Edwards, Daniel W.; and Yarvis, Richard M.: Stressful life events and community mental health center patients. Journal of Nervous and Mental Disease 166:16-24, 1978.

Subjects: 187 adults consecutively admitted to outpatient and day treatment clinics in community mental health centers and 321 normal control subjects drawn from the same community.

Method: Patients completed a modified Schedule of Recent Experience (for past 30 days) and a modified General Well-Being Schedule at two different times: before treatment began and about 3 months after treatment had ended. Control subjects completed the same instruments one time only. Life events data were analyzed in two ways: by categories of Undesirable/Desirable/Ambiguous and by independence from subject's psychological condition.

B31 Overbeck, Ann L.: Life stress antecedents to application for help at a mental health center: A clinical study of adaptation (Doctoral dissertation, Smith College School for Social Work, 1972). Dissertation Abstracts International 33:3782-A, 1973. [A report based on this project was published in the Smith College Studies in Social Work issue of June, 1977, pp. 192-233.]

Subjects: 20 new applicants to a mental health center.
Method: Subjects were administered a semistructured interview to obtain data on life events, coping patterns and adaptation styles, sources of social support, and help-seeking behavior. In addition, each subject was administered the Schedule of Recent Experience and Thurlow's Semantic Differential Scales of the Real Me and the World in Which I Live.

B32 Rahe, Richard H.; Biersner, R. J.; Ryman, David H.; and Arthur, Ransom J.: Psychosocial predictors of illness behavior and failure in stressful training. Journal of Health and Social Behavior 13:393-397, 1972.

Subjects: 194 U.S. Navy enlisted men who had been accepted into an Underwater Demolition Team training program.

Method: A few days before the start of training all subjects completed a modified Schedule of Recent Experience (with new unit scoring system) and the Cornell Medical Index (measure of perceived health status). During the course of UDT training, data were collected on number of dispensary visits made per week and severity of reported illnesses by reviewing illness logs kept by the dispensary. At the end of training each subject's success or his failure (approved medical withdrawal vs. voluntary drop out) was documented. Correlations of life change, symptom scores, dispensary visits, and training failure were examined in validation and cross-validation samples.

B33 Rahe, Richard H.; Gunderson, E. K. Eric; and Arthur, Ransom J.: Demographic and psychosocial factors in acute illness reporting. Journal of Chronic Diseases 23:245-255, 1970.

Subjects: 2,684 U.S. Navy and Marine Corps personnel aboard three cruisers on 6- to 8-month overseas deployment.

Method: All subjects completed a military version of the Schedule of Recent Experience (for past 6 months) at the beginning of the cruise. Dispensary records were reviewed at the end of the cruise to document number of visits, number of illnesses, type, and severity. Illness reporting was studied in relation to demographic factors (age, race, education, occupation), recent life change, ship's operational schedule (e.g., combat vs. noncombat periods), and job satisfaction.

B34 Roghmann, Klaus J., and Haggerty, Robert J.: Daily stress, illness, and use of health services in young families. Pediatric Research 7:520-526, 1973.

Subjects: 512 families (1,081 adults and 1,466 children)
Method: During an initial interview, mothers in each family were asked about demographic variables, recent illnesses in family, use of health services, and chronic or long-term "stress." Then each woman was asked to keep a diary for the whole family for 28 consecutive days, noting the following: "upsetting events" in the family, illness episodes (type, time of onset, length), and use of health services (mode, site, timing, frequency). Life

events were rated by investigators as "severe (weight 3)," "medium (weight 2)," and "mild (weight 1)."

B35 Satin, David George: (Help): Life stresses and psycho-social problems in the hospital emergency unit. Social Psychiatry 7:119-126, 1972.

Subjects: 257 people applying to a hospital emergency unit for help with health problems.
Method: Each subject was interviewed by a research psychiatrist for the following information: reasons for coming to emergency unit, factors leading up to admission, life changes in the past 6 months (general and upsetting events), and illness history (hospitalizations, major illnesses, operations). The interviewers listed the problems diagnosed; judged the presence and seriousness of psychosocial problems and judged whether the psychosocial problems influenced subject's decision to seek help at this time; and rated the mental status of subjects.

B36 Slaby, Andrew Edmund: Determinants and correlates of help-seeking behavior in a cohort of white male Yale College freshmen (Doctoral dissertation, Yale University, 1977). Dissertation Abstracts International 39:1703B-1704B, 1978.

Subjects: 188 white male freshmen at Yale.
Method: At the beginning of the academic year all subjects completed a demographic questionnaire, a modified Schedule of Recent Experience (for previous 3 months), 3 subscales of the Symptom Check List-90 (SCL-90), 3 subscales of Weissman's Social Adjustment Scale (SAS), and the Center for Epidemiologic Studies Depression scale (CESD). Three times during the course of the academic year, subjects completed questionnaires on help-seeking (medical, academic, and psychological) during the previous 5 weeks, gradepoint averages, drug use, personality traits (Maudsley Personality Inventory), and social matrix. They also provided current data on physical and psychological symptoms (SCL-90, CESD), life events (modified SRE), and social adjustment (SAS).

B37 Spilken, Aron Z., and Jacobs, Martin A.: Prediction of illness behavior from measures of life crisis, manifest distress and maladaptive coping. Psychosomatic Medicine 33:251-264, 1971.

Subjects: 92 male college students in good health and without a history of chronic symtomatology.

Method: Subjects completed a series of self-rating measures: the Life Change Inventory (recent role crises and failures), the Manifest Affect Rating Scale (current experience of unpleasant affect), and the Boston University Personality Inventory (for two indicators: manifest distress and faulty coping style of defiance, impulsivity, and danger-seeking). One year later 65 subjects were available for follow-up health interviews by telephone and postal questionnaire and were asked to report the following: illness during the past year, types of symptoms involved, and treatment-seeking (self-medication, professional care, no treatment). Those subjects who had not sought treatment (N=42) were compared to those who had sought treatment (N=23) on the basis of scores at initial testing for life change, affect, coping style, and manifest distress.

B38 Tucker, Charles W., and Smith, A. Emerson: Crisis, stress and psychiatric emergencies. Sociological Abstracts 19(1-2): E7976 (SSS 1971 0313), 1971.
Subjects: A random sample of 1,575 people requesting help from a psychiatric service in a metropolitan hospital. Method: The research examined the relationship between patient's life events and psychiatrist's judgment of the person's mental status. Patients were interviewed before seeing psychiatric staff members, and a special record-keeping system was devised to document psychiatric staff's evaluations of patient.

HMI.S67

B39 Ullman, W. Richard, and Garrison, S. Scott: Life stress events: An exploratory analysis of crisis line callers. Crisis Intervention 7:162-175, 1976.
Subjects: 56 callers to a "Help in Emotional Trouble" hotline during a 7-day period.
Method: A modified Schedule of Recent Experience (for past 6 months) was administered over the phone to callers by 15 trained hotline volunteers.

B40 Webb, Linda J.; Snodgrass, Donald; and Thagard, Jerry: Sex differences and life event experiences. Psychological Reports 43:47-53, 1978.
Subjects: 42 male and 48 female adults newly admitted to two psychiatric outpatient clinics.
Method: Subjects completed a modified Schedule of Recent Experience (for past 12 months). Differences in life event experiences of male and female subjects were examined.

PERFORMANCE:
Work and School
(B41 - B69)

B41 Adams, Daniel Wilson: Life change and counseling effectiveness (Doctoral dissertation, East Texas State University,
1976). Dissertation Abstracts International 37:4125-A, 1977.
Subjects: 54 master's level counselor trainees enrolled in
a practicum course.
Method: At the end of their semester course in counseling, the subjects completed Harris's modified Schedule of
Recent Experience [see B52] for college students (for past
12 months). Instructors in the counseling course and su-
pervisors in the field rated each trainee's effectiveness on
the Counselor Evaluation Rating Scale. Counseling effectiveness scores were studied in relation to high vs. low
life change scores.

B42 Arthur, Ransom J.: Success is predictable. Military Medicine 136:539-545, 1971.
The author reviews the literature and discusses the utility
of life change research in the prediction of illness and the
selection of military personnel.

B43 Bassetti, Roger Lee: Life change, trait anxiety, dogmatism,
and academic performance of college freshmen (Doctoral
dissertation, East Texas State University, 1973). Dissertation Abstracts International 34:5703A-5704A, 1974.
Subjects: 300 first-year college students.
Method: Subjects were divided into groups by level of
academic risk (high, medium, low). At the end of the fall
semester all subjects completed Harris's modified
Schedule of Recent Experience [see B52] for college students (for past 12 months), the State-Trait Anxiety Inventory (Form X-2), and the Dogmatism Scale (Form E).
At the beginning of the spring semester, academic records
were reviewed to obtain a grade point average for each
subject.

B44 Carranza, Elihu: The impact of teacher life changes and
performance on student dropouts. Educational Research
17:122-127, 1975.
Subjects: 110 high school teachers.
Method: Subjects completed the Schedule of Recent Experience in the middle of a school year. School records were

reviewed to determine number of students in each teacher's classes during the last year and a half who had dropped out of school. Selected teacher performance variables were also documented (number of illnesses, absenteeism, requests for transfer, job changes, number of classes and number of students taught, students' grades) and studied in relation to teacher's life changes and incidence of student drop outs, using pairwise and multiple correlation techniques.

B45 Carranza, Elihu: Life changes and teacher performance. California Journal of Educational Research 25:73-78, 1974.
Subjects: 110 high school teachers.
Method: Subjects completed the Schedule of Recent Experience in the middle of a school year. Various sources were reviewed to document selected teacher performance variables, including teacher's absenteeism (number of days, frequency, duration of illnesses), work history (requests for transfer, job changes), and grading patterns, as well as incidence of student drop outs, all in the previous year and a half. Pairwise, multiple, and canonical correlation procedures were used to analyze data.

B46 Carranza, Elihu: A study of the impact of life changes on high school teacher performance in the Lansing school district as measured by the Holmes and Rahe Schedule of Recent Experience (Doctoral dissertation, Michigan State University, 1972). Dissertation Abstracts International 33:4996A-4997A, 1973.
This is the original study upon which publications B44 and B45 were based.

B47 Clinard, John W., and Golden, Stanford, Jr.: Life-change events as related to self-reported academic and job performance. Psychological Reports 33:391-394, 1973.
Subjects: 105 undergraduate and graduate students who were also currently employed or had worked in the past year.
Method: All subjects completed a modified Schedule of Recent Experience (for the past three years). They also completed a checklist questionnaire concerning 16 academic and job-related performance variables (including grade point average; number of skipped classes, missed tests, and tardy arrivals; personal injury, illness and accidents in the past three years; number of promotions, raises, jobs previously held, and work days missed).

B48 Dickinson, Gary: Identifying adult learning needs through life change analysis. Literacy Discussion 5:639-648, 1974.
The author discusses possible uses of the Schedule of Recent Experience in adult basic education classes. One possibility is prevention of illness: focusing learning activities on life change events may help students avoid maladaptive consequences of life changes. Another use concerns direction of the course itself: Teachers might administer the Schedule of Recent Experience to identify individual students' social setting and concerns, and then choose class content and materials relevant to students' recent life change experiences.

B49 Dutton, LaVerne M.; Smolensky, Michael H.; Leach, Carolyn S.; Lorimor, Ronald; and Hsi, Bartholomew P.: Stress levels of ambulance paramedics and fire fighters. Journal of Occupational Medicine 20:111-115, 1978.
Subjects: 56 firefighters and 67 ambulance paramedics.
Method: All subjects completed a modified Schedule of Recent Experience (for the past 12 months) and a "job stress" questionnaire (to measure perception of job's arduousness, job satisfaction, and physical and emotional manifestations of overloading). Fifty-one of the subjects also provided two 24-hour urine samples (one work day, one off-day) for analysis of epinephrine, norepinephrine, and cortisol levels. The two occupational groups were compared.

B50 Dye, Bernice Julia: Investigation of life change unit scores in eighth grade students. Unpublished master's thesis, University of Washington, 1974.
Subjects: 85 eighth-grade students.
Method: All subjects completed a modification of Coddington's Schedule of Recent Experience for junior high school students. They also reported illnesses they had experienced in the past three months and estimated the "number of days absent" from school.

B51 Forester, Timothy Daniel: A description and evaluation of a life planning training program based on the self-empowerment construct: An exploratory study (Doctoral dissertation, University of Oregon, 1977). Dissertation Abstracts International 38:6010-A, 1978.
Subjects: 25 adults enrolled in a life training program called "Self-Empowerment."

Method: To evaluate the counseling system called "Self-Empowerment," all subjects completed a modified Schedule of Recent Experience, the Purpose-in-Life Test, and Rotter's Internal-External Locus of Control questionnaire before the course started; the Purpose-in-Life and locus of control instruments were readministered after the course was completed. At that time a structured interview schedule was also administered to examine subjects' perceptions of the course's applicability to and influence on their lives.

B52 Harris, Paul White: The relationship of life change to academic performance among selected college freshmen at varying levels of college readiness (Doctoral dissertation, East Texas State University, 1972). Dissertation Abstracts International 33:6665A-6666A, 1973.

Subjects: 300 first-year college students.
Method: Subjects were selected for study and divided into groups on the basis of college readiness (as determined by test scores): 100 students in the high readiness (low risk) group, 100 in the medium readiness (medium risk) group, and 100 in the low readiness (high risk) group. Near the end of the school year subjects completed the "Social and Collegiate Readjustment Rating Scale" (a modified Schedule of Recent Experience), and then after the school year academic records were reviewed to obtain each subject's grade point average. Harris's modification of the Schedule of Recent Experience for college students was derived from Bramwell's modifications of the SRE for college athletes [see B72, B73]. Harris's Social and Collegiate Readjustment Rating Scale is a 49-item checklist of life events in the past 12 months.

B53 Helton, Joseph Ralph, Jr.: The relationship of life change and risk taking to academic achievement (Doctoral dissertation, Oklahoma State University, 1976). Dissertation Abstracts International 37:5605A-5606A, 1977.

Subjects: 622 first-year college students who attended orientation sessions before the fall semester opened.
Method: Subjects completed the Choice Dilemma Procedure (a measure of risk-taking behavior) and Harris's modified Schedule of Recent Experience for college students [see B52] (for past 12 months). Each subject's location of residence and composite ACT (American College Test) score were also obtained. Twenty-one prediction models

for academic success (higher grade point averages) were tested by statistical analysis.

B54   Henard, Kay Fields: Life change and reading achievement as predictors of academic performance for selected community freshmen [Doctoral dissertation, Texas A & M University, 1975). Dissertation Abstracts International 36:5082-A, 1976.
Subjects: Entering first-year students at a 2-year community college [N not stated in abstract].
Method: Subjects completed the Nelson-Denny Reading Test during orientation sessions. Near the end of the academic year they were mailed a questionnaire packet containing a demographic data survey, the Attitude Survey (selected attitudes relevant to academic, personal, social, and career life), and Harris's modified Schedule of Recent Experience for college students [see B52]. Subjects were assigned to high or low life change groups and to high, moderate, or low reading achievement groups to study the value of life change and reading achievement as predictors of academic performance (grade point averages, course hour loads, attitudes).

B55   Herrman, Gerard; Schuckit, Marc A.; Hineman, Sherry; and Pugh, William: The association of stress with drug use and academic performance among university students. Journal of the American College Health Association 25:97-101, 1976.
Subjects: A cohort of 188 college sophomores.
Method: At the beginning of their sophomore year in college, all subjects were interviewed to collect self-report data on drug use (abstainers, marijuana only, multiple drugs) and academic performance (cumulative grade point average) during their first year of college (October 1971-October 1972). They also completed a modified Schedule of Recent Experience (for the past two years, i.e., senior year in high school and freshman year in college).

B56   Hoskins, Alice Lavonne: An assessment of the correlation between the magnitude of life change and the teacher behavior of the elementary intern teacher (Doctoral dissertation, Michigan State University, 1972). Dissertation Abstracts International 33:6217-A, 1973.
Subjects: 41 elementary intern teachers.
Method: All subjects completed the Schedule of Recent Experience. School and personnel records were reviewed to document four aspects of teacher performance: intern

teacher's absenteeism, student absenteeism, contact between intern and consultant (field supervisor), and student
referrals.

B57 Johnston, Robert G., and Masuda, Minoru: Medical school
class and illness history. Journal of Medical Education 45:
888-892, 1970.
Subjects: Over 240 medical students.
Method: Noting the common student belief that the third
and first years of medical school entail greater life change
and readjustment than the second and fourth years, the
authors examine the relationship between medical school
class and amount of illness experienced in two consecutive
years. During two survey years (1967 and 1968) an illness
history questionnaire was mailed to all University of Washington medical students asking for reports of any deviations
from usual healthy state in the previous 30 months (divided
into 3-month segments). Returned questionnaires (mean
return of 56%) were divided into groups according to medical school class, and illness reports were quantified using
Wyler's Seriousness of Illness Rating Scale.

B58 Larson, Olive: A nursing research study to explore the relationship between the magnitude of stressful life events and
absenteeism. Unpublished master's thesis, University of
Minnesota at Minneapolis, 1973.
Subjects: 54 Hamms Brewery workers.
Method: All subjects completed a modified Schedule of
Recent Experience (for past year). Company absenteeism
records were reviewed to document occurrences of and
reasons for absence over a 6-month period. Life change
magnitudes were divided into four levels of life crisis: no
life crisis (1-149 Life Change Units) and mild (150-199
LCU), moderate (200-299 LCU), and severe (300 and over
LCU) life crises. Data were analyzed by individual case
and by age groups (20-44 years, 45-59 years, 60-65 years
old).

B59 O'Meara, John Patrick: A study of relationships between
selected life events and school performance of eighth and
ninth grade students (Doctoral dissertation, Michigan State
University, 1977). Dissertation Abstracts International
39:98-A, 1978.
Subjects: 271 eighth- and ninth-grade students.

Method: A modified form of Coddington's Schedule of Recent Experience for junior high school students was administered. Six performance variables were examined: change in grade point average from 1974 to 1975 school year, change in citizenship grade average, change in number of absences, change in number of demerit points on the Conduct Code, change in total reading and in total mathematics scores on the Stanford Achievement Test.

B60 Paulucci, Joseph Anthony: The effects of life change upon the performance of preschool age children of varying temperament, physical health and development (Doctoral dissertation, Fuller Theological Seminary, 1976). Dissertation Abstracts International 38:373-B, 1977.

Subjects: 398 preschool children, ages 3-5.

Method: Mothers of subjects completed Coddington's Schedule of Recent Experience for preschool children. Teachers rated all children by rank order in (1) temperament and (2) physical health and development. A group of 36 children with either a great number of life changes or very few life changes was selected for further study and divided into subgroups by ratings of temperament/physical health and development: easy/above average, average/average, and difficult/below average. The McCarthy Scales of Children's Abilities were used to measure performance in the 36 children. The Shipley-Hartford Intelligence test was administered to parents of subjects, who also completed a modified Schedule of Recent Experience (for past 5 years). During an interview with parents, data were collected on the following: age, education, and employment of parents; ratings of their marriage and their parents' marriages; and family structures, points of tension, and coping strategies.

B61 Schuette, Clifford Gene: Life change, locus of control, needs, and academic performance of college freshmen (Doctoral dissertation, East Texas State University, 1975). Dissertation Abstracts International 36:5059A-5060A, 1976.

Subjects: 161 first-year college students.

Method: Subjects were drawn from a larger sample of students who had attended orientation sessions earlier in the year and were selected for study on the basis of having had high life change scores (measured by a version of Harris's modified Schedule of Recent Experience for college students [see B52]). They were further selected for having either high or low grades (documented by school records) at the end of the first academic semester. Subjects completed Rotter's Internal-External Locus of Control questionnaire and a measure of the need for academic recognition (Goal Preference Inventory).

B62 Secolsky, Stephanie: Behavioral adjustment of residentially-treated, acting-out adolescent males (Doctoral dissertation, University of Pennsylvania, 1977). Dissertation Abstracts International 38:3907-B, 1978.

> Subjects: 47 adolescent males who were residents at private treatment centers for emotionally disturbed youngsters and who had a history of acting-out behavior.
> Method: Clinical case records of subjects were reviewed to document 13 predictor variables for disruptive behavior while in the institution; one of the variables was the presence or absence of any of 8 specified life events. In addition, subjects were tested for two scores on the Means-Ends Problem-Solving Procedure. Three measures of disruptive behavior were selected: 5-month record of disciplinary actions in home-unit, 5-month record of school detentions, and staff ratings using the Devereux Adolescent Behavior Rating Scale.

B63 Simonton, Dean Keith: Creative productivity, age, and stress: A biographical time-series analysis of 10 classical composers. Journal of Personality and Social Psychology 35:791-804, 1977.

> Subjects: Bach, Beethoven, Mozart, Haydn, Brahms, Handel, Debussy, Schubert, Wagner, and Chopin.
> Method: The life of each composer was divided into 5-year segments from the beginning of productive activity to death; his works were then assigned to the appropriate 5-year period. Two measures of productivity were devised (a rating of total works and a rating of total themes produced) and applied to the composer's accomplished work. Using a multivariate cross-sectional time-series design, the quality and quantity of each composer's work were studied in relation to six variables: age, "biographical stress" (modified Schedule of Recent Experience), physical illness, social reinforcement (awards, honors, etc.), war intensity (international outbreaks and proximity), and internal disturbances (local and national upheavals and unrest). A variety of historical sources was consulted to collect life change data for each composer; life change scores were calculated for each 5-year period.

B64 Smith, Paul Edward: The relationship of life change, neuroticism, and academic performance among junior college
adults (Doctoral dissertation, Texas A & M University, 1976).
Dissertation Abstracts International 37:7475-A, 1977.
    Subjects: 201 junior college students aged 25 and older.
Method: At the end of the academic year, all subjects completed Harris's modified Schedule of Recent Experience
for college students [see B52] and the Neuroticism Scale
Questionnaire. Life change and neuroticism scores were
examined in relation to grade point averages from the fall
and spring semesters of that year.

B65 Vicino, Franco Luigi: Situational correlates of organizational
success (Doctoral dissertation, University of Rochester,
1978). Dissertation Abstracts International 39:1995B-1996B,
1978.
    Subjects: 140 managers in the Exxon organization.
Method: Company records were reviewed to document each
subject's predicted performance at time of hire by a battery of tests, and actual performance measured four years
later by another established test program developed by the
company. Four "correlates of organizational success"
were studied as variables which might account for differences between predicted and actual performance of managers: perceived challenge in subject's first assignment,
life change (modified Schedule of Recent Experience for
past two years), personality match of subject and first
supervisor, and success of first supervisor.

B66 Vicino, Franco L., and Bass, Bernard M.: Lifespace variables and managerial success. Journal of Applied Psychology
63:81-88, 1978.
    This article is based on the doctoral research reported
above in B65.

BF1.J55

B67 Wildman, Richard C.: The effects of life change on self-
attitudes, attitudes towards others, mental health, and role
performance in a college sample (Doctoral dissertation,
University of Nebraska, 1974). Dissertation Abstracts International 35:5541A-5542A, 1974-1975.
    Subjects: 156 college students.
25053.D57 Method: Subjects completed a modified Schedule of Recent
Experience (for past two years), Langner's 22-item index
(mental health inventory), and Berger's Acceptance of
Self and Acceptance of Others Scales. School records were

reviewed to document each subject's cumulative grade
point average and past semester's grade point average.
Eight control variables were also analyzed: age, sex,
college level, marital status, size of home community,
education of father, Scholastic Aptitude Test scores, and
conventionality (scores from a 36-item test).

B68 Wildman, Richard C.: Life change with college grades as a
role-performance variable. Social Psychology 41(1):34-46,
1978.
Subjects: 129 college students.
Method: This is a reanalysis of data collected in a doctoral
research project [see B67]. Life change data were gathered using a modified Schedule of Recent Experience (for
past year and year before) and performance data were
gathered from academic records (cumulative grade point
average, most recent semester GPA, and SAT scores).
Four life change scoring methods are tested and compared.
[See also C40 for a companion report on life change and
Langner's 22-item index scores.]

B69 Wilkins, Walter L.: Some relations of medical psychology
and military psychology. Military Medicine 137:311-316, 1972.
The author reviews life change research with military populations and discusses its relevance and applicability to
personnel planning in the areas of preventing illness, predicting performance, and facilitating adjustment in the
military.

PERFORMANCE:
Accidents
(B70 - B87)

B70 Alkov, Robert A.: Life changes and pilot error accidents.
Paper presented at the Fourth Annual Symposium on Psychology in the Air Force, United States Air Force Academy,
Colorado Springs, Colorado, April 25-27, 1974.
The author proposes development of a predictive measure
of accident liability based on life change measurement.
Susceptibility to pilot error accidents could be gauged using
life change analysis which takes into account not only the
pattern of life changes inherent in a pilot's occupation, but
also the recent life changes experienced by a given pilot.

B71   Barry, Patricia Z.: The relationship between stress and
      accidents: A preliminary investigation (Doctoral dissertation,
      University of North Carolina at Chapel Hill, 1972). Disserta-
      tion Abstracts International 34:743-B, 1973.
         Subjects: 309 drivers who had one automobile crash within
         the past year and another within the past three years, and
         147 drivers (matched for age and sex) with no crashes in
         past three years.
         Method: All subjects were interviewed by telephone. They
         were asked to provide demographic information (including
         illness experience), accident exposure data (e.g., amount
         of night driving), and life change data (Schedule of Recent
         Experience).

B72   Bramwell, Steven T.: Personality and psychosocial variables
      in college athletes. Unpublished medical thesis, University
      of Washington, 1971.
         This thesis presents three related papers: "Personality
         Variables in Football Players" (75 college football players
         and 203 nonplaying male college students completed the
         Edwards Personality Inventory); "The Black Athlete:
         Achievement or Frustration" (compares black and white
         college football players on educational performance, pro-
         fessional football performance, and eventual occupational
         status; also compares black and white players' expectations
         of their own performance at the beginning of a day's work-
         out); and "The Social and Athletic Readjustment Rating
         Scale" (describes the development of a life event scaling
         instrument based on the Social Readjustment Rating Ques-
         tionnaire and modified for college athletes). [The third
         study was incorporated into a larger project reported in
         publication B73.]

B73   Bramwell, Steven T.; Masuda, Minoru; Wagner, Nathaniel N.;
      and Holmes, Thomas H.: Psychosocial factors in athletic
      injuries: Development and application of the Social and
      Athletic Readjustment Rating Scale (SARRS). Journal of
      Human Stress 1(2):6-20, 1975.
         Part 1:
            Subjects: 79 college football players.
            Method: All subjects completed a modification of the
            Social Readjustment Rating Questionnaire called the
            Social and Athletic Readjustment Rating Questionnaire.
            Subjects' perceptions of the magnitude of readjustment

required by 57 life events were then scaled to produce the Social and Athletic Readjustment Rating Scale (SARRS). Differences between whites and blacks were examined, and the college athletes were compared to a white, middle-class American sample of young adults (below 30 years old) whose Social Readjustment Rating Questionnaire data were taken from Holmes and Rahe's original study [see H18].

Part 2:
    Subjects: 82 members of a university varsity football team.
    Method: All subjects completed the Athlete Schedule of Recent Experience at the beginning of a football season (for one and two years prior to this season). The ASRE is a modification of the Schedule of Recent Experience using life event items scaled in the Social and Athletic Readjustment Rating Scale. Three months later, at the end of the playing season, each player's injury record was obtained. Those players who missed three or more practices and/or one or more games due to a specific injury were assigned to the "injured" group; all others were put in the "noninjured" group. The relationship of life change to subsequent athletic injury was examined.

B74   Brown, George W., and Davidson, Susan: Social class, psychiatric disorder of mother, and accidents to children. Lancet 1:378-380, 1978.
    Subjects: 420 children living with their mothers (N=211) in the Camberwell district of London.
    Method: The subjects' mothers were drawn from a random sample of 458 women in the Camberwell community who were interviewed about life events (Brown and Birley method) and psychiatric disorders (Institute of Psychiatry schedule of questions to determine "caseness"). This subsample of mothers and their children was studied for differences in accident rates between children whose mothers were designated as psychiatric cases or borderline cases and children whose mothers had no psychiatric conditions. Accident rates of children at risk were compared by social class (working vs. middle class), mother's psychiatric status at the time of accident, recent life events (past year), mother's employment, and size of family.

B75 Davis, Sondra Nelson: The relationships between the incidence of accidents, locus of control, and life crisis. Unpublished master's thesis, University of Washington, 1977.

   Subjects: 91 hospital psychiatric staff members involved in direct contact with patients.

   Method: Subjects completed the Schedule of Recent Experience, Rotter's Internal-External Locus of Control questionnaire, and two self-report questionnaires on work history and on accidents. Work history information included amount of patient contact, previous experience in psychiatric staff work, and number of work days lost in past year. Accident data included both on-the-job and off-the-job incidents in the past year: cause of accident, place of occurrence, description of each incident.

B76 Huddleston, Charles T.: Life stress and industrial accidents. Unpublished master's thesis, North Texas State University, 1976.

   Subjects: 76 male employees of a petroleum servicing company: 38 with no record of job-related accidents and 38 with one or more job-related accidents (motor vehicle or personal injury) in the past 3 years.

   Method: All subjects completed a modified Schedule of Recent Experience. Two scoring methods were used to analyze the life change data: standard Life Change Unit scoring and a normative-ipsative technique.

B77 Levine, John B.; Lee, Jonathan O.; McHugh, William B.; and Rahe, Richard H.: Recent life changes and accidents aboard an attack carrier. Military Medicine 142:469-471, 1977.

   Subjects: 156 naval aviators and 879 aircraft support personnel aboard an aircraft carrier.

   Method: All subjects completed a modified Schedule of Recent Experience (for the year prior to the cruise). Accident reports made during the cruise were examined at the end of the cruise and organized by type (personal accidents among support personnel vs. aircraft accidents involving aviators). Correlations were examined between accidents and total life change scores, individual life change events, and job rating (specialist or nonspecialist occupational levels and pay grades of enlisted men).

B78 McGuire, Frederick L.: Personality factors in highway accidents. Human Factors 18:433-441, 1976.

58A2H8

This review of the literature describes personality factors of the "accident-haver" in both general and specific terms. The role of "external stress"—recent life changes and distressing life events—and the concept of accident-proneness are also discussed.

B79 Padilla, Eligio R.; Rohsenow, Damaris J.; and Bergman, Abraham B.: Predicting accident frequency in children. Pediatrics 58:223-226, 1976.

> Subjects: 103 boys in a junior high school physical education program.
> Method: Each subject was observed during gym class on four different occasions by five judges, and a rating on level of "risk-taking" was agreed upon by the judges for each subject. Each subject also completed Coddington's Schedule of Recent Experience for junior high school students (for the past 12 months). During the following five months, all subjects were interviewed weekly by telephone to obtain data on the frequency and severity of accidents experienced during the preceding week. Accident data included number of accidents; whether injury resulted and if it required treatment; and if so, what kind of treatment was required (first aid, medical attention, hospitalization).

B80 Plionis, Elizabeth Moore: Family functioning and childhood accident occurrence. American Journal of Orthopsychiatry 47:250-263, 1977.

> Subjects: 15 children hospitalized for accidental injury (burns, fractures, lacerations, concussions, etc.).
> Method: During a semistructured interview Geismar's scale of family functioning was used to assess each child's family. After a family functioning score had been assigned, medical records were reviewed to obtain the child's complete accident history. An accident rate was calculated for each child (number of accidents divided by child's age) and studied in relation to adequacy of family functioning. An alternative variable, "family stress," was also investigated by administering a modified Schedule of Recent Experience to the family (for the two years before child's index accident) and examining the relationship between accident occurrence and precipitating family stress.

B81 Selzer, Melvin L.: Alcoholism, mental illness, and stress in 96 drivers causing fatal accidents. Behavioral Science 14:1-10, 1969.

Subjects: 96 drivers responsible for fatal accidents and 96 matched control drivers.

Method: This is a further analysis of research first reported in B82. This report adds data on the prevalence of alcoholism and characteristic patterns of alcohol use, on driving and arrest records, and on social class of fatality drivers and controls.

B82 Selzer, Melvin L.; Rogers, Joseph E.; and Kern, Sue: Fatal accidents: The role of psychopathology, social stress, and acute disturbance. American Journal of Psychiatry 124:1028-1036, 1968.

Subjects: 96 drivers (surviving and deceased) responsible for fatal accidents and 96 matched control drivers.

Method: A variety of informants was interviewed to determine the emotional status of all drivers; the 25 surviving fatality drivers and all control drivers were also interviewed. Arrest and driving records of all subjects were also reviewed. Data were collected to assess psychopathology (paranoid thinking, suicidal inclination, depression, violence) and "social stress" in the 12 months prior to accident or control interview. Social stress included personal conflicts (disturbances in relationships with significant others), personal tragedies (death and illness of loved ones), vocational and financial crises (changes in work situation and financial affairs), and "acute preaccident disturbance" (upsetting events in the 6 hours before accident).

B83 Selzer, Melvin L., and Vinokur, Amiram: Life events, subjective stress, and traffic accidents. American Journal of Psychiatry 131:903-906, 1974.

Subjects: 532 male drivers (274 general drivers and 258 alcoholic drivers receiving inpatient or outpatient treatment).

Method: All subjects completed a self-administered questionnaire which collected data on the following: demographic information; driving history in the preceding 12 months (accidents, annual mileage, etc.); psychopathology and personality traits (aggression, paranoid thinking, depression, suicidal tendencies); "physical stress responses and subjective stress" (smoking, insomnia, headaches, etc., and serious disturbances in significant relationships); life changes (modified 1-year Schedule of Recent Experience, scored with a self-rating of adjustment required by reported events); concern with broad social issues; and alcohol use and abuse (self-report frequency and quantity data, plus the Michigan Alcoholism Screening Test). Data were analyzed to test variables predictive of accidents. [See also B84.]

B84   Selzer, Melvin L., and Vinokur, Amiram: Role of life events in accident causation. Mental Health and Society 2:36-54, 1975.

Subjects: 453 male drivers (237 general drivers and 216 alcoholic drivers).

Method: This is a more detailed analysis of research first reported in B83. Life change data were scored in four ways: number of life events experienced in past 12 months; total Life Change Unit scores based on Social Readjustment Rating Scale values; subjective readjustment rating (subject rated each reported event on a 4-point scale); and "subjective sum of life events stress" (subject rated on a 5-point scale the total "pressure" put on him by all reported life changes).

B85   Sobel, Raymond, and Underhill, Ralph: Family disorganization and teenage auto accidents. Journal of Safety Research 8:8-18, 1976.

Subjects: 496 adolescents (aged 16-19) who applied for driver licenses in two rural New Hampshire counties.

Method: The state highway safety department provided records of accidents involving all subjects from time of getting their licenses to time of interview. All subjects and their parents were interviewed at home using the Family Life Questionnaire (300 items addressed to teen-ager, with separate 200-item sections for parents). Data were collected on the following: family relationships and adjustment, risk-taking behavior, driving record and atti-tudes, life changes (Coddington's Schedule of Recent Ex-perience for high school students was completed by each subject; subjects' parents completed the Schedule of Recent Experience), health (including illness history, neurotic symptoms, depression, Langner's 22-item index, smoking and drug use), alcohol use, subject's attitudes and values, sexual adjustment, adjustment at work and school, and peer group relationships. All variables were examined for association with teenage auto accidents.

B86 Whitlock, F. A.; Stoll, J. R.; and Rekhdahl, R. J.: Crisis, life events and accidents. Australian and New Zealand Journal of Psychiatry 11:127-132, 1977.

> Subjects: 71 orthopedic patients with accidental injuries and 71 accident-free matched controls (students and patients undergoing minor surgery).
> Method: All accident patients were interviewed to document the circumstances surrounding their accidents, their medical and psychiatric histories in the 6 months preceding the accident, and their past accident histories. All accident patients and control subjects completed both the Schedule of Recent Experience and the Paykel et al. Recent Life Event interview (for the 6 months prior to accident or interview). Life events data were analyzed and compared in terms of number of reported events, Life Change Unit weightings, and quality of event (controllable, desirable, etc.).

B87 Yanowitch, Robert E.; Mohler, Stanley R.; and Nichols, E. A.: Psychosocial reconstruction inventory: A postdictal instrument in aircraft accident investigation. Aerospace Medicine 43:551-554, 1972.

> The authors describe the development of an interview inventory which they applied to the cases of 12 pilots who died in aircraft accidents. The pilots' spouses, parents, siblings, and mature children were interviewed, as well as airport personnel, close friends, business associates, and flying associates. Informants were asked about "Areas of Dynamic Influence" in the pilot's life (family, economic, social, and education history and physical and mental health), "Pre-Accident Influences" (symptoms of "psychosocial deterioration" such as depression, guilt feelings, etc.; and life events such as economic reverses, death of loved ones, marital disruption), and "Pre-Accident Behavior" (details of behavior immediately preceding flight).

PERFORMANCE:
Suicide
(B88 - B105)

B88 Bancroft, John; Skrimshire, Angela; Casson, Jeannette; Harvard-Watts, Olivia; and Reynolds, Frances: People who deliberately poison or injure themselves: Their problems and their contacts with helping agencies. Psychological Medicine 7:289-303, 1977.

Subjects: 130 cases of self-poisoning or self-injury.
Method: Subjects were interviewed shortly after the
suicide attempt. Data were gathered on the following:
personal history and relations with family and friends; life
events occurring in the week before (or anticipated to oc-
cur shortly after) the suicide attempt; psychiatric and
nonpsychiatric treatment history; hospitalizations in the
past year; perceptions of kinds of help needed; and contacts with helping agencies before the attempt.

B89   Bunch, Jane: Recent bereavement in relation to suicide.
Journal of Psychosomatic Research 16:361-366, 1972.
Subjects: 75 suicide cases and 150 living control subjects
matched for age, sex, marital status, and area of residence.
Method: Inquest testimony, medical records, and interviews with relatives and friends were obtained to document
each suicide's clinical state in the month prior to death,
previous personality, personal and family history, and
social circumstances. Similar data were collected by
interview with control subjects. Suicides and controls
were compared on bereavement of parent or spouse within
the past five years. Bereaved suicides and bereaved controls were studied for differences in sex, marital status,
social support, psychiatric history, and degree of disruption caused by bereavement.

B90   Bush, James A.: Similarities and differences in precipitating
events between Black and Anglo suicide attempts. Suicide and
Life-Threatening Behavior 8:243-249, 1978.
Subjects: 25 black and 25 Anglo patients who sought psychotherapy.
Method: Subjects were selected for study on the basis of
having considered, planned, or recently attempted suicide
and of having scored high on the depression section of the
Heimler Scale of Social Functioning. Mental health records
of each subject were reviewed to document precipitating
events for suicide attempts. In addition, ten mental health
practitioners were interviewed for their observations about
differences in events precipitating suicide attempts by
black and Anglo patients they treated.

B91   Cochrane, Raymond, and Robertson, Alex: Stress in the
lives of parasuicides. Social Psychiatry 10:161-171, 1975.
Subjects: 100 male parasuicides (attempted suicides) and
100 control subjects matched for age, sex, and social class.

Method: All subjects completed Cochrane and Robertson's Life Event Inventory [see H3] for the previous 12 months. They also were administered two subscales of the Hostility and Direction of Hostility Questionnaire, a modified Zung Depression Scale, and the Self-Anchoring Striving Scale (measure of perceived deprivation). Life events data were analyzed several ways: occurrence of specific events, number of reported events, sum of weighted values for events, and quality of events (pleasantness, controllability, etc.).

B92   Dizmang, Larry H.; Watson, Jane; May, Philip A.; and Bopp, John: Adolescent suicide at an Indian reservation. American Journal of Orthopsychiatry 44:43-49, 1974.
Subjects: 10 American Indians who committed suicide before the age of 25 and a matched control group of 40 members of the same tribe.
Method: Many sources (records and informants) were used to complete a 104-item data survey on each subject. Data were divided into five categories (family background, health, law and order record, education, personal data), and 35 variables were examined. Included in the variables were life events such as bereavements, parental divorce or desertion, and arrests in the past 12 months.

B93   Epstein, Lynn Chaikin; Thomas, Caroline Bedell; Shaffer, John W.; and Perlin, Seymour: Clinical prediction of physician suicide based on medical student data. Journal of Nervous and Mental Disease 156:19-29, 1973.
Subjects: 9 physicians who committed suicide, 18 matched control subjects (two for each suicide), and 6 "distractor" subjects.
Method: A psychiatrist reviewer, blind to the number of suicides and controls, rank ordered all 33 subjects for suicide potential. As medical students, all subjects had participated in a hypertension research project, and the extensive personal history data collected then was made available for this study, as were academic records of all subjects. The reviewer studied the voluminous files on each subject and assessed each for suicide potential on the basis of reviewer ratings using the Lorr Outpatient Mood Scale, modified Katz Adjustment Scales, the Minnesota-Hartford Personality Assay, a modified Schedule of Recent Experience (subject's known life changes through graduation from medical school), and reviewer's characterization of subject's psychopathology and coping styles.

B94 Henderson, A. S.; Hartigan, J.; Davidson, J.; Lance, G. N.;
Duncan-Jones, P.; Koller, K. M.; Ritchie, Karen; McAuley,
Helen; Williams, C. L.; and Slaghuis, W.: A typology of para-
suicide. British Journal of Psychiatry 131:631-641, 1977.
    Subjects: 350 parasuicide patients seen at two Australian
    hospitals.
    Method: Each subject was interviewed with a 6-part inter-
    view schedule to collect data on the following aspects of
    parasuicidal behavior: demographic characteristics; de-
    velopmental experiences and psychiatric illness in family;
    life events in the past 4 weeks and the preceding 11 months
    (items taken from the Schedule of Recent Experience and
    from the Paykel et al. Recent Life Events interview); cir-
    cumstances surrounding the parasuicidal act; facilitating
    factors (such as alcohol or drug use, or accessibility of
    agent used); and motivation for act (both subject's report
    and interviewer's judgment).

B95 Humphrey, John A.: Social loss: A comparison of suicide
victims, homicide offenders and non-violent individuals.
Diseases of the Nervous System 38:157-160, 1977.
    Subjects: 98 suicide cases, 62 homicidal offenders, and
    76 hospitalized patients with psychoneurotic complaints—
    all Caucasian males.
    Method: Detailed life histories were assembled for all
    subjects. The three subject groups were compared for
    loss in five social roles: childhood loss (death, divorce,
    or separation of parents; death of close sibling, relative,
    friend); student loss (age at end of schooling); occupational
    loss (permanent job loss, downward mobility, lengthy
    lay-off period, retirement); marital loss (death of spouse,
    divorce, separation); and parental loss (death of child,
    removal of child from home, child institutionalized, child
    reared by other parent/relative).

B96 Humphrey, John A.; French, Laurence; Niswander, G. Donald;
and Casey, Thomas M.: The process of suicide: The se-
quence of disruptive events in the lives of suicide victims.
Diseases of the Nervous System 35:275-277, 1974.
    Subjects: 160 completed suicides.
    Method: Psychological autopsies were collected for all
    subjects. A list of life events selected as specific "dis-
    ruptions of social relations" was applied to each case
    history, and data were analyzed using a scaling technique
    which measured sequential ordering of events in the lives

of the suicide subjects as a group. Life events selected
for study included bereavements in childhood and adulthood,
childhood institutionalization or placement in foster care,
abandonment by parents or spouse, loss of student role,
loss of occupational role, sexual incompatibility, psychiatric hospitalization or incarceration, death of or desertion
by a child, violent activity (assault or murder), onset of
alcoholism or drug abuse, suicide attempts and threats.

B97 Jacobs, Jerry, and Teicher, Joseph D.: Broken homes and
social isolation in attempted suicides of adolescents. International Journal of Social Psychiatry 13:139-149, 1967.
 Subjects: 50 adolescent suicide attempters and 32 control
 adolescents (matched for age, race, sex, and net family
 income).
 Method: Based on case histories and data from a number
 of sources, a life history chart was constructed for all
 subjects. The presence or absence and the sequential
 ordering of 19 kinds of life events were compared (change
 in residence, change in schools, parental separation or
 divorce, remarriage of parent, bereavements, suicide
 attempts, etc.).

B98 Jacobson, Gerald F., and Portuges, Stephen H.: Relation of
marital separation and divorce to suicide: A report. Suicide
and Life-Threatening Behavior 8:217-224, 1978.
 Subjects: 238 applicants to a crisis clinic who (1) had
 seriously discussed marital separation in the past 13
 months but were not separated from spouse or (2) were
 separated or divorced and not remarried.
 Method: Within a week of application to the crisis clinic,
 each subject was interviewed, and subjects were divided
 into groups by marital dissolution categories: "serious
 discussion," "recent separation or divorce," and "long-
 term separation or divorce." At that time a marital
 problem survey and a questionnaire to determine suicide
 potential were administered. The relation of marital dissolution category to suicidal status was examined. Subjects judged to be suicidal (N=39) were then administered
 the Suicide Prevention Center Assessment of Suicide
 Potential, and the relation of "marital process variables"
 (important events in the 2 weeks prior to interview) to
 suicide potential was examined.

B99   McQuade, Lorraine Lena Papa: Response to life event
       predictors of suicidal behavior (Doctoral dissertation, Uni-
       versity of Texas at Austin, 1978). Dissertation Abstracts
       International 39:1705-B, 1978.
           Subjects: 60 suicide attempters.
           Method: All subjects were administered the following in-
           struments: Beck's Suicide Intent and Hopelessness
           Scales, Rotter's Internal-External Locus of Control ques-
           tionnaire, the Schedule of Recent Experience, and the
           FIRO-B (a measure of preference for inclusion, control,
           and affection).

B100   Murphy, George E., and Robins, Eli: Social factors in
       suicide. Journal of the American Medical Association
       199:303-308, 1967.
           Subjects: 91 suicides in two diagnostic categories: 60
           affective disorder (depression) and 31 alcoholism.
           Method: The diagnosis of depression or alcoholism was
           based on extensive structured interviews with family,
           friends, and knowledgeable informants of each suicide
           subject. Those interviews also provided the data on which
           the two diagnostic groups were compared: age, marital
           status, living arrangements, and "disrupted affectional
           relationships" (marital separation, divorce, bereave-
           ments, and other significant life events) in the year be-
           fore suicide and in the 6 weeks before suicide.

B101   Newton, Eva Jeanne: The relationship between the occur-
       rence of suicidal attempts and life crisis events. Unpub-
       lished master's thesis, University of Washington, 1974.
           Subjects: 39 attempted suicide victims (21 female, 18
           male; mean age of 32).
           Method: All subjects completed the Schedule of Recent
           Experience. The life change data of suicide attempters
           were also compared to life change of fracture patients
           reported in another study [see A370].

B102   Paykel, Eugene S.; Prusoff, Brigitte A.; and Myers,
       Jerome K.: Suicide attempts and recent life events: A
       controlled comparison. Archives of General Psychiatry
       32:327-333, 1975.
           Subjects: 53 suicide attempters, 53 depressives, and 53
           general population control subjects (the depressives and
           general population control subjects were drawn from an
           earlier study and matched to suicide subjects).

Method: The suicide attempters and two control groups were administered similar but not identical life events interviews (for the 6 months prior to suicide attempt, onset of depression, or interview). To make the data comparable, the two instruments were condensed to a 32-item life events schedule. The life events data for each group were analyzed and compared in several ways: total number of reported life events, time patterns, frequencies of individual events, and quality of events (desirability, exit/entrance, area of activity, degree of upset, degree of control).

B103   Pokorny, Alex D., and Kaplan, Howard B.: Suicide following psychiatric hospitalization: The interaction effects of defenselessness and adverse life events. Journal of Nervous and Mental Disease 162:119-125, 1976.

Subjects: 40 male psychiatric inpatients: 20 who completed suicide following discharge and 20 controls who did not (matched for age, race, and time at risk in the community after discharge).

RC321.J83

Method: While hospitalized, all subjects had been administered the Brief Psychiatric Rating Scale; their scores on that instrument were used as a measure of defenselessness. The suicide and control groups were compared by diagnostic category, defenselessness score, and presence or absence of 1 or more of 8 adverse life events after discharge. The 8 life events were selected because all were undesirable, unlikely to have been initiated by subject, and rated at 30 or more Life Change Units on the Social Readjustment Rating Scale.

B104   Robertson, Alex, and Cochrane, Raymond: Attempted suicide and cultural change: An empirical investigation. Human Relations 29:863-883, 1976.

Subjects: 100 male attempted suicides and 100 controls in Edinburgh.

HI H8

Method: Subjects and controls were evenly distributed into subgroups by age (under 25 and over 40) and social class (working class or middle class). All subjects completed Cochrane and Robertson's Life Events Inventory [see H3], the Hostility and Direction of Hostility Questionnaire, the Zung Self-Rating Depression Scale, the Self-Anchoring Striving Scale (a measure of relative deprivation), and a newly designed "New Consciousness" questionnaire (a measure of value systems).

B105 Vigderhous, Gideon, and Fishman, Gideon: The impact of unemployment and familial integration on changing suicide rates in the U.S.A., 1920-1969. Social Psychiatry 13:239-248, 1978.

> The authors used a time series design to analyze the relation of suicide rates to unemployment and the ratio of divorce to marriage in the United States from 1920-1969. Data were extracted from government publications of vital statistics and economic growth statistics.

PERFORMANCE:
Family-Marital Functioning
(B106 - B113)

B106 Atkins, Howard Gray, Jr.: The relationship between family-marital functioning and chronic illness (Doctoral dissertation, University of Florida, 1975). Dissertation Abstracts International 36:6368B-6369B, 1976.

> Subjects: 51 chronically ill inpatients and 36 healthy controls.
> Method: All subjects completed the Schedule of Recent Experience and the Locke-Wallace Short Marital Adjustment Test. Life change in different activity areas (family-marital, personal-environmental, occupational-financial) and level of marital adjustment were studied in relation to measures of chronic illness episodes (severity of illness and immediacy of onset).

B107 Bain, Alastair: The capacity of families to cope with transitions: A theoretical essay. Human Relations 31:675-688, 1978.

> The author discusses the application of concepts from several areas of research—life change, social networks, coping styles, and role changes—to the study of families in crisis. He develops a four-factor formula to predict a family's capacity to cope. One of the factors, "transitional density," is a measure of life changes based on the work of Holmes, Rahe, and Masuda. The other factors are "role changes," "formal social container," and "social network."

B108 Cohler, Bertram J.; Grunebaum, Henry U.; Weiss, Justin L.; Robbins, Donna M.; Shader, Richard I.; Gallant, David; and Hartman, Carol R.: Social role performance and psychopathology among recently hospitalized and nonhospitalized mothers. II. Correlates with life stress and self-reported psychopathology. Journal of Nervous and Mental Disease 159:81-90, 1974.

> Subjects: 40 young mothers recently discharged from a psychiatric hospital and 41 matched, well control subjects. Method: Each subject was interviewed for the occurrence of 11 categories of life events for herself, her husband and children, and her extended family. She also completed the MMPI. The Social Role Performance Instrument was administered (a semistructured interview to collect and rate data on impairment of performance in role as housewife, wife, mother, friend and neighbor, and daughter in parental family). The effect of life events and symptoms of psychological distress on impaired role performance was examined for former patients and for control subjects. [See also A154 and A155.]

B109   Cowell, Daniel D.: The family dimension in medical practice. Military Medicine 143:249-255, 1978.

> The author reviews the literature and discusses the effects of illness on the family, the effect of the family on illness, and therapeutic considerations. He includes life change research as relevant information for the primary care physician in understanding the family's role in the onset and course of illness.

B110   Frederickson, Charles G.: Life stress and marital conflict: A pilot study. Journal of Marriage and Family Counseling 3(3):41-47, 1977.

> Subjects: 20 married couples (ages 22-56).
> Method: One or both partners in 10 of the couples were receiving marital counseling; the other 10 couples were not experiencing marital dysfunction. A modified Schedule of Recent Experience (for the past 12 months) was administered.

B111   Gilford, Rosalie Jonas: Social environment, self-concept, and social conduct: Sense of self as mediator of the relationship between life-change and marital interaction (Doctoral dissertation, University of Southern California, 1975). Dissertation Abstracts International 36:7651A-7652A, 1976.

> Subjects: 388 married couples (ages 18-90).
> Method: All subjects completed a self-administered questionnaire. Data were collected on the following variables

[no instrument names given in abstract]: social conduct (positive marital interaction), amount of recent life change, lifetime "success," lifetime "failure," number of years retired, self-concept (competence), sex, income, and health.

B112 Pless, I. Barry, and Roghmann, K. J.: Safety restraints for children in automobiles: Who uses them? Canadian Journal of Public Health 69:289-292, 1978.

Subjects: 150 families with children under 18 years old. Method: Parents were interviewed by telephone for reported use or nonuse of safety restraints to protect children in most recent car trip. A household interview-questionnaire completed by mothers during an earlier study was used to supply data on the following variables: education, religion, and age of mother; family income; number and ages of children. Another variable, "family stress," was divided into "long-term stress" (continuing problems in the past year) and "short-term stress" (life events recorded in a 28-day diary kept by mother).

B113 Schuman, Stanley H.; Jebaily, Gerard C.; and Samuelson, Dean C.: Life events in a family with life-threatening illness. Psychosomatics 18(2):34-39, 1977.

The authors describe six tools under study for use in analyzing the relationship of life events, "stress," and illness in individual families. The tools are "pedigree" charts (family risk factors), "psychofigures" (of emotional relationships), a "family tree" of known medical problems, "time flow charts" of life events and medical care, scheduled home visits, and computer-assisted life event interviews with different family members. A case history illustrates the use of these tools.

PERFORMANCE:
Child Abuse
(B114 - B119)

B114 Conger, Rand Donald: A comparative study of interaction patterns between deviant and non-deviant families (Doctoral dissertation, University of Washington, 1976). Dissertation Abstracts International 38:1660-A, 1977.

Subjects: 10 families with abused children, 10 families with neglected children, and 12 matched control families.

Method: Demographic and case history data were collected for each family. All families were observed at home for a total of 4 hours and assessed on behavioral interaction (coded as physical or verbal in nature). Three questionnaires were also administered to parents in each family: the Schedule of Recent Experience, the Cornell Medical Index (to measure emotional and physical disturbances), and the Survey on Bringing up Children (child-rearing attitudes and experiences).

B115 Gaines, Richard; Sandgrund, Alice; Green, Arthur H.; and Power, Ernest: Etiological factors in child maltreatment: A multivariate study of abusing, neglecting, and normal mothers. Journal of Abnormal Psychology 87:531-540, 1978.
Subjects: 80 known-abuse mothers, 80 neglectful mothers, and 80 normal control mothers (all with at least 1 child between 1 and 12 years old and all of lower socioeconomic status).

RC321.J7 Method: All subjects were administered the Michigan Screening Profile of Parenting (a measure of 8 personality variables), the Downstate Childrearing Questionnaire (abuse-proneness), the Schedule of Recent Experience, and the Family Life Form (32 negative life experiences associated with poverty and ghetto-living). A twelfth variable, "infant risk," was based on lengthy postnatal hospitalization of infant as reported by mother in interview.

B116 Garbarino, James: The human ecology of child maltreatment: A conceptual model for research. Journal of Marriage and the Family 39:721-735, 1977.
The author reviews the literature and presents a model for conducting and evaluating research on child maltreatment from an ecological perspective. He describes child
HQ1.J48 maltreatment as a problem in "family asynchrony" (a "mismatch" of parent to child and of family to community) and as a consequence of "stressful role transition." The research model includes collection of life events data by family interview.

B117 Justice, Blair, and Duncan, David F.: Child abuse as a work-related problem. Corrective and Social Psychiatry and Journal of Behavior Technology, Methods and Therapy 23:53-55, 1977.
RC321.J86 Subjects: 35 abusing parents and 35 matched controls (parents who were having trouble with their children but had never abused them).

Method: This is a more detailed analysis of some of the data first reported in B119. Particular attention is given to life change differences between abusing and non-abusing parents in the areas of work and related financial problems.

B118   Justice, Blair, and Duncan, David F.: Child abuse in terms of a public health model. Mental Health and Society 4:110-114, 1977.

The authors present a public health model for child abuse: The host is the parents who are responsible for abuse, the environment is the physical and social setting in which abuse occurred, and the agent is the child. Life change analysis is relevant both to retrospective research and to intervention by identifying high-risk parents, environments, and children.

B119   Justice, Blair, and Duncan, David F.: Life crisis as a precursor to child abuse. Public Health Reports 91:110-115, 1976.

Subjects: 35 abusing parents and 35 matched controls (parents who were having trouble with their children but had never abused them).
Method: All subjects completed a modified Schedule of Recent Experience (for the 12 months preceding first abuse incident or beginning of trouble with child, for controls). They also completed questionnaire items designed to elicit data about symbiotic relationships among family members.

PERFORMANCE:
Personal Habits and Behaviors
(B120 - B125)

B120   Dudley, Donald L.; Aickin, Mikel; and Martin, C. J.: Cigarette smoking in a chest clinic population—psychophysiologic variables. Journal of Psychosomatic Research 21:367-375, 1977.

Subjects: 240 patients in a private chest clinic.
Method: All subjects completed a 9-part physiologic test and completed a questionnaire on current and past smoking history (never/ever smoked, stopped/continued smoking, amount smoked, etc.). A symptom index was used to quantify cough, sputum production, wheeze, and

dyspnea. Psychosocial variables were assessed by the
following instruments: Berle Index (psychosocial assets),
the short form of the MMPI (10 scales), the Cornell Medical Index (symptoms and complaints), and the Schedule of
Recent Experience (life change).

B121 Hall, Sharon M.; Bass, Anthony; and Monroe, James: Continued contact and monitoring as follow-up strategies: A
long-term study of obesity treatment. Addictive Behaviors
3:139-147, 1978.
Subjects: 72 overweight women who completed a 10-week
course of behavioral self-management for obesity.
Method: Subjects were assigned to one of three follow-up
groups distinguished by degree of support: minimal contact, monitoring with minimal contact, and continued contact. At regular points through the following year subjects
were compared for weight loss (number of pounds and
percent overweight). Five variables in addition to follow-
up conditions were assessed: severity of obesity-related
health impairment; chronicity of obesity; socioeconomic
status; recent life change (modified Schedule of Recent
Experience administered at end of 52 weeks); and mood
disturbance (Profile of Mood States).

B122 Lindenthal, Jacob J.; Myers, Jerome K.; and Pepper,
Max P.: Smoking, psychological status and stress. Social
Science and Medicine 6:583-591, 1972.
Subjects: A community sample of 938 adults in New Haven,
Connecticut.
PER Method: All subjects were interviewed as part of a larger
study. Smoking data were collected for each subject:
frequency (often, sometimes, hardly ever, never) and
perception of smoking as a problem (very, somewhat, not
too serious). Life crises occurring in the previous year
were documented using the Paykel et al. Recent Life
Events interview method. For each reported event, subjects also indicated if there was a change in smoking rate
associated with that event. Psychological impairment
(very, moderately, not impaired) was assessed for each
subject using Gurin's modification of Macmillan's Health
Opinion Survey.

B123 Lindenthal, Jacob J.; Myers, Jerome K.; Pepper, Max P.;
and Stern, Maxine S.: Mental status and religious behavior.
Journal for the Scientific Study of Religion 9:143-149, 1970.

Subjects: A community sample of 938 adults in New Haven, Connecticut.

Method: All subjects were interviewed as part of a larger study. Data on religious behavior were collected for each subject: church affiliation, church attendance, changes in church attendance at times of crisis, prayer habits, and changes in prayer habits. Life crises during the previous year were documented using the Paykel et al. Recent Life Events interview method. Psychological impairment (very, moderately, or not impaired) was assessed for each subject using Gurin's modification of Macmillan's Health Opinion Survey.

B124   Mellinger, Glen D.; Balter, Mitchell B.; Manheimer, Dean I.; Cisin, Ira H.; and Parry, Hugh J.: Psychic distress, life crisis, and use of psychotherapeutic medications: National household survey data. <u>Archives of General Psychiatry</u> <u>35</u>:1045-1052, 1978.

RC321A66

Subjects: 2,552 United States adults selected in a national survey by a cross-sectional probability sampling.

Method: All subjects completed a modified Hopkins Symptom Check List (psychic distress) and a modified Schedule of Recent Experience (life change in the past year). They also provided data on prescription drug use (tranquilizers, daytime sedatives, and antidepressants) and on alcohol use.

B125   Thomas, Claudewell S.; Lindenthal, Jacob J.; and Myers, Jerome K.: Crisis, psychology and tranquilizer use. <u>Journal of Nervous and Mental Disease</u> <u>160</u>:359-364, 1975.

RC321.J83

Subjects: 720 adults in New Haven, Connecticut.

Method: All subjects were interviewed as part of a larger study. Subjects were asked if they had used tranquilizers "with any regularity" during the past year. Life crises during the past year were documented and analyzed using the Paykel et al. Recent Life Events interview method. Psychological impairment (very, moderately, or not impaired) was assessed for each subject using Gurin's modification of Macmillan's Health Opinion Survey.

PERFORMANCE:
Criminal Activity
(B126 - B129)

B126   Booth, Robert E., and Grosswiler, Ralph A.: Correlates and predictors of recidivism among drinking drivers. <u>International Journal of the Addictions</u> <u>13</u>:79-88, 1978.

Subjects: 47 former clients of an alcohol treatment program, all of whom had been arrested and convicted of driving while under the influence of alcohol.
Method: Follow-up interviews were held with all subjects at least 6 months after discharge from treatment. Recidivism was assessed three ways: by rearrest records, self-report driving-while-drinking behavior, and self-perceived changes in drinking behavior. Several predictors of recidivism were tested: time factors (of treatment and since treatment), demographic factors (age, employment status, etc.), and historical factors. Historical factors included specific events following arrest and before treatment and life events after leaving treatment (modified Schedule of Recent Experience).

B127   Chandler, Alvin, II: Correlates of violent and nonviolent criminal behavior among men (Doctoral dissertation, California School of Professional Psychology, 1975). Dissertation Abstracts International 38:4442-B, 1978.
    Subjects: Violent and nonviolent male criminals [number unstated].
    Method: All subjects were administered four instruments: the Eysenck Personality Inventory, Parnell's system of somatotyping, the Recent Life Changes Questionnaire, and Carney's Masculinity Rating Scales. Personality characteristics, somatotypes, life change, and ratings of masculinity were studied in relation to type and severity of criminal behavior.

B128   Masuda, Minoru; Cutler, David L.; Hein, Lee; and Holmes, Thomas H.: Life events and prisoners. Archives of General Psychiatry 35:197-203, 1978.
    Subjects: 176 male inmates of a federal prison and a state penitentiary.
    Method: All subjects completed the Schedule of Recent Experience (for past 10 years), thus providing life change data for five years prior to incarceration and up to five years after incarceration. Annual life change scores before and during incarceration were examined in relation to prisoners' age group, race, and education. Life event frequencies of prisoners were compared to frequencies in a "normative" sample of white, middle-class Americans

B129   Williams, C. L.; Henderson, A. S.; and Mills, Janet M.: An epidemiological study of serious traffic offenders. Social Psychiatry 9:99-109, 1974.

Subjects: 100 Australians convicted of serious traffic offenses (negligent, dangerous, and irresponsible driving) and 99 matched control subjects.

Method: All subjects completed a questionnaire on socioeconomic status, education, driving experience, personal and social variables, and "exposure to recent adversity" (adverse life events in the 4 weeks prior to the offense or, for controls, in the past 4 weeks). They also were administered the following instruments: the Standard Progressive Matrices (measure of nonverbal intelligence), the 16 Personality Factor Questionnaire, the Hostility and Direction of Hostility Questionnaire, the Eysenck Personality Inventory, and the General Health Questionnaire (a screen for nonpsychotic disorders).

PERFORMANCE:
Age-related Performance
(B130 - B133)

B130   Amster, Leslie Ellen, and Krauss, Herbert H.: The relationship between life crises and mental deterioration in old age. International Journal of Aging and Human Development 5:51-55, 1974.

Subjects: 25 mentally deteriorated and 25 normal elderly women.

Method: The Schedule of Recent Experience was modified for application to older subjects. A family member or close friend completed the Geriatric Schedule of Recent Experience for each subject. Magnitude and number of life crises were studied in relation to mental deterioration.

B131   Guttman, David: Life events and decision making by older adults. The Gerontologist 18:462-467, 1978.

Subjects: 410 elderly subjects living in the community (chosen by a stratified sampling procedure of seniors in Washington, D.C.).

Method: Subjects were interviewed about the occurrence of 34 life events in the past 6 months; each reported life event was assessed for who initiated it (subject, another person, or both self- and other-initiated) and whether it required some change in the personal or social condition of the subject. Data on decision making associated with each event were also gathered by interview, using a 7-step model of the decision-making process to organize data. Subjects evaluated their own satisfaction with their current life situation. The relation of life events, life satisfaction, and decision making was compared for action-takers and non-action-takers.

B132   Rubin, Karen Brown: Stressful life changes and adaptation among aging women (Doctoral dissertation, Ohio State University, 1977). Dissertation Abstracts International 38: 5548-B, 1978.
Subjects: 40 women living in retirement communities.
Method: A life change inventory to measure Perceived Stress and Objective Stress was developed and administered to all subjects. Adaptation was assessed with three measures: staff ratings of medical status, self-report of life satisfaction, and staff ratings of adaptive behavior.

B133   Sands, James Daniel: The relationship of the pattern of intellectual abilities and blood pressure to stress and coping style in elderly women (Doctoral dissertation, Emory University, 1978). Dissertation Abstracts International 39:997-B, 1978.
Subjects: 120 women aged 65-92.
Method: Intellectual functioning of all subjects was measured by five subtests of the Wechsler Adult Intelligence Scale. Decline in abilities was estimated by a formula based on the ratio of two subtest scores divided by two other subtest scores. A modified Schedule of Recent Experience was administered to all subjects, and a procedure for subjective life event ratings was added to the life change measurement. Coping style was evaluated using a locus of control scale designed for use with elderly subjects. Blood pressure was taken on two occasions and results were averaged.

PERFORMANCE:
Physical Performance
(B134 - B135)

B134   Biersner, Robert J.; Ryman, David H.; and Rahe, Richard H.; Physical, psychological, blood serum, and mood predictors of success in preliminary underwater demolition team training. Military Medicine 142:215-219, 1977.
Subjects: 148 trainees in a preliminary UDT training program.

Method: All subjects completed the Schedule of Recent Experience, the Cornell Medical Index (illness symptom recognition), and an attitude survey (motivation) at the beginning of training. They also completed physical testing: push-ups, pull-ups, a 300-yard swim, and a 1-mile run. In addition, 76 of the subjects also took part in measurements of blood serum (weekly analysis of uric acid and cholesterol levels) and moods (Mood Questionnaire at weekly blood-drawing appointment) during training. Mean predictor values for each variable were examined and compared for those who passed and those who failed the training program.

B135   Popkin, Michael K.; Stillner, Verner; Pierce, Chester M.; Williams, Michael; and Gregory, Paul: Recent life changes and outcome of prolonged competitive stress. Journal of Nervous and Mental Disease 163:302-306, 1976.

Subjects: 25 men competing in the Alaskan Iditarod Trail Sled Dog Race (an annual long-distance event taking 2 to 6 weeks).

RC321.J83

Method: The day before the race began, all subjects completed the Schedule of Recent Experience (for past 12 months) and a biographical questionnaire (demographic variables). After the race subjects were divided into "Finisher" and "Nonfinisher" groups, and then adjusted order of finish was calculated for each subject. Correlations of life change scores to finishing order were examined.

PERFORMANCE:
Political Activity and Attitudes
(B136 - B137)

B136   Geigle, Ray A.: Psychobiological adaptation and political response prediction. Paper presented at the 1977 Annual Meeting of the American Political Science Association, Washington, D.C., September 1-4, 1977.

Subjects: A random sample of 250 voters in Bakersfield, California.

Method: In this pilot project all subjects completed two instruments: the Schedule of Recent Experience and a measure of conservatism and cynicism toward government. Correlations of life change scores to the two political attitudes were examined.

B137　Keith, Pat M.: A comparison of general and age-specific factors associated with political behavior. Experimental Aging Research 3:289-304, 1977.

Subjects: 169 men and women aged 65 and older.

Method: A structured interview was conducted with each subject. Voting and political interest were the measures of political activity. The following independent variables were examined: efficacy (attitudes toward effectiveness of political activity); life change and continuity (changes in income, health, organizational participation, activities outside the home, marital status); age-related dimensions (attitudes toward old age, participation in age-specific organizations, age identification, belief in old age intervention); and demographic characteristics (amount of volunteer work, years of education, income, sex).

LIFE CHANGE EVENTS
AND PSYCHOLOGY

PSYCHOLOGY:
Symptoms
(C1-C42)

C1   Andrews, Gavin; Tennant, Christopher; Hewson, Daphnc M.;
     and Vaillant, George E.: Life event stress, social support,
     coping style, and risk of psychological impairment. Journal
     of Nervous and Mental Disease 166:307-316, 1978.
          Subjects: A representative sample of 863 suburban Aus-
     tralians.
          Method: All subjects completed a questionnaire which in-
     cluded the following: the General Health Questionnaire, a
     20-item measure of psychological health (symptom changes
     in "past few weeks"); the Tennant and Andrews 63-item life
     events inventory (for past 12 months); a modified form of
     Vaillant's measure of coping style (maturity of ego defense
     mechanisms); and a measure of social support (the indi-
     vidual's "social health" as indicated by available crisis sup-
     port, neighborhood interaction, and community participa-
     tion). Psychologically impaired subjects were compared
     to nonimpaired subjects according to single and combined
     measures of life events, coping style, and social support.

C2   Coates, D. B.; Moyer, S.; Kendall, L.; and Howat, M. G.:
     Life-event changes and mental health. In Stress and Anxiety
     (Vol. 3). Irwin G. Sarason and Charles D. Spielberger (Eds.),
     pp. 225-250. New York: Wiley, 1976.

Subjects: 197 residents of a suburb of Toronto (ages 18-59).
Method: All subjects had been interviewed 1 year earlier
as part of the larger Yorklea Study [C3]. At the initial interview they had provided data on life events in the past
year (Modified Life Events List, a survey asking for occurrences of 24 life events taken from the Social Readjustment
Rating Scale, household member involved, and if outcome
was "for better, for worse, or the same"); mental health
(Yorklea Mental Health Scale to measure distress, symptoms, ego strength, anxiety, and self-esteem); and personal problems (Problems List of 11 problems experienced
in life and in past year). At reinterview a year later, the
Modified Life Events List and the Yorklea Mental Health
Scale were readministered.

C3   Coates, Donald; Moyer, Sharon; and Wellman, Barry: The
Yorklea study of urban mental health: Symptoms, problems
and life events. Canadian Journal of Public Health 60:471-481,
1969.

Subjects: 845 adults living in a suburb of Toronto.
Method: All subjects were administered a questionnaire interview to collect data on demographic characteristics,
close relationships, usual activities, problems and satisfactions, recent life events, and nature of recent help-
seeking. This preliminary report presents data on the relationship of symptom scores (18-item checklist of psychophysiological symptoms) to selected demographic variables
(age, sex, marital status, etc.), life events in the past year
(occurrence of 26 life events from the Social Readjustment
Rating Scale, household member involved), and recent and
lifetime personal problems (timing and duration of 11 problems, and to whom subject turned for assistance).

C4   Cochrane, Raymond, and Stopes-Roe, Mary: Psychological
and social adjustment of Asian immigrants to Britain: A community survey. Social Psychiatry 12:195-206, 1977.

Subjects: 100 Asian immigrants (50 born in India, 50 born
in Pakistan) and 100 matched native British controls, all
residents of Birmingham, England.
Method: All subjects were interviewed using a community
survey questionnaire which included a modification of
Langner's 22-item scale (symptoms of psychological disturbance); the Cochrane and Robertson Life Events Inventory (for past 12 months); and questions on housing and employment history, personal and family relationships, satisfaction with living conditions, and demographic variables.

C5 Comstock, George W., and Helsing, Knud J.: Symptoms of
depression in two communities. Psychological Medicine 6:
551-563, 1976.
Subjects: 3,845 randomly selected rural and urban adults
residing in two study communities.
Method: All subjects were interviewed using a structured
questionnaire to collect data on demographic characteristics, health status (with emphasis on depressed mood), and
psychosocial factors (including a modified Schedule of Recent Experience). The Center for Epidemiologic Studies
Depression (CES-D) Scale was used to measure symptoms
of depression. Symptom scores were examined and adjusted for a number of independent variables (including recent life events). Rural and urban subjects' adjusted scores
were compared by age, sex, race, marital status, education, employment, and household income.

C6 Diehl, Luther Albert: The relationship between demographic
factors, MMPI scores and the Social Readjustment Rating
Scale (Doctoral dissertation, Ohio University, 1977). Disser-
tation Abstracts International 38:2360-B, 1977.
Subjects: A community sample of 423 adults living in sev-
eral small cities.
Method: All subjects were administered the following in-
struments: a questionnaire of demographic variables, the
Shipley Institute of Living Scale, a modified Schedule of
Recent Experience (for past 6 months), and the MMPI.

C7 Eastham, Katherine; Coates, Donald; and Allodi, Federico:
The concept of crisis. Canadian Psychiatric Association
Journal 15:463-472, 1970.
The authors review the literature on "crisis" with the purpose of clarifying the concept for use in the Yorklea Study
(see C3) of life events, symptoms, and problems of urban
subjects. The emphasis of this study is on theory and
methodology.

C8 Eaton, William W.: Life events, social supports, and psy-
chiatric symptoms: A re-analysis of the New Haven data.
Journal of Health and Social Behavior 19:230-234, 1978.
Subjects: 720 adults in New Haven, Connecticut, who were
interviewed in 1967 and 1969 by Myers, Lindenthal, and
Pepper.
Method: The data originally reported by Myers, Lindenthal,
and Pepper (C22, C23, C24, and C25) is reanalyzed using a

different method—the panel regression technique. Three analytic questions are addressed: whether life events are statistically independent over time, whether the level of symptoms reported at Time 1 has an influence on reported life events at Time 2, and whether the availability of social supports lessens the impact of life events on risk for mental disorder.

C9   Factor, Robert M.: Life events and minor health changes in college students (Doctoral dissertation, University of Pennsylvania, 1975). Dissertation Abstracts International 36:6052-B, 1976.
        Subjects: 20 college students.
        Method: All subjects filled out a structured daily diary each evening for 3 weeks. The 3-part diary contained a checklist of 27 life events commonly experienced by students (subject rated each reported event for magnitude of emotional arousal, amount of pleasure/displeasure experienced, and degree to which event was anticipated); a checklist of 7 topics of chronic worry or concern (also rated for emotional arousal and amount of pleasure/displeasure); and a checklist of 23 symptoms and moods.

C10   Gersten, Joanne C.; Langner, Thomas S.; Eisenberg, Jeanne G.; and Simcha-Fagan, Ora: An evaluation of the etiologic role of stressful life-change events in psychological disorders. Journal of Health and Social Behavior 18:228-244, 1977.
        Subjects: 732 children in Manhattan who were available for a 5-year follow-up to a study of 1,034 children aged 6-18.
        Method: Mothers of subjects had been interviewed 5 years earlier (Time 1) using a structured questionnaire about the child and family. At Time 2 the same interview was administered and data about intervening life events were collected. Six factors of child behavior were assessed to rate child's psychological impairment at Time 1 and 2, and 21 social and family variables were assessed at Time 1 and 2. Life event measures included the frequency of 34 events and objective and subjective ratings of events in terms of change and desirability.

C11   Hagberg, Richard Arthur, Jr.: Personality trait and symptom correlates of stressful life events (Doctoral dissertation, Washington State University, 1978). Dissertation Abstracts International 39:2754-A, 1978.

Subjects: A group of security guards at a large industrial facility [number unspecified].
Method: All subjects were administered the "Life Change Index" and the MMPI. One year later the same instruments were readministered to examine the relationship of life change patterns and personality traits to the development of (or changes in) psychopathological symptoms.

C12 Hashimi, Joan Kay: Explorations of stressful life events in their relationship to mental disorder and social status variables (Doctoral dissertation, Washington State University, 1978). Dissertation Abstracts International 39:6971-A, 1979.
Subjects: 161 subjects from another study.
Method: Data on subjects were obtained from the files of a research center and based on subjects' responses to extended questionnaires administered as part of an earlier research project. The relationship of life events (modified Schedule of Recent Experience) and "social status characteristics" to "mental distress" was examined in groups of subjects ("formed in Q-type factor analyses").

Z5053.D57

C13 Hendrie, H. C.; Lachar, D.; and Lennox, K.: Personality trait and symptom correlates of life change in a psychiatric population. Journal of Psychosomatic Research 19:203-208, 1975.
Subjects: 295 psychiatric patients (109 inpatients, 186 outpatients) seen consecutively at a clinic over a 6-month period.
Method: All subjects completed the Schedule of Recent Experience (for the year prior to illness onset, when known, or prior to initial clinic visit). They also completed the MMPI. The relationship of life change scores to diagnostic group, demographic variables, and scores on the 13 Wiggins Content Scales of the MMPI was examined for males and for females.

C52.J6

C14 Holzer, Charles Elmer, III: The impact of life events on psychiatric symptomatology (Doctoral dissertation, University of Florida, 1977). Dissertation Abstracts International 38: 2939-B, 1977.
Subjects: 517 respondents available in 1973 for a follow-up study to a 1970 epidemiological survey of 1,645 people.
Method: All subjects had been administered the Health Opinion Survey in 1970; it was readministered in 1973. Life events data (for the intervening 3 years) were also

collected using the Paykel et al. method. Changes in symptom scores over the 3-year period were studied in relation to socioeconomic status and to intervening life events (frequency of individual events, weighted distress scores, category of events, area of social activity, dependence of event on previous symptomatology).

C15 Hornstra, Robijn K., and Klassen, Deidre: The course of depression. Comprehensive Psychiatry 18:119-125, 1977.
Subjects: 473 respondents to a Kansas City survey of 1,171 adults who were available for a 1-year follow-up interview. Method: At initial interview and at a 1-year follow-up interview all subjects completed the following measures of depression and symptomatology: Center for Epidemiologic Studies Depression (CES-D) Scale (for "past week"); Langner's 22-item scale (symptoms "in the last year"); questions on emotional problems ("during last month"), enjoyment of life, and general happiness; Depression Adjective Checklist (feelings "right now, today"); and Bradburn Happiness Scale (psychological well-being "in the past week"). They also completed a 40-item life events questionnaire covering the past year. Data were analyzed for subgroups divided according to life events and depression scores at initial interview (e.g., low events/low depression, low events/high depression, etc.). Changes over time in life events and depression were examined for all subgroups.

C16 Ilfeld, Frederic W., Jr.: Current social stressors and symptoms of depression. American Journal of Psychiatry 134:161-166, 1977.
Subjects: A probability sample of 2,299 adults (aged 18-65) in the Chicago area.

Method: All subjects were interviewed using a structured questionnaire to collect data on background and demographic factors, indicators of "current social stressors" in 5 social contexts (neighborhood, job, finances, parenthood, marriage), coping strategies, and psychological status. The paper reports data on the relation of current social stressors to depressive symptoms (measured by 10 items on the Psychiatric Symptom Index) and compares these findings to research on past social stressors (life events).

C17 Justice, Blair; McBee, George W.; and Allen, Richard H.: Life events, psychological distress and social functioning. Psychological Reports 40:467-473, 1977.

Subjects: 39 new outpatients admitted to adult psychiatric clinics (Symptom Relief; Personality; Marriage and Family) at a mental health center.
Method: All subjects completed a modified Schedule of Recent Experience (past 12 months), the Denver Community Mental Health Questionnaire (psychological distress and social functioning), and the MMPI Mini-Mult (personality disruptions).

C18 Lichtenstein, Larry: The effects of temporal and spatial patterns of life events on general well-being and depression (Doctoral dissertation, George Peabody College for Teachers, 1978). Dissertation Abstracts International 39:5566-B, 1979.
Subjects: Not identified in abstract.
Method: Data were collected on "recent" and "remote" life events [instrument not named] and "health-risk" (as measured by the Dupuy General Well-Being Scale and the Zung Depression Scale). Changes in number of life events over time were examined in the analysis of temporal patterns; "dispersion of life events over life space categories" was examined in the analysis of spatial patterns of life events.

Z5053.D57

C19 Markush, Robert E., and Favero, Rachel V.: Epidemiologic assessment of stressful life events, depressed mood, and psychophysiological symptoms—a preliminary report. In Stressful Life Events: Their Nature and Effects. Barbara Snell Dohrenwend and Bruce P. Dohrenwend (Eds.), pp. 171-190. New York: Wiley, 1974.
Subjects: A combined community sample of over 2,100 adults living in Kansas City, Missouri, and Washington County, Maryland.
Method: All subjects were interviewed using a structured questionnaire as part of the larger Community Mental Health Assessment project. This paper reports data collected using the Center for Epidemiologic Studies Depression (CES-D) Scale (mood scale for feelings during the week preceding interview), a version of Langner's 22-item scale (psychophysiological symptoms during the past year), and a list of weighted life events (based on Dohrenwend's modification of the Schedule of Recent Experience and using geometric mean values from the Social Readjustment Rating Scale). High, middle, and low levels of life change, depressed mood, and symptoms were examined in subjects grouped according to sex, age, race, education, and home community.

BF575.S75
C641973

C20 Micklin, Michael, and Leon, Carlos A.: Life change and psychiatric disturbance in a South American city: The effects of geographic and social mobility. Journal of Health and Social Behavior 19:92-107, 1978.
Subjects: 681 adults in a large Colombian city.
Method: All subjects were interviewed to collect the following data: age, sex, level of education attained, detailed residential and occupational history, and a measure of psychiatric disturbance (Langner's 22-item index of psychophysiological symptoms). Geographic mobility (migration experience) was assessed by number of changes of residence in 6 life cycle periods; social mobility was assessed by comparing occupational status of subject and his or her father.

C21 Murphy, H. B. M.: The meaning of symptom-check-list scores in mental health surveys: A testing of multiple hypotheses. Social Science and Medicine 12A:67-75, 1978.
Subjects: 160 women living in two districts of Montreal and chosen for income, residence (inner or outer city), and having scored high or low on Langner's 22-item symptom checklist.
Method: All subjects were administered a standardized interview which included Langner's 22-item symptom checklist. Half the subjects were also administered an open-ended interview to collect data on satisfaction with neighborhood; coping strategies; self-report illness and health-care-seeking; and ideals, needs, and goals (including self-actualization and awareness of higher needs as well as basic needs for security, shelter, etc.). One quarter of the subjects also completed several psychological tests and a modified Schedule of Recent Experience (including self-rating of adverse vs. beneficial events). Differences in mean symptom scores between the inner and outer city groups were examined in relation to a number of variables.

C22 Myers, Jerome K.; Lindenthal, Jacob J.; and Pepper, Max P.: Life events and psychiatric impairment. Journal of Nervous and Mental Disease 152:149-157, 1971.
Subjects: A community sample of 938 adults in New Haven, Connecticut.
Method: All subjects were interviewed to collect the following data: demographic variables, physical health status, psychological impairment (Gurin's modification of Macmillan's Health Opinion Survey), and life events in the past

year (62-item interview plus open-ended questions to elicit
other events). Subjects also provided data on changes in
social role performance and in physical or mental health
status associated with each reported life event. Life events
data were analyzed by frequency of occurrence and by category and quality of event (area of social activity, changes
in social field, and desirability). [See also B122, B123,
C23, C24, and C25.]

C23   Myers, Jerome K.; Lindenthal, Jacob J.; and Pepper, Max P.:
Life events, social integration and psychiatric symptomatology.
Journal of Health and Social Behavior 16:421-427, 1975.
Subjects: 720 adults living in New Haven, Connecticut.
Method: Subjects were interviewed in 1967 and again in
1969 to collect data on demographic variables, physical
and mental health status, help-seeking behavior and health
care utilization, and life events in the past year [see C22].
Using a multiple regression analysis, changes in number
of life events (few/many) and level of symptomatology (low/
high) from 1967 to 1969 were studied in relation to social
integration (16 variables including sociodemographic factors, social and instrumental role performance factors,
and treatment status).

C24   Myers, Jerome K.; Lindenthal, Jacob J.; and Pepper, Max P.:
Social class, life events, and psychiatric symptoms: A longitudinal study. In Stressful Life Events: Their Nature and Effects. Barbara Snell Dohrenwend and Bruce P. Dohrenwend
(Eds.), pp. 191-205. New York: Wiley, 1974.
Subjects: 720 adults living in New Haven, Connecticut.
Method: Subjects were interviewed in 1967 and again in
1969 to collect data on demographic variables, physical
and mental health status, help-seeking behavior and health
care utilization, and life events in the past year [see C22].
Hollingshead's Two Factor Index of Social Position was
used to determine each subject's social class. The effect
of life events on the relationship of social class to level of
symptoms at Time 1 and Time 2 was studied using a new
Desirability-Change Life Events Index scoring method (combined weights derived from modifications of the Social Readjustment Rating Scale).

C25   Myers, Jerome K.; Lindenthal, Jacob J.; Pepper, Max P.;
and Ostrander, David R.: Life events and mental status: A
longitudinal study. Journal of Health and Social Behavior 13:
398-406, 1972.

Subjects: 720 adults living in New Haven, Connecticut.
Method: Subjects were interviewed in 1967 and again in
1969 to collect data on demographic variables, physical
and mental health status, help-seeking behavior and health
care utilization, and life events in the past year [see C22].
This is the preliminary report on the relationship of changes
in life events to changes in symptoms between Time 1 and
Time 2. Life events data are analyzed by frequency of
occurrence and by category of event (area of social activity, changes in social field, degree of desirability).

C26   Oliver, Sandra L.; Comstock, George W.; and Helsing,
       Knud J.: Mood and lithium in drinking water. Archives of
       Environmental Health 31:92-95, 1976.
       Subjects: A random sample of 384 people living in Wash-
       ington County, Maryland.
       Method: As part of the larger Community Mental Health
       Assessment program, subjects were interviewed using the
       following questionnaires: the Lubin Depression Adjective
       Checklist, the Center for Epidemiologic Studies depression
       scale and functioning scale, a question on general happi-
       ness, an aggression scale, and the Cantril ladder for self-
       rating of present status. A modified Schedule of Recent
       Experience was administered as part of the "demographic
       characteristics" section of the questionnaire. Samples of
       drinking water were collected at each subject's home and
       were analyzed for lithium content.

C27   Payne, R. L.: Recent life changes and the reporting of psycho-
       logical states. Journal of Psychosomatic Research 19:99-103,
       1975.
       Subjects: 192 employed British males, aged 30-60, most
       of whom held supervisor-level jobs.
       Method: All subjects were interviewed for biographical
       data, recent patterns of social relationships, and reports
       of recent physical and mental health (including an index of
       13 symptoms and two scales to measure recent positive
       and negative affect). Subjects also completed a slightly
       modified Schedule of Recent Experience (for past year) and
       questionnaires measuring psychological well-being (modi-
       fied Bradburn scales), self-esteem, and job satisfaction.
       The effects of age, marital status, and psychological states
       on life change scores were examined, and the ability of the
       Schedule of Recent Experience to predict illness prospec-
       tively and retrospectively was evaluated.

C28   Pressman, Marcia Lee: An investigation of psychological
      and physical health in college freshmen (Doctoral disserta-
      tion, Brigham Young University, 1977). Dissertation Ab-
      stracts International 38:711-A, 1977.
         Subjects: A random sample of 338 first-year college stu-
         dents.
         Method: All subjects completed the following instruments:
         the Cornell Medical Index (CMI), the MMPI Depression
         Scale (D-Scale), the Manifest Affect Rating Scale (MARS),
         the Tennessee Self-Concept Scale (TSCS), the Boston Uni-
         versity Personality Index (BUPI), and the Schedule of Re-
         cent Experience (SRE). The relation of measures of psy-
         chological well-being (D-Scale, MARS, TSCS, BUPI, and
         SRE) to CMI scores was examined for males and females.

C29   Smokvina, Gloria Jacqueline: Life events as stressors: Re-
      lationship to health status in the aged (Doctoral dissertation,
      Wayne State University, 1977). Dissertation Abstracts Inter-
      national 38:5282B-5283B, 1978.
         Subjects: 90 elderly subjects living in a senior citizen
         complex.
         Method: Each subject was interviewed and then the follow-
         ing instruments were administered: the Schedule of Recent
         Life Events for the Elderly (frequency of life change events
         in the past 5 years and subjective ratings of magnitude of
         readjustment required by each event); the Guttman Health
         Scale for the Aged; and the Cornell Medical Index. The re-
         lation of number of life change events, perception of adjust-
         ment required, and health status to adaptive ability was ex-
         amined.

C30   Steele, Robert Emanuel: Race, sex, and social class differ-
      ences in depression among normal adults (Doctoral disserta-
      tion, Yale University, 1975). Dissertation Abstracts Interna-
      tional 36:2485B-2486B, 1975.
         Subjects: 134 employed adults (34 black and 31 white fe-
         males, 32 black and 37 white males) in selected social
         classes (upper, upper-middle, and lower-middle class).
         Method: All subjects completed a 19-page questionnaire
         which included the following sections: basic sociodemo-
         graphic data; 3 clinical measures of depression (Zung Self-
         Rating Depression Scale, Wessman-Ricks Mood Inventory,
         and Osgood's Semantic Differential); 2 measures of guilt;
         a dependency measure; the Depressive Experience Ques-
         tionnaire; a modified Schedule of Recent Experience; and

25053.D57

Rotter's Internal-External Locus of Control Scale. The relation of social, psychological, and life event variables to depression was studied in terms of race, sex, and social class differences. [See also C31.]

C31 Steele, Robert E.: Relationship of race, sex, social class, and social mobility to depression in normal adults. Journal of Social Psychology 104:37-47, 1978.
This article is based on data originally reported in the author's doctoral dissertation [see C30].

HM251. A1J6

C32 Stuart, Daniel Maxwell: The relation between stressful life events, age, personality and illness (Doctoral dissertation, University of Southern California, 1977). Dissertation Abstracts International 38:3950-B, 1978.
Subjects: 100 female college students and 100 older women living in Leisure World (a California retirement community). Method: All subjects completed a 5-part questionnaire which contained the following: a section on demographic variables; the Zung Self-Rating Depression Scale (divided into the Clinical Depression and the Self-Satisfaction subscales); the Schedule of Recent Experience (for past year); the Cornell Medical Index; and Byrne's Repression-Sensitization Scale. Each subject was assigned two illness scores by dividing the Cornell Medical Index into "Objective" items (recalled medical diagnoses) and "Subjective" items (symptoms). The effects of life change, age, and psychological defense mechanisms on objective-subjective illness rates and depression were studied.

C33 Tennant, Christopher, and Andrews, Gavin: The cause of life events in neurosis. Journal of Psychosomatic Research 22: 41-45, 1978.
Subjects: 150 neurotic adults and a matched group of 150 nonneurotic adults, all drawn from a community survey of suburban Australians.
Method: Subjects had been deemed "impaired" or "unimpaired" on the basis of General Health Questionnaire scores obtained in a community survey [see C34]. They had also marked the occurrences of 63 life events (in the past year) listed in a questionnaire. Differences in the life event experience of impaired and unimpaired subjects were compared in terms of distress experienced and the causes of the reported events. Two life event scores were calculated for each subject: a "distress" score using the Tennant and

RC52.J6

Andrews life event scalings developed for Australian populations [see H29] and a "contingency" score using another set of Tennant and Andrews's life event scalings [see H28] which rate life events by the degrees to which they are caused by "Chance," "Self," and "Others."

C34 Tennant, Christopher, and Andrews, Gavin: The pathogenic quality of life event stress in neurotic impairment. Archives of General Psychiatry 35:859-863, 1978.
Subjects: A community survey of 863 suburban Australian adults.
Method: All subjects completed a questionnaire which included a list of 63 life events (for occurrences in the past year) and the 20-item version of the General Health Questionnaire (symptoms of neurotic impairment). Three life events scores were calculated for each subject: an "event" score (cumulative number of reported events) and "distress" and "life change" scores calculated using the Tennant and Andrews life event scalings [see H29] developed for use with Australian populations. The relation of the three life events scores to neurotic impairment was examined.

C35 Thoits, Peggy Ann: Life events, social integration, and psychological distress (Doctoral dissertation, Stanford University, 1978). Dissertation Abstracts International 39:3869-A, 1978.
Subjects: A subsample of married men, married women, and formerly married women taken from a longitudinal study of 4,332 participants in an income-maintenance experiment in Denver, Colorado.
Method: As part of the larger study, data were collected periodically on life events (changes in marital status, family composition, employment, income, health and education) and psychological distress (using a version of the Macmillan Health Opinion Survey) of subjects following their enrollment in an income-maintenance experiment. Two possible mediators of the relationship between life events and psychological distress—"social integration" and "self-esteem"—were tested by comparing the effects of life events on psychological distress in subjects whose initial integration and self-esteem were high or low. [See also C36.]

C36 Thoits, Peggy A., and Hannan, Michael T.: The impact of an income maintenance experiment on psychological distress. Sociological Abstracts 26(3):78S09013 (SSSP 1978 1042),

1978. [This study was later published as "Income and psychological distress: The impact of an income-maintenance experiment" in Journal of Health and Social Behavior 20:120-138, 1979.]

> Subjects: 7,500 adult heads of household participating in an income-maintenance experiment in Seattle and Denver.
> Method: Subjects were assigned to one of a number of experimental treatment groups or to the control (no payment) group. All subjects were interviewed every 4 months during the experiment (for reports on health and on other life events accompanying the financial change in situation). A version of the Macmillan Health Opinion Survey was administered twice, at Time 1 and again 16 months later at Time 2. The effect of income maintenance on psychological distress was examined in relation to 12 background variables including sex, marital status, and race (white, black, Chicano).

C37 Uhlenhuth, Eberhard H.; Lipman, Ronald S.; Balter, Mitchell B.; and Stern, Martin: Symptom intensity and life stress in the city. Archives of General Psychiatry 31:759-764, 1974.

> Subjects: A probability sample of 735 urban adults.
> Method: All subjects were interviewed about their life situations, health problems, and coping methods. A 54-item symptom checklist was administered, and subjects rated each symptom experienced in the past week on a 4-point scale ("not at all" to "extremely bothered by"). A mean symptom score was calculated for each subject as a measure of overall symptom intensity. Life events data were collected using a shortened version of the Paykel et al. questionnaire (for events in the past 12 months); weighted values for undesirable events were used to calculate "life stress" scores. The relation of life events to symptom intensity was studied in relation to a number of demographic variables such as age, sex, and reported health care status (under care/needs care/does not need care). [See also C39, C38.]

C38 Uhlenhuth, Eberhard H., and Paykel, Eugene S.: Symptom configuration and life events. Archives of General Psychiatry 28:744-748, 1973.

> Subjects: 146 psychiatric outpatients and 21 psychiatric day patients.
> Method: This is the companion article to publication C39. Data collected using a 72-item symptom checklist were

organized into a 5-factor symptom profile (irascibility, somatization, compulsiveness, anxiety, depression) that was used as an index of symptom configuration. Each of the factor scores was compared to the mean score (used in C39 as a measure of symptom intensity), and symptom profiles were studied in relation to the following independent variables: weighted life events score, mean symptom checklist score, age, social class, sex, marital status, religion, race, and patient group (day or inpatient).

C39 Uhlenhuth, Eberhard H., and Paykel, Eugene S.: Symptom intensity and life events. Archives of General Psychiatry 28: 473-477, 1973.

Subjects: 45 psychiatric inpatients, 21 psychiatric day patients, 146 psychiatric outpatients, and 155 nonpatients (relatives of other clinic patients).

RC321A66 Method: All subjects completed a questionnaire concerning demographic variables and life events in the past 12 months (a 61-item inventory including individual ratings on a 20-point scale of distress/upset associated with each event). All patients also completed a 72-item symptom checklist (covering the past 7 days), reporting how much each symptom bothered them (4-point scale ranging from "not at all" to "extremely"). The relationship of weighted life events scores to overall symptom intensity (the mean of 5 dimensions derived by factor analysis) was examined in relation to a number of independent variables such as sex, race, age, and subject group. [See also C38 and C37.]

C40 Wildman, Richard C., and Johnson, David Richard: Life change and Langner's 22-item mental health index: A study and partial replication. Journal of Health and Social Behavior 18:179-188, 1977.

Subjects: In Study 1, 156 college students; in Study 2, a probability sample of 237 urban adults.

RII.J687 Method: In Study 1, all subjects completed a modified Schedule of Recent Experience for college students; they also completed Langner's 22-item index (as a measure of psychological distress). In Study 2, all subjects completed a modified Recent Life Changes Questionnaire (64 items covering the past 2 years, and including subjective ratings on a 10-point readjustment scale); they also completed Langner's 22-item index. The relation of life change unit scores (LCU) to psychological distress scores was examined; the two studies were also compared. [See also B68.]

C41 Zautra, Alex, and Beier, Ernst: The effects of life crisis on psychological adjustment. <u>American Journal of Community Psychology</u> <u>6</u>:125-135, 1978.

> Subjects: A probability sample of 454 suburban adults.
> Method: This is the companion report to publication C42. Data were analyzed using multivariate analyses of variance and stepwise regression in order to examine the relation of "life crisis" (12-month Schedule of Recent Experience), five social conditions (income, education, age, marital status, and religious participation), and ratings of quality of life (Perceived Quality of Life Scale) to psychological adjustment (Langner's 22-item index and reported utilization of mental health clinic services).

C42 Zautra, Alex; Beier, Ernst; and Cappel, Lawrence: The dimensions of life quality in a community. <u>American Journal of Community Psychology</u> <u>5</u>:85-97, 1977.

> Subjects: A probability sample of 454 suburban adults.
> Method: All subjects were interviewed to collect data on the following: happiness and life satisfaction (using a modified Perceived Quality of Life Scale), psychiatric symptoms (the Bradburn Negative Affect Scale, Langner's 22-item index, and questions on use of professional helping agencies), and participation in life concerns (personal, family, and community activities and quality of involvement). Subjects also completed the Schedule of Recent Experience (for past year). Factor analysis was performed on selected variables to define groups of "quality of life" factors. The effects of 6 demographic variables (age, sex, marital status, income, education, and religious participation) on dimensions of life quality were examined. [See also C41.]

PSYCHOLOGY:
Coping Styles and Methods
(C43-C58)

C43 Antonovsky, Aaron: Conceptual and methodological problems in the study of resistance resources and stressful live events. In <u>Stressful Life Events: Their Nature and Effects</u>. Barbara Snell Dohrenwend and Bruce P. Dohrenwend (Eds.), pp. 245-258. New York: Wiley, 1974.

> This study was based on interviews with 391 Jewish Israelis living in Jerusalem and receiving medical care in a family practice center of a medical school. The author describes

the development of an interview instrument to measure both life crises and resistance resources. The questionnaire that was developed includes several sections: a life crisis history (frequency and duration of 20 life crisis items); a measure of current tensions (using Cantril's technique in the Self-Anchoring Striving Scale); a measure of past resistance resources (self-rating of residual effect of reported life crises); and a measure of current resistance resources (3-part section to measure flexibility, ties to others, and community ties).

C44 Bell, Janice M.: Stressful life events and coping methods in mental-illness and -wellness behaviors. Nursing Research 26:136-141, 1977.

 Subjects: 30 newly admitted psychiatric inpatients matched to 30 well control subjects.

 Method: All subjects completed two questionnaires: a modified Schedule of Recent Experience (for the past 6 months) and an 18-item coping scale (subject rated his or her own likelihood of using each coping method on a 5-point scale ranging from "never" to "always"). The relation of life change scores and coping methods to mental-illness or -wellness status was examined in terms of age and sex, and use of short-term coping methods was compared to use of long-term coping methods.

C45 Cohen, Frances, and Lazarus, Richard S.: Active coping processes, coping dispositions, and recovering from surgery. Psychosomatic Medicine 35:375-389, 1973.

 Subjects: 61 adult surgical patients admitted for elective operations (22 hernia, 29 gall bladder, 10 thyroid conditions).

 Method: The day before surgery each subject was briefly interviewed about his or her emotional state and knowledge about the coming operation, and subject was rated by the interviewer on (1) use of avoidant and vigilant coping mechanisms and (2) anxiety. Subjects were also administered the Goldstein coper-avoider Sentence Completion Test (a measure of coping disposition). They were then asked to complete two instruments: the Epstein and Fenz modified Repression-sensitization scale (another coping disposition measure) and the Schedule of Recent Experience (for a total 2-year life change score). Five recovery variables were documented (e.g., number of days in hospital, minor complications) and used as an index of recovery.

RTI.N8

C46 Cohen, Judith Blackfield: Health care, coping, and the counselor. <u>Personnel and Guidance Journal</u> <u>56</u>:616-620, 1978.

This review discusses definitions of "stress," "coping theory," and their relation to disease. The role of social support in mediating the effects of "breakdown" and in aiding recovery is discussed in terms of the counselor's role. Life events research is included in the section on "stress."

C47 Engel, George L.: A life setting conducive to illness: The giving-up-given-up complex. <u>Annals of Internal Medicine</u> <u>69</u>: 293-300, 1968.

The author reviews his research with colleagues at the University of Rochester leading to the development of the giving-up-given-up complex, a state of psychological disturbance that signals a "temporary failure of mental coping mechanisms" in response to overwhelming environmental demands and that can contribute to the onset of disease. He reviews examples of life settings conducive to illness, many of them falling into the category of what Engel calls the "personal dramas and tragedies of everyday life"—deaths of family and friends, personal illness or injury, loss of home, job, or possessions, financial setbacks, and other common life events.

C48 Fontana, Alan F.; Dowds, Barbara Noel; Marcus, Jonathan L.; and Rakusin, John M.: Coping with interpersonal conflicts through life events and hospitalization: predictive validity of the model. <u>Journal of Nervous and Mental Disease</u> <u>162</u>:88-98, 1976.

Subjects: A subsample of 60 male psychiatric inpatients drawn from a larger study of 171 consecutive admissions to a VA hospital.

Method: These subjects (taken from the 1973 replication study reported in C50) were followed to test the validity of the coping model first described in a 1972 study (C49) for the posthospitalization period. During hospitalization each subject was rated for personal adjustment and role skills by himself, the nursing staff, his therapists, and his significant others; similar ratings at 1 and 6 months after discharge were collected from subjects and their significant others. The outcome (rehospitalization or recovery) of subjects who had resolved their conflicts during hospitalization was compared to the outcome of subjects who had not resolved their conflicts while hospitalized.

C49   Fontana, Alan F.; Marcus, Jonathan L.; Noel, Barbara; and
      Rakusin, John M.: Prehospitalization coping styles of psychi-
      atric patients: The goal-directedness of life events. Journal
      of Nervous and Mental Disease 155:311-321, 1972.
         Subjects: 99 recently admitted male psychiatric inpatients
         and 99 matched, nonhospitalized control subjects.
         Method: All subjects completed a questionnaire about the
         occurrence of 54 life events in the past year (divided into
         quarters). An interview was held with a subsample of 17
         patients and their significant others to obtain detailed infor-
         mation about reported life events, other sources of help
         tried before hospitalization, the circumstances surrounding
         hospitalization, and the effects of hospitalization on others
         in the patient's life. Life events data collected by question-
         naire were divided into categories by quality of event: posi-
         tive (10), indeterminate (17), and negative (27) events.
         Data collected by interview were also analyzed by two addi-
         tional categories: "contingent" or "noncontingent" events
         (whether event's occurrence depended on some action by
         patient) and "involved" or "not involved" events (whether
         event was involved in the problem for which patient was
         hospitalized). Each patient was also rated for severity of
         pathology (staff ratings combined with patient's own esti-
         mate and explanation of his situation). The relation of num-
         ber of life events to severity of pathology was examined for
         patients. The number, pattern, and quality of life events
         were compared for patients and control subjects to test a
         model of coping in which life events and hospitalization are
         seen as attempts at indirect coping. [See also C50 and C48.]

C50   Fontana, Alan F.; Rakusin, John M.; Marcus, Jonathan L.;
      and Dowds, Barbara: Coping, stress, and life events. Pro-
      ceedings of the American Psychological Association (81st An-
      nual Convention) 8:367-368, 1973.
         Subjects: 171 consecutive male admissions to a hospital's
         psychiatry service and 99 nonhospitalized control subjects.
         Method: This work reports the results of a replication of
         the study described in C49. The same procedures were
         used to collect life events data by questionnaire for all sub-
         jects and by interview for a subsample (60 patients and their
         significant others). The same control group of 99 nonpa-
         tients was used in both studies. [See also C48.]

C51   Hamburg, David A., and Adams, John E.: A perspective on
      coping behavior: Seeking and utilizing information in major

transitions. Archives of General Psychiatry 17:277-284, 1967.

> The authors review one aspect of coping—the seeking and utilizing of information—in a series of coping studies conducted over the course of 16 years by one of the authors. The subjects described here were faced with one of three major life events: severe personal injury (burns, poliomyelitis), fatal childhood illness (parents of leukemia patients), and going away to college (students during their first year away from home).

C52 Hibler, Russell James: Life events and coping ability: A problem solving approach (Doctoral dissertation, Ohio State University, 1975). Dissertation Abstracts International 36: 4158-B, 1976.

> Subjects: 154 fifth- and sixth-grade children (79 boys, 75 girls).
> Method: All subjects completed a modified version of Coddington's Schedule of Recent Experience for children (self-report of occurrence, frequency, and subjective feelings of 39 life events). The State-Trait Anxiety Inventory for Children (measure of anxiety) and the Purdue Elementary Problem Solving Inventory (measure of coping ability) were administered. The relation of life events to coping ability was examined, and the effect of A-trait anxiety as a mediator of that relationship was also studied.

C53 Lazarus, Richard S.: Psychological stress and coping in adaptation and illness. International Journal of Psychiatry in Medicine 5:321-333, 1974.

> This theoretical discussion of coping processes emphasizes the role of cognitive appraisal and of self-regulatory processes as mediators of the individual's response to "stressful transactions," thereby influencing "somatic outcome." The life change research of Holmes and Rahe is discussed.

C54 Marx, Martin B.; Garrity, Thomas F.; and Somes, Grant W.: The effect of imbalance in life satisfactions and frustrations upon illness behavior in college students. Journal of Psychosomatic Research 21:423-427, 1977.

> Subjects: 56 college seniors, selected specifically for their history of high life change (all had originally participated in a study during their freshman year of college).
> Method: All subjects were interviewed to assess health status (number of health problems, number of episodes,

number of disability days) in the past 60 days. They also completed Anderson's College Schedule of Recent Experience, Langner's 22-item index of psychophysiological symptoms, and the Heimler Scale of Social Functioning (as a potential index of coping skill). The relation of high recent life change to measures of psychophysiological strain and health status was examined, and the effect of coping ability on those relationships was studied.

C55 McNeil, Jo, and Pesznecker, Betty L.: Keeping people well despite life change crises. Public Health Reports 92:343-348, 1977.
Subjects: A community survey of 536 adults.
Method: All subjects completed a postal questionnaire which collected data on the following: health habits (19 items as a measure of "good" or "poor" health practices); social assets (past social support and present social support measures); psychological well-being (Bradburn's 8-item index of positive and negative experience); life change (Schedule of Recent Experience for the past 2 years); and health status (report of "major change in health during past 2 years"). The effects of health habits, psychological well-being, and social supports on the relationship between life change and health change were examined.

C56 Sedney, Mary Anne: Use and effectiveness of rumination as a cognitive strategy following stressful life events in middle-aged women (Doctoral dissertation, University of Massachusetts, 1976). Dissertation Abstracts International 38:380-B, 1977.
Subjects: 40 women, aged 45-57.
Method: Each subject was interviewed with open-ended questions and was also administered quantitative measures [unnamed in abstract] to collect data on recent life events (in the past 18 months), distress-related symptoms, self-rating of coping, recent use of psychotherapy, and reported rumination ("frequent stress-related thoughts") in response to two life events (frequency and effectiveness of rumination at 1 week, 3 months, and 6 months after the event).

C57 Strong, Catherine: The relationship of life event interpretations to helping interactions: A case study. American Journal of Community Psychology 6:455-464, 1978.
The author presents a case study of a woman facing divorce as an example of interpretation of a life event as an impor-

tant "mediate point" in the pathway from onset of "stressful event" to its resolution or outcome. This case history illustrates the relationship between interpretation of a life event and the decision to seek help to cope with the event.

C58 Wild, Bradford S., and Hanes, Carolyn: A dynamic conceptual framework of generalized adaptation to stressful stimuli. Psychological Reports 38:319-334, 1976.
The authors present a multifactor paradigm of the relationship of external, environmental demands ("stress") to internal, psychological demands ("strain") in the adaptation (coping) process. They present their model as a synthesis of definitions and theoretical arguments in the literature they review, which includes the life events research of Brown and Birley, Cobb and Kasl, and Dohrenwend and Dohrenwend.

PSYCHOLOGY:
Social Supports
(C59-C67)

C59 Cassel, John: The contribution of the social environment to host resistance. American Journal of Epidemiology 104:107-123, 1976.
In this study, originally presented as the Fourth Wade Hampton Frost Lecture, the author reviews the literature and discusses the role of environmental factors in resistance and susceptibility to disease. Particular attention is given to the effects of social supports, which the author describes as the "protective factors buffering or cushioning the individual from the physiologic or psychologic consequences of exposure to the stressor situation."

C60 Cobb, Sidney: Social support as a moderator of life stress. Psychosomatic Medicine 38:300-314, 1976.
The author begins by defining "social support" and then examines the literature for evidence of the degree to which social support can protect individuals during a variety of life phases and life crises. Beginning with Nuckolls's study of life change, social supports, and complications of pregnancy, the author goes on to review studies of social support in relation to the following life events and life crises: birth and early life experiences, transitions to adulthood, hospitalization, recovery from illness, the risk of stopping

drinking, the risk of depression at times of high life change, loss of job, bereavement, aging and retirement, and threat of death.

C61 Dean, Alfred, and Lin, Nan: The stress-buffering role of social support: Problems and prospects for systematic investigation. Journal of Nervous and Mental Disease 165:403-417, 1977.

The authors present a critical review of the literature and research issues (key concepts, representative findings, major issues for future research, theoretical limitations, measurement, and research design). They offer detailed proposals for approaching those issues in future research by formulating three hypotheses to identify the buffering function of social support and then outline the methodology to test the hypotheses. The list of references contains 121 items.

C62 Dickey, Elizabeth Dunbar: Life events, social support, and adjustment in women: A field study (Doctoral dissertation, University of Massachusetts, 1977). Dissertation Abstracts International 38:1876-B, 1977.

Subjects: 200 female residents of northern New England. Method: All subjects completed a postal questionnaire which included measures [unnamed in abstract] of the following: life events, social support, personality adjustment, and general life satisfaction. A subsample (23 women) was administered individual interviews to provide a "qualitative point of view" to the quantitative data collected by questionnaire.

C63 Gore, Susan: The effect of social support in moderating the health consequences of unemployment. Journal of Health and Social Behavior 19:157-165, 1978.

Subjects: 100 stably employed, married men (aged 40-59) who lost their jobs when their company plants were permanently shut down.
Method: The analyses in this article are based on data originally reported in the author's doctoral dissertation (see C64). This report does not include the original control subjects in its analyses.

C64 Gore, Susan: The influence of social support and related variables in ameliorating the consequences of job loss (Doctoral dissertation, University of Pennsylvania, 1973). Dissertation Abstracts International 34:5330A-5331A, 1974.

Subjects: 100 stably employed, married men (aged 40-59) who lost their jobs when their company plants were permanently shut down and 76 control subjects who were continuously employed in comparable jobs at other workplaces. Method: All subjects were followed during 5 stages of the job loss experience: 6 weeks before shutdown, 1 month after closing, and then at 6 months, 1 year, and 2 years after job loss. A public health nurse made the 5 home visits to collect the following: blood and urine specimens (for analysis of cholesterol and other physiologic changes); measures of "stress" related to job loss (number of weeks unemployed, economic deprivation); health data (measures of depression, self-blame, illness symptoms, number of days with illness, disease); and measure of social support (a 13-item interview index).

C65 Gourash, Nancy: Help-seeking: A review of the literature. American Journal of Community Psychology 6:413-423, 1978.
This review covers three aspects of help-seeking: who seeks help, role of the social network, and the outcomes (satisfaction with and effectiveness of helping interactions). Particular attention is directed to the role of the social network as a mediating factor between distressing life events and help-seeking behavior.

C66 Henderson, Scott; Duncan-Jones, Paul; McAuley, Helen; and Ritchie, Karen: The patient's primary group. British Journal of Psychiatry 132:74-86, 1978.
Subjects: 50 new patients with a nonpsychotic psychiatric disorder and 50 matched, well control subjects. Method: Patients were administered the Present State Examination to determine diagnostic category. All subjects were administered the General Health Questionnaire (measure of morbidity for patients, a screening instrument for controls); the Social Interaction Schedule (numerical size, duration of contact, and "affective quality" of interactions with primary group and with more diffuse social bonds; index of perceived social support); and a Life Event Inventory (a modification of instruments developed by Holmes and Rahe, Paykel et al., and Tennant and Andrews). Patients and control subjects were compared for size and nature of primary group, indicators of social support, and duration and perceived quality of social transactions.

C67   Kaplan, Berton H.; Cassel, John C.; and Gore, Susan: Social support and health. Medical Care 15 (Supplement, No. 5):47-58, 1977.

The authors review the literature pointing to the importance of social support in the etiology of disease (including several life change studies), and they assess the research evidence on the mechanisms of social support. Their assessment of the current state of knowledge is accompanied by suggestions for the direction and design of future research.

RIIM437X

PSYCHOLOGY:
Locus of Control
(C68-C75)

C68   Beisheim, Sandra Tiernan: The magnitude of life change events, locus of control and reported health change. Unpublished master's thesis, University of Washington, 1978.

Subjects: 60 military personnel newly assigned as students to a training facility.

Method: All subjects completed the Schedule of Recent Experience and Rotter's Internal-External Locus of Control scale. Health change was determined by yes or no responses to Schedule of Recent Experience question #13 (occurrence of "major personal illness or injury").

C69   Bryant, Brenda K., and Trockel, Jennifer F.: Personal history of psychological stress related to locus of control orientation among college women. Journal of Consulting and Clinical Psychology 44:266-271, 1976.

Subjects: 34 female undergraduate students.

Method: All subjects were administered the Norwicki-Strickland Personal Reaction Survey (a general measure of locus of control) and modified versions of Coddington's Schedule of Recent Experience for preschool, elementary, junior high, and senior high students. The modifications to Coddington's instruments were made to collect retrospective childhood and adolescent life change data from subjects. Subjects were given a list of life change events for each of the age periods and were asked to mark (1) whether the event occurred to her then and, if so, (2) whether she remembered her "affect" as being positive, negative, or neutral. The relation of "remembered affective significance" to recalled life changes was compared at

BFI.JS75

each age period for subjects with internal vs. external control orientation in adulthood.

C70 Crandall, James E., and Lehman, Robert E.: Relationship of stressful life events to social interest, locus of control, and psychological adjustment. Journal of Consulting and Clinical Psychology 45:1208, 1977.

Subjects: 46 male and 35 female undergraduate students. Method: All subjects completed the following measures: a modified Schedule of Recent Experience (including subject rating of reported events as pleasant/unpleasant/neutral); Crandall's Social Interest Scale (a personality variable important to adjustment); Rotter's Internal-External Locus of Control Scale; and Langner's 22-item index (symptoms of maladjustment). The relation of recent life change to social interest, locus of control, and psychological adjustment was compared for total life change scores and for life change scores based only on unpleasant events.

C71 Gilbert, Lucia A.: Situational factors and the relationship between locus of control and psychological adjustment. Journal of Counseling Psychology 23:302-309, 1976.

Subjects: In Experiment 1, 123 students who requested counseling at a university's counseling service (clients) and 422 volunteer student subjects (nonclients); in Experiment 2, 23 clients and 24 nonclients.

Method: In Experiment 1, all subjects completed 10 items drawn from Rotter's Internal-External Locus of Control scale (5 items on "luck" factor, 5 on "blame" factor) under two instructional conditions: they answered the set of items in relation to "how they had been feeling or thinking lately" (situational I-E) and then in relation to "what they considered to be typical of themselves" (characteristic I-E). Characteristic and situational perceptions of control were compared for clients and nonclients. In Experiment 2, clients and nonclients were administered the following measures before counseling began (or initial contact, for nonclients): Harris's modification of the Schedule of Recent Experience for college students (events "in your immediate past"); a modification of Rotter's Internal-External Locus of Control scale ("chance" and "powerful others" scales) for two instructional conditions (situational and characteristic I-E); and a short form of Taylor's Manifest Anxiety Scale. Several months later a follow-up questionnaire containing the locus of control and anxiety measures was mailed to all subjects for completion. Clients were also asked to rate their satisfaction with the counseling experience. Pre- and posttreatment measures were compared for clients and nonclients.

C72   Johnson, James H., and Sarason, Irwin G.: Life stress, depression and anxiety: Internal-external control as a moderator variable. Journal of Psychosomatic Research 22:205-208, 1978.

RC52.J6

Subjects: 124 undergraduate students in psychology courses. Method: All subjects completed the following instruments: the Life Experiences Survey (a 54-item inventory of life events experienced in the past year, with subject rating of reported events' desirability and degree of impact); Rotter's Internal-External Locus of Control scale; the State-Trait Anxiety Inventory; and the Beck Depression Scale. The relation of positive and negative life change scores to measures of anxiety and depression was compared for subjects with internal vs. external locus of control.

C73   Kilmann, Peter R.; Lavel, Ramon; and Wanlass, Richard L.: Locus of control and perceived adjustment to life events. Journal of Clinical Psychology 34:512-513, 1978.
Subjects: 164 university students.
Method: All subjects were administered two instruments:

RC321.J74 Rotter's Internal-External Locus of Control scale and a modified Schedule of Recent Experience (43-item checklist of events in the past 2 years plus subject rating on a 6-point scale of his or her difficulty in adjusting to reported event). "Internal scorers" were compared to "external scorers" on number of experienced life events and perceived adjustment to life events.

C74   Manuck, Stephen B.; Hinrichsen, James J.; and Ross, Elizabeth O.: Life stress, locus of control, and state and trait anxiety. Psychological Reports 36:413-414, 1975.
Subjects: 129 undergraduate students.
Method: All subjects completed the following instruments: the Jacobs, Spilken, and Norman Life Change Inventory (Category A); Rotter's Internal-External Locus of Control scale; and Spielberger's State-Trait Anxiety Inventory. The relationship of life change, locus of control, and anxiety measures were examined. [See also B24 for a follow-up study of these subjects.]

C75 Wyatt, Gail Elizabeth: The relationship of life changes and locus of control attributions to cognitive aspects of the black mother-child interaction (Doctoral dissertation, University of California, Los Angeles, 1973). Dissertation Abstracts International 34:7059A-7060A, 1974.

Subjects: 40 black mothers and their 4- to 5-year-old children enrolled in Head Start.

Method: A number of home observations of mother and child were made to assess four parent behaviors (suggestions, commands, manual intrusions, facilitations) in cognitively oriented learning situations (playing with three toys demanding different degrees of parental involvement). Life changes and locus of control measures [unnamed in abstract] were also obtained and studied in relation to each mother's "general approval" and "specific approval" of her child's task-oriented behavior.

PSYCHOLOGY:
Anxiety
(C76-C82)

C76 Justice, Blair; McBee, George; and Allen, Richard: Social dysfunction and anxiety. The Journal of Psychology 97:37-42, 1977.

Subjects: 44 new outpatients admitted to adult psychiatric clinics (Symptom Relief; Personality; Marriage and Family) at a mental health center.

Method: All subjects completed the following instruments: the Denver Community Mental Health Questionnaire (measure of personal and social functioning); the MMPI Mini-Mult; a modified Schedule of Recent Experience (for past 12 months); and the Taylor Manifest Anxiety Scale. The relation of manifest anxiety scores to measures of social functioning, personality, and life change was examined for males and females.

C77 Lauer, Robert H.: Rate of change and stress: A test of the "Future Shock" thesis. Social Forces 52:510-516, 1974.

Subjects: 648 university students drawn in a 5% sample of summer classes at a U.S. university.

Method: All subjects completed the following instruments: the Schedule of Recent Experience (measure of personal changes); the short form of the Taylor Manifest Anxiety Scale; and a series of 7 statements asking for Likert-type responses to measure perceived rate of, desirability of, and control over social change, and perceived desirability of and control over personal changes. All measures were subdivided into high vs. low scores, and the relationships among all variables were examined. [See also C79.]

C78   Lauer, Robert H.: The Social Readjustment Rating Scale and anxiety: A cross-cultural study. Journal of Psychosomatic Research 17:171-174, 1973.

     Subjects: 648 U.S. university students and 130 U.K. university students.

RC52.J6   Method: All subjects completed a questionnaire containing the Schedule of Recent Experience and the short form of the Taylor Manifest Anxiety Scale. Data were analyzed by dividing life change scores into low, medium, and high ranges and by dividing anxiety scores into low and high ranges. The relation of anxiety scores to life change scores was compared for U.S. and U.K. subjects.

C79   Lauer, Robert H., and Thomas, Rance: A comparative analysis of the psychological consequences of change. Human Relations 29:239-248, 1976.

     Subjects: 648 U.S. university students and 130 U.K. university students.

H1H8   Method: This report compares data collected on U.S. subjects and analyzed in C77 to data collected following the same procedures with a U.K. sample. The U.S. and U.K. subjects are here compared on the relation of anxiety and life change scores to perceived rate of, desirability of, and control over personal and social change.

C80   Reavley, William: The relationship of life events to several aspects of "anxiety." Journal of Psychosomatic Research 18: 421-424, 1974.

     Subjects: 40 U.K. adults (aged 18-60) who were students in evening classes or clerical workers.

     Method: All subjects completed the following instruments: the Schedule of Recent Experience, the short form of the Taylor Manifest Anxiety Scale, the IPAT (Institute for Personality and Ability Testing) Anxiety Questionnaire, and the SRT (symptom rating test). This research was designed to replicate Lauer's study [C78] of life events and anxiety but using measures of anxiety hypothesized to be more appropriate measures of "state" as opposed to "trait" anxiety. The relation of life change and anxiety scores was examined for subscales of each anxiety measure.

RC52.J6

C81 Salib, Samir Boulos: Life change events and adjustment in children (Doctoral dissertation, St. Louis University, 1975). Dissertation Abstracts International 36:4408A-4409A, 1976.
    Subjects: 361 6-year-old children in the St. Louis Baby Study.
    Method: The following instruments were used to collect data on each child: Coddington's Schedule of Recent Experience for preschool children, the Test for General Anxiety, and the Test for Defensiveness. The relation of life change scores to measures of anxiety and defensiveness was examined. The life change data were then divided into three categories (events related to parents and grandparents, events related to siblings, events related to index child), and the relation of each category of events to anxiety and defensiveness was studied using rank order correlations.

C82 Westbrook, Mary T., and Viney, Linda L.: The application of content analysis scales to life stress research. Australian Psychologist 12:157-166, 1977.
    The authors review their earlier studies of affective responses of subjects undergoing 1 of 5 life events (200 women in a childbearing year, 48 students beginning university, 52 women undergoing relocation, 29 people newly hospitalized for psychiatric care, and 32 students settling into their second year at university). They use their work with the Gottschalk-Gleser content analysis scales (7 anxiety subscales, 3 hostility subscales, and subscales for positive affect and cost ratio) to illustrate a discussion of methods for studying affective reactions over time and methods for collecting verbal samples for retrospective research.

PSYCHOLOGY:
Miscellaneous Personality Measures
(C83-C91)

C83 Branson, David Howard: Individuation-transcendence of Jungian types, life change and illness (Doctoral dissertation, University of Washington, 1975). Dissertation Abstracts International 36:3499A-3500A, 1975.
    Subjects: 187 college students.
    Method: All subjects completed three instruments: the Schedule of Recent Experience, the Cornell Medical Index (measure of health status), and the Myers-Briggs Type Indicator (measure of Jungian constructs). The dynamics of

the Jungian typology (individuation and transcendence) was studied in relation to life change (in high, medium, and low risk groups) and health status (high vs. low Cornell Medical Index scores).

C84   Burchfield, Susan Renee: Personality characteristics of extremely healthy people (Doctoral dissertation, University of Washington, 1978). Dissertation Abstracts International 39: 2488-B, 1978.

       Subjects: 356 members of a prepaid group health organization who were undergoing their annual physical examination. Method: In addition to the physical examination, all subjects completed the following instruments: the Interval (health status in past 6 months) and Past Medical Histories (diseases, surgery, family history); a modified Schedule of Recent Experience (a checklist of events in the past year and events anticipated in the next year); the Heimler Scale of Social Functioning (satisfactions and frustrations in life); and the Assessment of Current Life Conditions (a new measure of personality characteristics). Subjects were divided according to diagnostic category and other defined criteria into groups representative of the spectrum of a "normal" healthy population: extremely healthy (101), healthy (89), general population (81), and sick but still maintaining employment (85).

C85   Chan, Kwok Bun: Individual differences in reactions to stress and their personality and situational determinants: Some implications for community mental health. Social Science and Medicine 11:89-103, 1977.

PER   The author reviews the literature and discusses concepts of "stress" and "stressful life events" in order to posit some personality constructs (e.g., self-esteem, locus of control, learned helplessness) which might account for individual variations in response to the same "stressful" stimulus. He places his discussion in the context of intervention and prevention strategies relevant to community mental health programming.

C86   Costantini, Arthur F.; Braun, John R.; Davis, Jack; and Iervolino, Annette: Personality and mood correlates of Schedule of Recent Experience scores. Psychological Reports 32:1143-1150, 1973.

      Subjects: 262 university students.

Method: All subjects completed three instruments: the
Schedule of Recent Experience, the Profile of Mood States,
and the Psychological Screening Inventory. The relation
of life change scores to mood and personality measures
was examined.

C87 Daly, Elizabeth Ballas: Life change adjustments, ego energy
and field-dependent perception in older adults (Doctoral dissertation, Boston University School of Nursing, 1978). Dissertation Abstracts International 39:4274-B, 1979.
Subjects: 120 older (age 55-75) subjects living in a small
Cape Cod community.
Method: The following instruments were administered to
all subjects: the Schedule of Recent Experience (for past
year), the Ego Permissiveness Scale of the Experience
Questionnaire (to measure ego energy), and the Children's
Embedded Figures Test (to determine field dependent-
independent perception).

Z5053.D57

C88 Garrity, Thomas F.; Somes, Grant W.; and Marx, Martin B.:
Personality factors in resistance to illness after recent life
changes. Journal of Psychosomatic Research 21:23-32, 1977.
Subjects: 250 first-year college students.
Method: All subjects completed Anderson's College Schedule of Recent Experience (for past year) and the Omnibus
Personality Inventory. At least 3 months later each subject was interviewed to collect data on five health variables:
number of health problems, illness episodes, illness days,
and disability days in the past 60 days; and score on Langner's 22-item index (symptoms of psychiatric impairment).
Data from the personality inventory's 14 scales were reduced to three dimensions (social conformity, liberal intellectualism, and emotional sensitivity) which were studied
as possible intervening variables between life change and
health change.

RC52.J6

C89 O'Donnell, Michael Joseph: Stress: Incidence, mediation
and adaptation among college students (Doctoral dissertation,
University of New Mexico, 1975). Dissertation Abstracts
International 36:3126B, 1975.
Subjects: 129 college students.
Method: All subjects completed the following question-
naires: a modified Schedule of Recent Experience (for
past year); the Pittsburgh Manifest Anxiety Scale; the
Myers-Briggs Type Indicator (a personality measure);

Z5053.D57

O. J. Harvey's "This I Believe" instrument (an indicator of conceptual systems); a 10-item "future shock" measure (derived from statements by Alvin Toffler); a questionnaire on 8 demographic variables; and a pathology measure (self-report of visits to physician). The effects of personality type and conceptual systems on the relationship of life change, pathology, "future shock," and anxiety were examined.

C90 Phillips, Walter Mills: Life change events, adjustment and personal construct systems (Doctoral dissertation, University of South Dakota, 1975). Dissertation Abstracts International 36:4175-B, 1976.
     Subjects: Not described in abstract.
     Method: "Standardized adjustment and readjustment scores" [unnamed] were used in this "empirical investigation of the relationship of readjustment stress, adjustment and selected aspects of the personal construct system" based on George Kelly's Personal Construct Theory. The dependent variables were two types of personal construct scores, "structural scores" and "label ratings."

C91 Wall, Thomas William: Life change, illness, and ego-functioning (Doctoral dissertation, University of Washington, 1974). Dissertation Abstracts International 35:5140A-5141A, 1974-75.
     Subjects: 187 college students.
     Method: All subjects completed the following instruments: the Schedule of Recent Experience, the Cornell Medical Index (measure of health status), the Barron Ego-Strength Scale, and the Jacobs Ego-Strength-Ego-Weakness bipolarity measure. The relationship of life change (high, medium, and low risk groups) to health status (high vs. low Cornell Medical Index scores) was studied in relation to the two measures of ego-functioning.

PSYCHOLOGY:
Other Topics
(C92-C111)

C92 Allen, Bem P., and Potkay, Charles R.: The relationship between ACT self-description and significant life events: A longitudinal study. Journal of Personality 45:207-219, 1977.
     Subjects: 49 college students.

Method: All subjects completed a log sheet for 47 consecutive days by recording five adjectives describing themselves and listing any "significant events" that had occurred that day. The Adjective Generation Technique list of 1,700 words was used to assign "favorability" values to subjects' self-descriptions, and an independent sample of raters reviewed the reported events and ranked each on a 6-point favorable-unfavorable scale. Variations in favorability of self-descriptions were studied in relation to favorability of reported life events.

C93 Bourque, Linda B., and Back, Kurt W.: Life graphs and life events. Journal of Gerontology 32:669-674, 1977.
Subjects: 371 adults aged 45-70 (divided into age-sex cohorts of 5-year intervals).
Method: All subjects drew a life graph, a projective technique which reveals subject's life satisfactions and expectations by its pattern and peaks, at Time 1 and again 4 years later at Time 2. At Time 2 they also completed a modified Schedule of Recent Experience (for inclusive Time 1-Time 2 period). Frequency data were tabulated for four kinds of events: child leaving home, bereavement, retirement or major work change, and personal illness. The effect of anticipated vs. unanticipated life events on subjects' personal life satisfaction was studied by comparing Time 1 and Time 2 life graphs for age-sex cohorts.

HQ1060.J6

C94 Dohrenwend, Barbara Snell: Social stress and community psychology. American Journal of Community Psychology 6: 1-14, 1978.
In order to define what community psychologists do and how they differ from clinical psychologists, the author presents a model of the process by which psychosocial "stress" leads to psychopathology. Central to the model is the concept of "stressful life events," and the author reviews the controversies and issues surrounding their definition. Strategies for reducing the rate of psychopathology in the community are also discussed.

RA790A1A47

C95 Horowitz, Mardi, and Wilner, Nancy: Stress films, emotion, and cognitive response. Archives of General Psychiatry 33: 1339-1344, 1976.
Subjects: 75 college students.
Method: All subjects rated themselves on expected emotional response to films with themes portraying horror,

RC321A66

tragedy, and eroticism; they were then randomly assigned to 1 of 4 groups of mixed high- and low-responders. Each subgroup viewed 1 of 4 different silent films based on themes of "separation," "bodily injury," "erotic arousal," and "neutral." Subjects then performed a number of tests and tasks designed to measure affect, "mental content" (thoughts while performing signal detection tasks), and cognitive styles. They also completed a 38-item life events inventory (for the past 2 years) as a measure of "presumptive stress" (amount of "stress" one might still be experiencing). Each subgroup saw a second film and completed further tests and tasks to measure affect, mental content, cognitive styles, and self-reports of intrusive and repetitive thoughts. Data were analyzed by comparing the effects of the different kinds of positive and negative arousal films on subjects' affect, performance of tasks, cognitive response.

C96 Jenks, Letitia Chambers: Change and the individual: The relationship between the amount of change in the life of a student and his self-concept (Doctoral dissertation, Oklahoma State University, 1973). Dissertation Abstracts International 34: 6357-A, 1974.
Subjects: 10th-, 11th-, and 12th-grade students from two high schools [number unstated].
Method: All subjects completed Coddington's Schedule of Recent Experience for high school students (past 12 months) and the Tennessee Self-Concept Scale.

Z5053.D57

C97 Kaplan, Howard B.: Self-derogation and adjustment to recent life experiences. Archives of General Psychiatry 22:324-331, 1970.
Subjects: A random sample of 500 adults in Harris County, Texas.
Method: All subjects were interviewed at home according to a structured 23-page schedule of questions which included a 10-item measure of self-derogation (responses on a 4-point scale ranging from "strongly agree" to "strongly disagree") and an 11-item life events inventory (occurrence during the past 12 months). The relation of number of recent life experiences requiring behavioral adaptation to low vs. high self-derogation was examined. The effect of age, sex, race, and social class on the relationship of specific recent life events to self-derogatory attitudes was also studied.

RC321A66

C98   Keith, Pat M.: Life changes, stereotyping, and age identi-
       fication. Psychological Reports 41:661-662, 1977.
           Subjects: 169 subjects aged 65 and over.
           Method: All subjects were administered a structured in-
           terview to collect data on the following: life changes (indi-
           cating "declined," "remained same," or "improved"
           changes in health, income, organizational participation,
           marital status, getting out of the house, and performance
           of enjoyed activities); stereotypes of old age (13-item mea-
           sure developed by Tuckman and Lorge); and age identifica-
           tion (thinking of self as "old," "elderly," or "middle-
           aged"). The effects of life changes and stereotypes of old
           age on age identity were examined.

C99   Klassen, Deirdre; Hornstra, Robijn K.; and Anderson,
       Peter B.: Influence of social desirability on symptom and
       mood reporting in a community survey. Journal of Consult-
       ing and Clinical Psychology 43:448-452, 1975.
           Subjects: A community sample of 976 adults in Kansas
           City, Missouri.
           Method: All subjects completed a survey instrument of
           over 300 questions which included a section of demographic
           characteristics; a measure of social desirability (short-
           ened Marlowe-Crowne Social Desirability Scale); a variety
           of mental health, mood, and physical health measures
           (e.g., Langner's 22-item index, Bradburn's happiness
           scales, the Depression Adjective Checklist, questions on
           satisfaction and general happiness, number of disability
           days in past week); and a 40-item life events inventory
           (for past year) concerning subject's experience and the
           experience of significant others in subject's life. Differ-
           ences in social desirability scores were examined in
           terms of demographic characteristics, and the relation of
           social desirability scores to mental health measures was
           studied.

C100   Lahr, Jessica Jo: Relationship between experience in trans-
       cendental meditation and adaptation to life events and related
       stress. Unpublished master's thesis, Ohio State University,
       1974.
           Subjects: 44 beginning meditators, 48 experienced medita-
           tors, and 142 nonmeditating matched control subjects (all
           age 18-33 and with at least a college education).
           Method: All subjects completed the Schedule of Recent
           Experience and a 1-year illness history based on items in

the Seriousness of Illness Rating Scale. Differences were examined in amount of life change and seriousness of illness experienced by beginning and advanced meditators and nonmeditators.

C101   Luborsky, Lester; Todd, Thomas C.; and Katcher, Aaron H.: A self-administered social assets scale for predicting physical and psychological illness and health. Journal of Psychosomatic Research 17:109-120, 1973.

BC52.J6

The authors describe the development and application of the Social Assets Scale, a self-administered questionnaire which is scored with weighted values demonstrated to have a high degree of consensus among judges. The success of the Social Assets Scale in predicting illness and health is compared to that of longer and better known instruments such as the Schedule of Recent Experience, the Cornell Medical Index, and the Phipps Psychiatric Clinic symptom checklist. [See also A121.]

C102   Marx, Martin B.; Barnes, Graham; Somes, Grant W.; and Garrity, Thomas F.: The Health Script: Its relationship to illness in a college population. Transactional Analysis Journal 8:339-344, 1978.

Subjects: 56 college seniors who reported high life change in a study conducted at the beginning of their freshman year. Method: All subjects were restudied in 1975 and asked to complete Anderson's College Schedule of Recent Experience (for past year), the Heimler Scale of Social Functioning (used as index of coping ability), Langner's 22-item index (measure of psychophysiological strain), and the Health Script, a new 13-item questionnaire designed to identify childhood impressions and current feelings and beliefs about health and illness. Subjects' responses to the Health Script questionnaire were tape-recorded and also later transcribed; three Transactional Analysis therapists, blind to all other data, independently assigned each subject to either the Positive or Negative Health Script group based on content and affect of responses. Future health and illness patterns for the 1975-1976 school year were predicted based on Health Script categories, and health change data were collected at the end of the school year by interview.

C103   Milman, Jeffrey Alan: Life changes and sensation seeking in hospitalized and previously hospitalized patients (Doctoral dissertation, Adelphi University, 1975). Dissertation Abstracts International 36:3579B-3580B, 1976.

> Subjects: 168 subjects from two settings, a hospital and an evening school (21 hospitalized medical patients and 14 healthy visitors to the hospital, and 14 recently hospitalized students, 15 recently injured students, and 104 control students without recent hospitalization or injury). Method: All subjects completed the Schedule of Recent Experience (for 1 year), the Sensation Seeking Scale (measure of level of sensation seeking), and the "Weighted Illness Scale." The relation of life change and sensation-seeking to serious illness or injury was compared for ill or injured subjects and their comparison groups, and for subjects in the hospital setting vs. subjects in the school setting.

C104 Rethinger, Paul Joseph: The relationship between six scales of the Missouri Children's Picture Series and the psychological parameters measured by three objective children's instruments (Doctoral dissertation, Ohio University, 1975). Dissertation Abstracts International 36:6485A-6486A, 1976.

> Subjects: 32 third-grade boys and 49 fifth-grade boys. Method: All subjects were administered the following objective instruments: Coddington's Schedule of Recent Experience for school children (for past school year, about 9 months), the General Anxiety Scale for Children, the Children's Social Desirability Questionnaire, and the Missouri Children's Picture Series ("a nonverbal instrument with several scales"). The relation of life change to psychological dysfunction in children was examined, and the effect of life change, anxiety, and social desirability on the 6 scales of the Picture Series was also studied in order to evaluate the usefulness of that instrument.

C105 Roskin, Michael: Life change and emotional health: A demonstration project focused on primary intervention (Doctoral dissertation, University of Illinois at Chicago Circle, 1978). Dissertation Abstracts International 39:3809-B, 1979.

> Subjects: Individuals [number unstated] who had experienced two or more major life changes in the past year. Method: Subjects were considered at "high risk" of developing emotional difficulties because of their recent life change. Half the subjects received intervention (6 sessions combining information about life changes, social supports and personal health with group support and dis-

cussion of coping skills) and were compared to the other half who did not. All subjects completed the Symptom Checklist 90 as a measure of health status. After the experimental group's intervention was completed, the control group received intervention. Differences in health status between experimental (intervention) and control (nonintervention) groups were examined, and then differences in the control group pre- and postintervention were also studied.

C106 Smith, Ronald E.; Johnson, James H.; and Sarason, Irwin G.: Life change, the sensation seeking motive, and psychological distress. Journal of Consulting and Clinical Psychology 46: 348-349, 1978.
Subjects: 75 college students.
BFI.J575 Method: All subjects were administered the following instruments: the Sensation-Seeking Scale (a 22-item measure by Zuckerman et al.); the Life Experiences Survey [see H13] (a 12-month checklist of life events with subject rating of positive or negative quality of reported events); and the Discomfort scale of Lanyon's Psychological Screening Inventory (as a measure of psychological distress). The relation of positive, negative, and total life change scores to psychological distress was examined for high vs. low sensation seekers.

C107 Streifer, Richard Joseph: Life events, cognitive-affective states, and adjustment: Students in transition (Doctoral dissertation, Arizona State University, 1978). Dissertation Abstracts International 39:3008B-3009B, 1978.
Subjects: 138 undergraduate students (new-to-community and hometown freshmen and nonfreshmen).
Method: Early in the semester all subjects were assessed for two "person variables," Positive Affect (PA) and Cognitive Anxiety (CA), through "content analysis of verbal self-reports." Three months later four self-administered "measures of psychological and somatic well-being" were obtained to measure adjustment of psychosocial transition. Life events data were collected but not analyzed. The author discusses methodological problems that obstructed the intended study of the combined predictive power of PA, CA, and life change for near-future adjustment problems.

C108 Sundberg, Norman D.; Snowden, Lonnie R.; and Reynolds, William M.: Toward assessment of personal competence and incompetence in life situations. Annual Review of Psychology 29:179-221, 1978.

The authors review the literature from 1974 through early 1977 on concepts of "competence" and "competence building" and methods for assessing competency. They discuss life change research as a "promising approach" for investigations of competency when combined with evaluations of coping styles.

C109 Townes, Brenda D.; Ferguson, William D.; and Gillam, Sandra: Differences in psychological sex, adjustment, and familial influences among homosexual and nonhomosexual populations. Journal of Homosexuality 1:261-272, 1976.

Subjects: 12 homosexual cross-dressers and 38 homosexual non-cross-dressers, 8 applicants for sex change surgery, and 10 heterosexuals—all males between the ages of 18 and 49.

Method: All subjects completed the following questionnaires: the Sexual Identification and Life-Style Questionnaire (current living situations, jobs, sexual relationships, and attitudes); Winch's Family Life Inventory (subject's perception of the potency of his family members during childhood); and the Schedule of Recent Experience (for past 10 years). Questionnaire data were used to evaluate and compare 11 variables (such as gender role and gender identity, homosexual adjustment, social adjustment, past adaptation, parental nurturance relationships) for each subgroup.

C110 Wong, Elwyn Louie: Role of recent life changes upon participants in group psychotherapy (Doctoral dissertation, United States International University, 1976). Dissertation Abstracts International 37:1934-B, 1976.

Subjects: Individuals [number unstated] attending group therapy sessions in a community college.

Method: "Self-concept at termination of group therapy" was the measure used to study the relation of high vs. low recent life change to the outcome of group psychotherapy. [No instruments are named in the abstract.]

C111 Zubin, Joseph: Abnormal psychology: Use and misuse. Annals of the New York Academy of Sciences 309:98-113, 1978.

The author evaluates the current state of success in determining the etiology of mental disorders, reviewing six scientific models for the etiology of psychopathology which he sees as having "ground to a halt." He proposes the "vulnerability model"—in which life events are seen as having a triggering effect on vulnerability, eliciting episodes of disorder—as the most useful conceptual framework to adopt for future etiological research as well as for therapeutic intervention.

LIFE CHANGE EVENTS
AND PHYSIOLOGY

D1   Barthrop, R. W.; Luckhurst, E.; Lazarus, L.; Kiloh, L. G.;
and Penny, R.: Depressed lymphocyte function after bereavement. Lancet 2:834-836, 1977.

     Subjects: 26 bereaved spouses and 26 matched control
subjects.

     Method: All bereaved subjects had blood samples taken
within three weeks after bereavement and again six weeks
later; matched controls had samples taken at the same
times. The laboratory analysis of samples included
lymphocyte transformation tests, other measures of T and
B cell function, and hormone assays. Immunological function was compared for bereaved and control subjects.

D2   Cobb, Sidney: Physiologic changes in men whose jobs were
abolished. Journal of Psychosomatic Research 18:245-258,
1974.

     Subjects: 100 men whose jobs were abolished because of
permanent plant closures and 74 control subjects in similar jobs at other plants.

     Method: Terminated subjects were visited at home during
five phases: anticipation of job termination, shortly after
plant shutdown, and 6, 12, and 24 months after plant
closure. Controls were visited at comparable times for
12 months. The same set of physiological, psychological,
social, and economic data was collected at each visit by
public health nurses. This report describes the physiological data based on blood and urine analysis for norepinephrine excretion, serum creatine, serum uric acid,

serum urea nitrogen, and serum cholesterol. Physiologic changes were compared through the five phases for subjects divided into subgroups according to: high vs. low psychological defenses (Gough's flexibility-inflexibility scale, Crowne and Marlowe's need for approval scale, Block's ego resilience scale, and the Lazarus et al. orality scale); high vs. low social support (13-item measure of supportive relationships); coffee vs. no coffee drinking; and life events in the 12 months after job termination (modified Schedule of Recent Experience). [See also D6 and D7, C63, C64, G30, G32, G33.]

D3   Hofer, Myron A.; Wolff, Carl T.; Friedman, Stanford B.; and Mason, John W.: A psychoendocrine study of bereavement. Part I. 17-Hydroxycorticosteroid excretion rates of parents following death of their children from leukemia. Psychosomatic Medicine 34:481-491, 1972.
      Subjects: 36 parents (15 fathers, 21 mothers), whose children died from leukemia.
      Method: Approximately 6 months after death of their child, parents returned for several days to the hospital for the following procedures: careful medical history, review of systems and physical exam, 2-5 hours of interviewing, and consecutive 24-hour urine collections. About 2 years after bereavement, 21 of the parents made a second return visit and the same data were collected. Using preloss data collected during an earlier study, investigators compared the group mean excretion rates of 17-hydroxycorticosteroid at first and second return visits. They also compared at-home urine collection data (done by some of the parents and mailed in) to in-hospital collections. Intraindividual changes in mean rates were also examined and compared to group mean rates. [See also Part II (D4).]

D4   Hofer, Myron A.; Wolff, Carl T.; Friedman, Stanford B.; and Mason, John W.: A psychoendocrine study of bereavement. Part II Observations on the process of mourning in relation to adrenocortical function. Psychosomatic Medicine 34:492-504, 1972.
      Subjects: 36 parents whose children had died from leukemia.
      Method: This is the companion report to D3 above. Psychologic data collected by interview were compared for subjects divided into groups (highest vs. lowest quartiles) by 17-hydroxycorticosteroid excretion rate at return visit. In addition, intraindividual differences were examined, and three illustrative case histories are presented.

D5   Kalucy, R. S.; Brown, D. G.; Hartmann, Margot; and Crisp,
A. H.: Sleep research and psychosomatic hypotheses. Post-
graduate Medical Journal 52:53-56, 1976.
> The authors review their own and others' research on sleep
> as it relates to psychosomatic disorders. They propose
> the study of sleep and its processes as a focal point for
> psychosomatic medicine and research, providing a way to
> study specific psychosomatic events as well as a way to
> test and illuminate more general "psychosomatic hypothe-
> ses" such as Engel and Schmale's "giving-up-given-up"
> formulation and Holmes and Rahe's "life crisis" model.

D6   Kasl, Stanislav V., and Cobb, Sidney: Can one extrapolate
chronic changes from reactivity to acute stress? Psychosomatic Medicine 39:55-56, 1977. (Abstract)
> Subjects: 100 men undergoing job loss because of per-
> manent plant closure.
> Method: Data were collected for subjects at Time 1 (when
> all were anticipating job loss), Time 2 (when subjects ex-
> perienced either prompt reemployment or unemployment),
> and Time 3 (when some stabilized on new job, some went
> from unemployment to reemployment, and some remained
> unemployed). The Time 1-Time 2 period reflected "reac-
> tivity to acute stress" and was compared to Time 2-Time 3
> which reflected "chronic stress" situations. Data included
> indexes of economic well-being, deprivation in the work
> role, indices of mental health and physical well-being, and
> physiologic variables (serum uric acid and cholesterol,
> blood pressure, pulse rate).

D7   Kasl, Stanislav V.; Cobb, Sidney; and Brooks, George W.:
Changes in serum uric acid and cholesterol levels in men
undergoing job loss. Journal of the American Medical Association 206:1500-1507, 1968.
> Subjects: About 150 men whose jobs were abolished because
> of permanent plant closure and 50 control subjects with
> similar jobs at other plants.
> Method: Subjects were visited at home during five phases
> of the job loss experience: anticipation of job loss, shortly
> after termination, 4-8 months later, and 1 and 2 years
> later. Controls were visited at comparable times. A
> standardized set of psychological, physiological, social,
> and economic data was collected at each visit by public
> health nurses. This report describes changes in uric acid
> and cholesterol levels in terms of the employment expe-
> rience of terminated subjects (employment; loss of job;

unemployment for some, probationary reemployment for others, and stable employment on a new job) and of controls who remained continuously employed. [See also C63, C64, D2, D6, G30, G32, and G33.]

D8   Kiritz, Stewart, and Moos, Rudolf H.: Physiological effects of social environments: A review article. Psychosomatic Medicine 36:96-114, 1974.

The authors review the literature: they summarize evidence relating physiological changes to perceived social environment dimensions (e.g., support, cohesion, involvement) and examine the interaction of individual and environmental variables (including life change studies). They present a conceptual model for the relationship between social environmental stimuli and observable physiologic changes.

D9   Mueller, Ernst F.; Kasl, Stanislav V.; Brooks, George W.; and Cobb, Sidney: Psychosocial correlates of serum urate levels. Psychological Bulletin 73:238-257, 1970.

The authors begin their review of the literature with background information about uric acid (biochemistry, metabolic pathways, relationship with central nervous system), methodological problems in determining urate levels (measurement, age and sex effects, genetic influences), and variables which can alter uric acid levels in the blood (e.g., body size, alcohol, diet). They then focus on psychological and social correlates of uric acid levels: social class (with a historical note on gout), achievement and achievement-oriented behavior, and "stress" (including life change studies). They conclude with a discussion of problems and directions for future research.

D10   Parker, David M.; Wilsoncroft, William E.; and Olshansky, Ted: The relationship between life change and relative autonomic balance. Journal of Clinical Psychology 32:149-153, 1976.

Subjects: 67 undergraduate students.
Method: All subjects followed rules on food and drink restrictions for the 24 hours before they were administered the $\overline{A}$ series of physiological tests. The $\overline{A}$ score is a measure of "physiological stress" which reveals the relative dominance of the sympathetic and parasympathetic components of the autonomic nervous system. After the $\overline{A}$ series, subjects were administered a modified Schedule

of Recent Experience. Correlations were examined between
A̲ scores (8 variables) and life change scores (calculated
3 ways).

D11 Rahe, Richard H., and Arthur, Ransom J.: Biochemical
correlates of behavior. Diseases of the Nervous System
29:114-117, 1968.
The authors selectively review studies of changes in neuro-
endocrine metabolites in the setting of various life situations, emotions, and behaviors. Major emphasis is given
to studies of 17-hydroxycorticosteroids; studies of
catecholamines, serum lipids, and uric acid are also
included.

D12 Rahe, Richard H.; Rubin, Robert T.; and Arthur, Ransom J.:
The three investigators study: Serum uric acid, cholesterol,
and cortisol variability during stresses of everyday life.
Psychosomatic Medicine 36:258-268, 1974.
Subjects: 3 male medical investigators.
Method: Two subjects were followed on a semiweekly basis
for six months; the third subject was followed for three
months. Each kept a diary of daily life events and noted
moods and feelings associated with each event. Blood
drawn at the semiweekly session was analyzed for serum
uric acid, serum cholesterol, and serum cortisol levels.
The relation of life events and emotions to biochemical
variability was studied.

D13 Rahe, Richard H.; Rubin, Robert T.; Arthur, Ransom J.;
and Clark, Brian R.: Serum uric acid and cholesterol variability: A comprehensive view of Underwater Demolition
Team training. Journal of the American Medical Association
206:2875-2880, 1968.
Subjects: 32 members of a U.S. Navy UDT training class.
Method: All subjects were followed through graduation (or
dropout) from the 16-week course. At the beginning they
all completed a military version of the Schedule of Recent
Experience. Blood samples were drawn several times a
week, and at that time each subject completed a standardized mood and attitude questionnaire. Variations in serum
uric acid and cholesterol were studied in relation to type
of activity and associated moods and attitudes and were
compared for subjects who graduated and those who with-
drew from the course.

D14   Rubin, Robert T., and Rahe, Richard H.: U.S. Navy under-
water demolition team training: biochemical studies. In Life
Stress and Illness. E. K. Eric Gunderson and Richard H.
Rahe (Eds.), pp. 208-226. Springfield, Illinois: Charles C
Thomas, 1974.

RC49.G85

> Subjects: 32 trainees in a U.S. Navy UDT training program.
> Method: The authors summarize and discuss their re-
> search on uric acid, cholesterol, and cortisol variability
> in relation to the extreme physical and psychological de-
> mands of underwater demolition team training. (See B32,
> B134, and D13 for original reports of research.)

D15   Volicer, Beverly J., and Volicer, Ladislav: Cardiovascular
changes associated with stress during hospitalization. Journal of Psychosomatic Research 22:159-168, 1978.

> Subjects: 463 hospitalized medical and surgical patients.
> Method: On Day 3, 4, or 5 of hospitalization all subjects
> were interviewed for the following: demographic charac-

RC52.J6

> teristics, life change scores (2-year modified Schedule of
> Recent Experience), and prior hospitalizations data. They
> were also administered the Hospital Stress Rating Scale
> [see H54] in which they indicated the occurrence of any of
> 49 events since hospitalization. A "total hospital stress"
> score and 9 "factor" scores (clusters of items) were de-
> rived for each subject. Patient charts were reviewed to
> collect data to calculate mean systolic and mean diastolic
> blood pressure and mean heart rate for each of the first
> five days of hospitalization and the day before discharge.
> Mean blood pressure, mean stroke volume, and mean
> cardiac output were also calculated. Data relating hospital
> stress scores to cardiovascular changes were analyzed
> separately for subjects divided into 4 patient groups by type
> of hospitalization (medical vs. surgical) and seriousness
> of illness (high vs. low on Seriousness of Illness Rating
> Scale).

LIFE CHANGE EVENTS
AND ECONOMICS

E1   Brenner, M. Harvey: Economic changes and heart disease
      mortality. <u>American Journal of Public Health</u> 61:606-611,
      1971.
           The author hypothesized that "the various types of stress
      inherent in an economic downturn might lead to an increase
      in heart disease mortality." This study examined the re-
      lationship between economic changes and changes in heart
      disease mortality rates from 1900-1967 in New York State
      and in the United States as a whole. The author used the
      Employment Index for Nonagricultural Industries as the
      measure of economic change, superimposing peaks and
      troughs in mortality rates on peaks and troughs of unem-
      ployment levels. Four different techniques to measure
      inverse relationships were used to analyze the data.

E2   Brenner, M. Harvey: Fetal, infant, and maternal mortality
      during periods of economic instability. <u>International Journal</u>
      <u>of Health Services</u> 3:145-159, 1973.
           The author hypothesized that for industrialized societies
      "the problem of adapting to economic change concerns less
      the level of economic growth than whether that growth is
      relatively smooth or chaotic." This study investigated the
      role of "environmental change associated with economic
      fluctuations" in fetal, infant, and maternal mortality in the
      past 45 years in the United States. Three different methods
      of time series analysis were used to analyze data on "eco-
      nomic instability" (as measured by U.S. trends in unem-
      ployment rates, periods of economic upturn and downturn)

and four categories of infant and fetal mortality (by race and age at death).

E3   Brenner, M. Harvey: Patterns of psychiatric hospitalization among different socioeconomic groups in response to economic stress. <u>Journal of Nervous and Mental Disease</u> 148:31-38, 1969.

The author investigated the impact of short-term economic change (using the manufacturing employment index as a measure) on changes in the level of mental hospital first-admissions in New York State from 1910 to 1960. Hospitalization data were analyzed for differences (in frequency, diagnosis, sex) between four socioeconomic groups (determined by level of education attained) in times of economic adversity.

E4   Brenner, M. Harvey: Personal stability and economic security. <u>Social Policy</u> 3:2-4, 1977.

The author examined the impact of changes in the unemployment rate on seven indices of "social stress" in the United States from 1940 to 1974: total mortality rate, specific rates of homicide, suicide, and cardiovascular-renal disease mortality, total state imprisonment rates and state mental hospital admission rates. The author also computed the "human toll" (number of attributable deaths) and the "cost in dollars" (lost income, unemployment-related government expenditures) for the 5 years following a sustained 1.4 percent rise in unemployment during 1970.

E5   Brenner, M. Harvey: Reply to Mr. Eyer. <u>International Journal of Health Services</u> 6:149-155, 1976.

This is the author's response to Joseph Eyer's review of his book <u>Mental Illness and the Economy</u> (see E13). Brenner answers the questions raised by Eyer about the methods, procedures, and research design of studies reported in the book.

E6   Brenner, M. Harvey: Trends in alcohol consumption and associated illnesses: Some effects of economic changes. <u>American Journal of Public Health</u> 65:1279-1292, 1975.

Using a variety of statistical techniques to measure time-lag correlations, the author examined the relation of long-term trends and short-term fluctuations in alcohol consumption to cirrhosis mortality rates and fluctuations in the national economy of the United States. He divided changes in alcohol consumption by type (beer and wine vs. distilled spirits) and compared their relation to short-term vs. long-term economic patterns (e.g., "stress-related use" during and following economic downturn vs. prosperity-related use during period of growth and stability) and to cirrhosis mortality (within a 2-year time lag).

E7   Catalano, Ralph: Community stress: A preliminary conceptualization. Man-Environment Systems 5:307-310, 1975.
The author proposes uniting two areas of research—life events and illness research and studies of the economy as stressor—in order to study "community stress." He hypothesizes that a community's rates of "stress-related disorders" vary over time in relation to changes in the local economy and changes in the proportion of its members at risk because of life change experience. Life events research tools could be adapted for application to communities as a whole, using demographic characteristics data and factor analysis of life events to determine high risk cohorts within the population. He outlines four research design elements to test the hypothesis: prospective rather than retrospective monitoring; definition of communities by economic system rather than political borders; use of survey as well as archival measures of outcomes; and study of coping strategies to clarify intervening variables.

E8   Catalano, Ralph, and Dooley, C. David: Economic predictors of depressed mood and stressful life events in a metropolitan community. Journal of Health and Social Behavior 18:292-307, 1977.
The authors studied the relation of survey measures of depressed mood (Center for Epidemiologic Studies-Depression scale) and frequency of life events (Dohrenwend and Dohrenwend's 40-item Life Events Schedule) to seven measures of change in economic conditions (including unemployment rates, inflation as measured by the Consumer Price Index for food, and changes in the size and structure of local economy). They used archival data for the Kansas City Standard Metropolitan Statistical Area (an economically defined community) to determine monthly economic change, and they used data from an NIMH epidemiological survey over 16 months (1,173 Kansas City adults) to assess changes in mood and life events. Single and multiple regression analyses were performed for no-lag, and 1-, 2-, and 3-month time lags.

E9   Dooley, David, and Catalano, Ralph: Money and mental dis-
       order: Toward behavioral cost accounting for primary pre-
       vention. American Journal of Community Psychology 5:217-
       227, 1977.

           The authors review the literature relating changes in the
           economy to fluctuations in suicide rates and rates of first-
           admissions to mental hospitals. They summarize the pro-
           cedures and findings of a survey they conducted to assess
           93 community mental health workers' attitudes and percep-
           tions concerning the effects of economic change and social
           status on mental health care utilization. They discuss
           their survey in relation to needed tools for primary pre-
           vention and intervention, and they suggest future research
           to develop predictive models and measures for the effects
           of economic changes on behavior and mental health.

E10   Ellison, Patricia H.: Neurology of hard times: Economic
       depression as related to neurologic illness in children.
       Clinical Pediatrics 61:270-274, 1977.

           The author presents five case histories illustrating the
           occurrence of neurologic illness in children whose families
           experienced significant changes in their economic circum-
           stances.

E11   Eyer, Joseph: Does unemployment cause the death rate peak
       in each business cycle? A multifactor model of death rate
       change. International Journal of Health Services 7:625-662,
       1977.
           In this companion study to E12 below, the author analyzed
           the proportional contribution of a number of causal factors
           to death rate-business cycle fluctuations. Causal factors
           under study included unemployment, housing conditions,
           nutrition, alcohol and tobacco consumption, and "social
           stress" (changes in social relationships associated with
           the modern economy: for example, life events signaling
           family disintegration and community disruption, most of
           which are ranked highest on the Social Readjustment Rating
           Scale).

E12   Eyer, Joseph: Prosperity as a cause of death. International
       Journal of Health Services 7:125-150, 1977.
           Using time series correlation techniques, the author
           studied the relation of fluctuations of the general death
           rate in the United States in the nineteenth and twentieth
           centuries to fluctuations in the business cycle (booms,

depressions, changes in unemployment rate). He compared causes of death in older historical data to twentieth-century data, and he hypothesized that "social stress" in the twentieth century probably accounts for most of the rise in death rate associated with business cycle booms in the modern economy. [See also E11.]

E13 Eyer, Joseph: Review of Mental Illness and the Economy, by M. Harvey Brenner. International Journal of Health Services 6:139-148, 1976.

This review of Mental Illness and the Economy (published in 1973 by Harvard University Press) summarizes Brenner's work on the relation of mental hospital admissions to employment cycles in New York State in the nineteenth and twentieth centuries. The reviewer also discusses problems he sees in Brenner's methods and research design. [See E5 for Brenner's response.]

E14 Frank, Jeanine Amy: Economics and mental health in Hawaii. Unpublished master's thesis, University of California, Irvine, 1978.

The author studied the relation of macroeconomic fluctuations (using seven measures of economic change) to monthly admissions (inpatient and outpatient) to all state mental health facilities in Hawaii from September 1972 through December 1975. No life events data were collected, but life events were defined as the "intervening link" between economic change and disorders in the model upon which the study was based.

E15 Pierce, Albert: The economic cycle and the social suicide rate. American Sociological Review 32:457-462, 1967.

Citing Durkheim's theories relating suicide rates to the economy, the author hypothesized that rate of economic change (both up and down) is associated with variation in the suicide rate. He used a time-series design to study the relation of U.S. suicide rates (white males) to differences in the index of common stock prices (which was chosen as an index of the public's perception of the economic situation) for the years 1919-1940.

LIFE CHANGE EVENTS
AND SOCIOLOGY

F1   Dohrenwend, Barbara Snell: Social status and stressful life
      events. Journal of Personality and Social Psychology 28:225-
      235, 1973.
          Subjects: A cross-sectional survey of 124 heads of house-
      hold.
HM251.J56 Method: All subjects were interviewed to collect data on
      demographic characteristics (sex, social class, ethnic
      group), life change (27-item checklist of events experienced
      in past 12 months and/or anticipated to occur in next 12
      months), and psychological symptoms (Langner's 22-item
      screening instrument). Life change scores were calculated
      using ratings from the Social Readjustment Rating Scale,
      and life events were also divided into four categories by
      "locus of responsibility" (controllable vs. uncontrollable).
      The relation of life change scores to psychological symp-
      tom scores was studied in relation to sex, social class,
      and ethnicity (3 relatively advantaged ethnic groups vs.
      2 disadvantaged ethnic groups).

F2   Dohrenwend, Bruce P.: Sociocultural and social-psychologi-
      cal factors in the genesis of mental disorders. Journal of
      Health and Social Behavior 16:365-392, 1975.
          The author reviews and analyzes the major issues raised
      in three areas of research: epidemiological studies of
R11.J687 "true prevalence" of psychiatric disorders, studies of the
      individual's responses to extreme or catastrophic life
      situations, and studies of life events and psychopathology.
      He reports the progress of an ongoing study to resolve one

219

of the major research issues—social class differences—and outlines innovative methodological strategies for future research into the role of sociocultural and social-psychological factors in the occurrence and distribution of mental disorders.

F3   Graves, Forrest W., Jr.: Psychosomatic symptoms associated with vital-life crises: An exploratory analysis of self-perceived neighborhood contexts. Unpublished master's thesis, Eastern Michigan University, 1975.

Subjects: A survey of 766 adults living in 8 suburban communities in the Detroit Standard Metropolitan Statistical Area (SMSA).

Method: All subjects were interviewed to collect data on life change (modified Schedule of Recent Experience for past 12 months, for respondent and all household members); psychosomatic symptomatology (checklist of symptoms and indication of time of occurrence); and perceived neighborhood networks (three questions). The neighborhood networks data were used to develop six self-perceived neighborhood types—integral, parochial, diffuse, stepping-stone, transitory, and anomic. Subjective neighborhood types were studied as intervening variables in the relationship between life crises and development of psychosomatic symptoms.

F4   Liem, Ramsay, and Liem, Joan: Social class and mental illness reconsidered: The role of economic stress and social support. Journal of Health and Social Behavior 19:139-156, 1978.

The authors review research from several disciplines in order to assess the role of social class in the development and mediation of psychological impairment. Life events research is considered in detail. Evidence from studies of economic change and psychological dysfunction is combined with evidence from studies of social support and psychological well-being to produce an integrated model of psychological function within a social framework. The authors propose a theory of linked "stress factors" and "support factors" within social classes, thereby relating membership in a social class to psychological functioning.

F5   Syme, S. Leonard, and Berkman, Lisa F.: Social class, susceptibility and sickness. American Journal of Epidemiology
104:1-8, 1976.

The authors review the literature to find "a more satisfactory hypothesis" to account for the observed association of higher morbidity and mortality rates in lower class groups. They attempt to identify risk factors that affect general susceptibility to disease, and one of the factors they propose for further study is life change events.

STUDIES OF SPECIFIC
LIFE CHANGE EVENTS

SPECIFIC EVENTS:
Bereavement
(G1-G26)

G1   Bornstein, Philipp E.; Clayton, Paula J.; Halikas, James A.;
Maurice, William L.; and Robins, Eli: The depression of
widowhood after thirteen months. British Journal of Psychiatry 122:561-566, 1973.
      Subjects: 92 bereaved spouses (65 widows, 27 widowers)
available for follow-up 1 year after bereavement.
      Method: This is a follow-up study of 109 bereaved subjects
initially studied approximately 13 months earlier (see G7).
Subjects were reevaluated for depression using the same
criteria, and the original structured interview was slightly
modified and readministered. Depressed (N=16) and not
depressed (N=76) subjects were compared using 185 variables, including psychological symptoms and signs, physical health, and social support. The relation of normal depression in widowhood to the primary affective disorder
was examined.

RC321
B856X

G2   Clayton, Paula J.: The effect of living alone on bereavement
symptoms. American Journal of Psychiatry 132:133-137, 1975.
      Subjects: 109 bereaved spouses (76 widows, 33 widowers)
and 109 matched, married control subjects.
      Method: Bereaved subjects were interviewed for symptoms
of depression at 1 month after death of spouse and were
compared on the basis of living alone or living with others.

RC321A52

223

After 1 year, 89 subjects and 89 matched controls were interviewed for the following: depressive symptoms, physical symptoms, medical treatment, and medication use. Bereaved subjects were again compared to each other on the basis of current living arrangements, and then subjects and controls were compared on the basis of living alone or living with others.

G3   Clayton, Paula J.: Letter to the editor. Psychosomatic Medicine 40:435-438, 1978.

The author comments on "An epidemiological review of the mortality of bereavement" by Jacobs and Ostfeld (Psychosomatic Medicine 39:344-357, 1977) [see G11]. She reviews the literature associating bereavement with risk of mortality and discusses methodological problems and possibly spurious conclusions in the research. Jacobs and Ostfeld reply.

G4   Clayton, Paula J.: Mortality and morbidity in the first year of widowhood. Archives of General Psychiatry 30:747-750, 1974.

RC321A66

Subjects: 109 bereaved spouses and 109 married control subjects, matched for age and sex.
Method: Subjects and controls were followed prospectively and were compared for mortality at approximately 13 months after bereavement of subjects. At 13 months, 90 bereaved subjects and 90 married controls were interviewed and compared on the following: 26 psychological symptoms, 15 physical symptoms, medical and psychiatric care-seeking, and medication use during the past year.

G5   Clayton, Paula J.; Desmarais, Lynn; and Winokur, George: A study of normal bereavement. American Journal of Psychiatry 125:168-178, 1968.

RC321A52

Subjects: 40 relatives of 30 patients who had recently died in St. Louis hospitals.
Method: Each subject was interviewed 2-26 days after death of relative; 27 subjects were reinterviewed 3 months later. The systematic interview included previous mental illness and family history and a symptoms-and-feelings inventory. The inventory covered primarily depressive symptoms but also included diagnostic inquiries for anxiety, neurosis, schizophrenia, alcoholism, and acute brain syndrome. Data were collected for three time periods: "ever before," "during the terminal illness," and "since the

death." Bereavement symptoms were examined in relation to age, sex, length of deceased's illness, and subject's relation to deceased (spouse vs. parent or child). Follow-up symptom reports were compared to symptoms at first interview for the subsample of 27.

G6 Clayton, Paula J.; Halikas, James A.; and Maurice, William L.: The bereavement of the widowed. Diseases of the Nervous System 32:597-604, 1971.
Subjects: 109 bereaved spouses (76 widows, 33 widowers).
Method: All subjects were interviewed about their experiences during the first month of bereavement. A structured interview was used to collect data on the following: assessment of marriage, survivor's physical and mental health, and social network and support available to subject. Bereavement symptoms were examined and compared according to subject's age and sex, and length of deceased's illness. Medical treatment (physician care and hospitalization) and medication use (particularly tranquilizers) were also studied.

G7 Clayton, Paula J.; Halikas, James A.; and Maurice, William L.: The depression of widowhood. British Journal of Psychiatry 120:71-78, 1972.
Subjects: 109 recently bereaved spouses (76 widows, 33 widowers).
Method: All subjects were interviewed within 1 month of bereavement. Each subject was diagnosed as "depressed" or "not depressed" according to predetermined mood and symptom criteria. The depressed group (N=38) was compared to the not depressed group (N=71) on 53 demographic, social, and physical variables, including the following: age, sex, religion, and socioeconomic status; assessment of marriage; previous psychiatric history of subject and family; subject's symptoms and medical actions after death of spouse; problems subsequent to the death (e.g., loneliness, money worries, concern for deceased's suffering); and social support (available from first-degree relatives). [See also G1.]

G8 Clayton, Paula J.; Herjanic, Marijan; Murphy, George E.; and Woodruff, Robert, Jr.: Mourning and depression: Their similarities and differences. Canadian Psychiatric Association Journal 19:309-312, 1974.

Subjects: 34 recently bereaved spouses and 34 patients hospitalized for depression (primary affective disorder), matched for age and sex.

Method: All subjects were administered a similar structured interview to collect data on 37 psychiatric and medical symptoms (past and present). The numbers and frequencies of symptoms of depression in the bereaved subjects were compared to symptoms of hospitalized patients.

G9   Crisp, A. H., and Priest, R. G.: Psychoneurotic status during the year following bereavement. Journal of Psychosomatic Research 16:351-355, 1972.

Subjects: 777 adults (aged 40-65) registered with a medical group practice in South West London.

Method: All subjects completed two questionnaires: a brief questionnaire concerning bereavements in the past year, and the Middlesex Hospital Questionnaire (measures on six scales: anxiety, phobic, obsessional, somatic, depressive, hysteria). Subjects were divided into subgroups by sex and bereaved status: 64 bereaved and 286 nonbereaved males, and 65 bereaved and 362 nonbereaved females. Differences in Middlesex Hospital Questionnaire scale scores were examined for bereaved and nonbereaved subjects according to sex and age of subject, and relation to deceased (mother, father, spouse, child, other).

G10   Frost, Nicholas R., and Clayton, Paula J.: Bereavement and psychiatric hospitalization. Archives of General Psychiatry 34:1172-1175, 1977.

Subjects: 249 consecutively admitted psychiatric inpatients and 249 matched controls (nonpsychiatric inpatients), plus a psychiatric hospital survey group of 95 inpatients.

Method: All subjects and controls were interviewed to collect data on bereavements in the year (0-6 months and 6-12 months) prior to hospitalization. Bereaved subjects were asked to specify their relation to the deceased, to assess their subjective reaction to the loss, and whether they believed the loss was related to their present illness and hospitalization. Subjects, controls, and the survey group were compared for the following: incidence of recent bereavement, time of death, relation to deceased (first-degree relative, or spouse vs. second-degree relative, close friend, or other), diagnosis and subjective reaction (degree and effect on illness).

G11 Jacobs, Selby, and Ostfeld, Adrian: An epidemiological review of the mortality of bereavement. Psychosomatic Medicine 39:344-357, 1977.

The authors review more than a dozen studies of mortality associated with conjugal bereavement published from 1959 to 1976. They summarize the methods and findings of cohort studies (direct observation over time) and studies using data from secondary sources (death certificates, vital statistics). They discuss and evaluate the basic epidemiological findings in several contexts: the basic pattern of mortality, specific risk factors, methodologic issues, and problems of interpretation. [See G3 for a comment by Paula J. Clayton on this review and a reply by Jacobs and Ostfeld.]

G12 Maddison, David, and Viola, Agnes: The health of widows in the year following bereavement. Journal of Psychosomatic Research 12:297-306, 1968.

Subjects: 375 widows (132 in Boston, 243 in Sydney, Australia) and 199 married control subjects (98 in Boston, 101 in Sydney).

Method: All subjects completed a questionnaire on demographic, personal, and social variables, and on health during the 13 months since bereavement ("past year" for controls). The self-report health measure (a 57-item inventory of new or exacerbated symptoms and complaints as well as treatment sought) produced weighted illness scores for each subject. Health deterioration in widows and controls was studied in relation to personal and social variables, and the prevalence of individual symptoms was compared within and between samples of widows and control subjects.

G13 Maddison, David, and Walker, Wendy L.: Factors affecting the outcome of conjugal bereavement. British Journal of Psychiatry 113:1057-1067, 1967.

Subjects: 132 widows of men aged 45-60 in Boston.
Method: All subjects completed a comprehensive questionnaire which collected data on demographic, personal, and social variables, and health during the 13 months since bereavement (a 57-item self-report inventory of new or exacerbated complaints and treatment-seeking). A weighted illness score was calculated for each subject. The relationship of outcome (illness score) to personal and social characteristics was then examined in a subgroup of 57 "good outcome" (low illness score) and 28 "bad outcome" (high illness score) subjects. A further subsample was selected

to match 20 "good outcome" to 20 "bad outcome" subjects on personal and social characteristics: Each widow was then interviewed about the social support network available to her and about the perceived helpfulness of 59 kinds of interactions with those people.

G14 Parkes, C. Murray: Components of the reaction to loss of limb, spouse or home. Journal of Psychosomatic Research 16:343-349, 1972.

The author compares findings from studies of reactions to "losses": amputation of a limb (N=45 amputees interviewed 1 month and 13 months after amputation), death of close relative (N=23 London widows interviewed five times during the first year of bereavement), and forced relocation (N=473 Boston women interviewed 1 month before relocation and 2 years later). He examines the ways in which the loss reactions are similar and different in order to discuss the nature of changes we identify as "losses" and the reaction process associated with them.

G15 Parkes, C. Murray: Determination of outcome following bereavement. Proceedings of the Royal Society of Medicine 64: 279, 1971. (Abstract)

Subjects: 68 young widows and widowers.
Method: Subjects were interviewed soon after death of spouse and again 1 year later to collect data on possible predictors (e.g., socioeconomic status, length of spouse's terminal illness, life crises, marital discord, emotional reactions to bereavement) of 1-year outcome. Subjects with poor 1-year outcome were studied in more detail to identify specific patterns of reaction associated with poor outcome 1 year after bereavement. [See also G20.]

G16 Parkes, Colin Murray: The first year of bereavement: A longitudinal study of the reaction of London widows to the death of their husbands. Psychiatry 33:444-467, 1970.

Subjects: 22 London widows (under age 65).
Method: Each subject was interviewed 1 month after death of her spouse for information about the circumstances of his terminal illness and death, her reactions at the time and since, and her life situation and family history. Followup interviews were held at 3, 6, 9, and 13 months after bereavement for information about events and reactions since previous interview, and at the final interview each subject was also rated on her psychological, social, and physical

adjustment. Data were compared in order to document the process of grief and its changes over the course of 13 months.

G17 Parkes, C. Murray: Psycho-social transitions: A field for study. Social Science and Medicine 5:101-115, 1971.

P & R

The author combines ideas from three fields ("stress" research, crisis studies, and "loss" research) to develop a new conceptual field for study, Psychosocial Transitions. He defines psychosocial transitions as "major changes in life space" which meet three criteria: their effects are long lasting, they take place relatively quickly, and they affect major areas of one's "assumptive world." Death of spouse, loss of limb, and involuntary relocation (change in residence) are discussed as examples of such psychosocial transitions.

G18 Parkes, C. Murray: Recent bereavement as a cause of mental illness. British Journal of Psychiatry 110:198-204, 1964.

RC321
B856X

Subjects: All admissions (N=3,245 patients) to the psychiatry units at two English hospitals from 1949 to 1951.
Method: All subjects' case summaries (made at discharge) were reviewed to collect data on the following: age, sex, and psychiatrist's diagnosis on discharge; incidence of death of first-degree relative (spouse, parent, sibling, child) in the 6 months prior to illness onset and amount of social interaction with deceased. Bereaved patients (N=94) were compared to the nonbereaved patients in terms of expected vs. observed incidence of bereavement and by age, sex, and diagnosis differences.

G19 Parkes, C. Murray; Benjamin, B.; and Fitzgerald, R. G.: Broken heart: A statistical study of increased mortality among widowers. British Medical Journal 1:740-743, 1969.

R31 B83

Subjects: 4,486 men (older than 54) whose wives died in 1957.
Method: Subjects were identified in a search of women's death certificates and were then followed for 9 years through National Health Service Central Register reports of death. When a widower's death was reported, the following data were collected from his death certificate: age, occupation (as indicator of social class), and certified cause of death. Rate of mortality of widowers was compared during each year (1-9) since bereavement, and causes of death for widowers were compared to their dead wives'. Social class, mortality rates, and causes of death were also compared

for widowers and for married men in the same age in the
general population.

G20   Parkes, C. Murray, and Brown, R. J.: Health after bereave-
       ment: A controlled study of young Boston widows and widowers.
       Psychosomatic Medicine 34:449-461, 1972.
           Subjects: 49 widows and 19 widowers under age 45 whose
           spouses had died 14 months earlier and 68 matched control
           subjects.
           Method: Bereaved and nonbereaved subjects were inter-
           viewed and compared using a structured questionnaire
           which collected data on health in the preceding year: utili-
           zation of health services; psychologic health (changes in
           sleep, appetite, habits; 15 symptoms of depression; 11
           other symptoms and personality attributes); and physical
           health (acute symptoms, chronic symptoms, autonomic re-
           actions, and other physical symptoms). In addition, 59
           subjects and controls were administered follow-up inter-
           views 2 to 4 years after bereavement, and changes in de-
           pression and symptom scores were examined and compared.

G21   Raphael, Beverley: Preventive intervention with the crisis of
       conjugal bereavement. Unpublished medical thesis, University
       of Sydney, 1974.
           Subjects: 194 recently bereaved widows (under age 60).
           Method: Each subject was interviewed within 7 weeks after
           death of her husband and was assessed on the basis of four
           indices predictive of "bad outcome." Those subjects found
           to be at high risk (N=64) were randomly assigned to an inter-
           vention group (N=31) or to the control group (N=33). Inter-
           vention consisted of 1-9 home visits by a psychiatrist dur-
           ing which the subject was given "selective ego support of
           relevant bereavement processes." All intervention was
           completed within three months of husband's death. Thirteen
           months after bereavement a follow-up health change ques-
           tionnaire [see G12] was mailed to available subjects, and
           differences in morbidity (good vs. bad outcome) were com-
           pared for intervention (N=27) and control (N=29) groups.

G22   Raphael, Beverley: Preventive intervention with the recently
       bereaved. Archives of General Psychiatry 34:1450-1454, 1977.
           Subjects: 194 recently bereaved widows (under age 60).
           Method: This publication is based on data first reported in
           the author's 1974 medical thesis (see G21).

G23   Rees, W. Dewi, and Lutkins, Sylvia G.: Mortality of bereave-
      ment. British Medical Journal 4:13-16, 1967.
         Subjects: 903 close relatives of 371 people who died in a
         6-year period and 878 close relatives of 371 matched living
         control subjects from the same semirural area of Wales.
         Method: Investigators used death certificates and medical
         registers of the county medical officer to compare risk of
         mortality for the survey group of bereaved close relatives
         (spouse, parent, sibling, child) and the control group of
         nonbereaved close relatives living in the same community.
         The survey group and the control group were compared for
         death following bereavement or matched nonbereavement
         in relation to the following: length of bereavement (1-6
         years); relationship to the deceased or control (spouse,
         parent, child, sibling); age and sex of deceased or control
         and relatives; site of deceased's death.

G24   Shepherd, Daphne, and Barraclough, B. M.: The aftermath
      of suicide. British Medical Journal 2:600-603, 1974.
         Subjects: 44 spouses (27 widows, 17 widowers) of people
         who committed suicide.
         Method: Subjects were traced 5 years after the suicide of
         their spouses. Death certificates were obtained for the 10
         who had died in the intervening years, and they were com-
         pared to the general population and to people widowed by
         other causes for risk of mortality and cause of death. In-
         terviews were held with the 34 surviving subjects about
         their reactions to the inquest process, experience of stigma
         associated with spouse's suicide, and outcome (better off,
         worse off, indeterminate). Rates of remarriage for the 34
         subjects were compared to remarriage rates among those
         widowed by causes other than suicide.

G25   Ward, Audrey W. M.: Mortality of bereavement. British
      Medical Journal 1:700-702, 1976.
         Subjects: 279 widows and 87 widowers.
         Method: Subjects were originally known as survivors of
         366 patients studied earlier in a terminal care study. Two
         years after the death of their spouses the subjects were
         traced to collect mortality data: actual number of deaths
         vs. expected number (based on life tables); number of
         months between bereavement and death of subject; cause
         of bereaved subject's death; site of ill spouse's death.
         Data were compared to findings of Rees and Lutkins [G23],
         Clayton [G4], and others.

G26 Williams, W. Vail; Lee, John; and Polak, Paul R.: Crisis intervention: Effects of crisis intervention on family survivors of sudden death situations. Community Mental Health Journal 12:128–136, 1976.

Subjects: 105 families who lost a family member by sudden death and 56 families with no bereavements in the past 2 years.

Method: Bereaved families were divided into two groups: the experimental bereaved group (39 families) received preventive crisis services soon after the sudden death, while the control bereaved group (66 families) received no intervention. Six months after the sudden death, both bereaved groups and the nonbereaved control group were interviewed to assess each family on five areas of outcome (using a variety of measures): medical illness, psychiatric illness, family functioning, crisis coping, and social cost. Bereaved and nonbereaved families were compared, and the effect of intervention on 6-month outcome was examined for the two groups of bereaved families.

RA790.A1C53

SPECIFIC EVENTS:
Work, Unemployment, and Retirement
(G27–G38)

G27 Andersson, Lars: Retirement, psychosocial factors and health: An annotated bibliography. Report No. 52b, Laboratory for Clinical Stress Research. Stockholm: Karolinska Institute, 1978. [Available from the Laboratory for Clinical Stress Research, Box 60205, S-104 01 Stockholm, Sweden.]

A 37-page review of the literature (originally published in Swedish in 1976) precedes the bibliography, and in it the author discusses general conceptions and theories of social gerontology, retirement planning programs, effects and consequences of retirement, and two groups of Swedish investigations. The bibliography itself contains 651 references organized in the following seven areas: Preparation for retirement, education; Evaluation of retirement planning programs; Retirement and working life; Age of retirement; The transitional stage—role change and attitudes; Evaluation of effects—adjustment; Evaluation of effects—morbidity, mortality; Retirement and leisure time, activities; and Miscellaneous.

G28   Baker, Ellen K.: Relationship of retirement and satisfaction
      with life events to locus of control (Doctoral dissertation, Uni-
      versity of Wisconsin-Madison, 1976). Dissertation Abstracts
      International 37:4748-B, 1977.
         Subjects: A group of males over 55 years old who had been
         surveyed by the Survey Research Center at the University
         of Michigan in their national "Quality of Life Study" [N is
         not stated].
         Method: Subjects were divided into subgroups by retirement
         status (preretired, transitional, retired) and were compared
         on the basis of locus of control orientation [unnamed mea-
         sure] and life satisfaction ("cumulative measure of past suc-
         cess and failure experiences in terms of noted life events").

G29   Berger, Michael; Wallston, Barbara Strudler; Foster, Martha;
      and Wright, Larry: You and me against the world: Dual-
      career couples and joint job seeking. Journal of Research
      and Development in Education 10(4):30-37, 1977.
         Subjects: 160 married couples in which one spouse had re-
         cently received a Ph.D. (in psychology, biochemistry,
         microbiology, or physiology) and the other also had pro-
         fessional training.
         Method: Each subject completed a 10-page questionnaire
         concerning the couple's past and future job-seeking strate-
         gies and experiences, the problems involved in accommo-
         dating two careers and family life, and the special con-
         straints each believed to be operating on him or her during
         the job-seeking process. Each subject was also asked to
         rate the "stressfulness" ("amount of adjustment required
         for coping") of the job-seeking process on a 100-point scale,
         using the following anchor points: 1=change in sleeping
         patterns, 50=marriage, and 100=death of spouse.

G30   Cobb, Sidney; Brooks, George W.; Kasl, Stanislav V.; and
      Connelly, Winnifred E.: The health of people changing jobs:
      A description of a longitudinal study. American Journal of
      Public Health 56:1476-1481, 1966.
         In this initial study the authors describe the design, theo-
         retical framework, purposes, methods, and procedures for
         their study of blue-collar workers changing jobs. The
         study began while the men were anticipating job loss be-
         cause of permanent plant closure and was designed to fol-
         low them for 2 years through unemployment and reemploy-
         ment. Findings are reported in later publications focusing

on health changes and illness behavior (G32 and G33), on physiological changes (see D2, D6, D7), and on the moderating effects of social support (C63, C64).

G31 Crawford, Marion P.: Retirement as a psycho-social crisis. Journal of Psychosomatic Research 16:375-380, 1972.
Subjects: 53 British married couples of retirement age.
Method: Husbands and wives were separately (but at the same time) administered a semistructured interview 6 months before and 12 months after retirement. The interviews collected data to assess attitudes toward retirement and perceptions of health changes (general health, frequency of visits to physician, occurrence of "minor conditions"; changes in appetite, weight, or sleep). Pre- and post-retirement reports were compared for men, women, and couples.

RC52.J6

G32 Kasl, Stanislav V.; Cobb, Sidney; and Gore, Susan: Changes in reported illness and illness behavior related to termination of employment: A preliminary report. International Journal of Epidemiology 1:111-118, 1972.
Subjects: 113 blue-collar male workers whose jobs were abolished due to permanent plant closure and 76 employed control subjects working at similar jobs in other plants.
Method: Subjects were visited at home during six phases of the job loss experience: anticipation of job loss, shortly after termination, three times during the year following job loss (when some were unemployed, others on probationary employment, and others stably reemployed), and 2 years after job loss. Controls were visited at comparable times. A standardized set of psychological, physiological, social, and economic data was collected at each visit by public health nurses. This preliminary report describes the changes in self-reported illness and illness behavior collected during all phases: number of Days Complaint (not feeling as well as usual) and Days Disability (not carrying out usual activities); health diaries (kept for 2-week periods); symptom checklists; self-report drug use; and 3-month retrospective reports. [See also G30, G33.]

RA421A37

G33 Kasl, Stanislav V.; Gore, Susan; and Cobb, Sidney: The experience of losing a job: Reported changes in health, symptoms and illness behavior. Psychosomatic Medicine 37:106-122, 1975.

Subjects: 113 blue-collar male workers whose jobs were
abolished due to permanent plant closure and 76 employed
control subjects working at similar jobs in other plants.
Method: This is a more detailed description and analysis
of findings first reported in G32. The measures reported
here include the following: days complaint, days disability,
percent days complaint that are also disability days, days
saw doctor, days used drugs (all based on self-report data
from 2-week health diaries); an index based on number of
changes in employment status (Job Changes Index) and an
index of life changes (modified Schedule of Recent Experience); subjective assessment of severity of the experience
of losing a job (made during last two phases of study); a
symptom checklist and a depression scale; and a "sense of
social support" scale (5 items). [See also G30, G32.]

G34   Lynch, Kathleen: Stressful life change and satisfaction during
       retirement (Doctoral dissertation, Wayne State University,
       1978). Dissertation Abstracts International 39:6099B-6100B,
       1979.
           Subjects: 100 retired people.
           Method: All subjects were interviewed to collect data on the
           following: demographic characteristics (including income
           level before and after retirement), life change experience,
           perceptions of adjustment required by life change events,
           coping styles, and present life satisfaction. [No instrument
           names are given in the abstract.]

G35   Manuso, James S. J.: Coping with job abolishment. Journal
       of Occupational Medicine 19:598-602, 1977.
           Subjects: 16 computer operators whose jobs were scheduled
           for abolishment in 3 months and a comparison group of 91
           fellow employees who had experienced only a "precipitous
           change" in their working conditions (change in management,
           job responsibilities, or methods).
           Method: All subjects worked for the same insurance com-
           pany and used the same Employee Health Center. The com-
           pany sponsored a "stress management" workshop as part of
           a larger program to help the 16 computer operators to pre-
           pare themselves for finding and getting new jobs. Each
           workshop member completed the Thematic Apperception
           Test before and after the workshop, and the test responses
           were compared on five dimensions of possible psychological
           change. Health center records were reviewed to compare
           the number and nature of visits during the 3 months before

and the 3 months after job abolishment was announced or "precipitous change" was experienced in order to examine the effects of the intervention program and to compare differences in the experiences of those undergoing job loss and those undergoing changes in working conditions.

G36   Renshaw, Jean R.: An exploration of the dynamics of the overlapping worlds of work and family. Family Process 15: 143-165, 1976.

Subjects: 50-60 managers in a large multinational corporation and their wives.

Method: All subjects were interviewed about the effects on themselves, their spouses, and their families resulting from one of three job changes recently experienced: husband's acceptance of international transfer, husband's extensive business traveling, or husband's new job role as a consultant for organizational changes ("staff facilitator of change"). Data were analyzed using grounded theory methodology and a systems theory approach. Illustrative case histories are presented.

G37   Williams, Carolyn Antonides: The relationship of occupational change to blood pressure, serum cholesterol, a specific overt behavior pattern, and coronary heart disease (Doctoral dissertation, University of North Carolina at Chapel Hill, 1969). Dissertation Abstracts International 30:4234B-4235B, 1969-1970.

Subjects: 3,269 working men aged 39-59 at the beginning of a 5-year prospective study of coronary heart disease.

Method: During the course of a larger study, questionnaires [unnamed] and physical examinations were administered to obtain data on the following: Behavior Types A and B, social status, blood pressure and serum cholesterol, and experience of occupational changes (e.g., change in job locale, change in employer, other changes in job situation). The relation of status inconsistency (discrepancies among education, occupation, and income) to Behavior Type A, blood pressure, and cholesterol was examined. Subjects with Behavior Type A were compared to those with Type B for differences in blood pressure and cholesterol at intake to the study and for incidence of subsequent occupational changes. Changes over time in blood pressure and cholesterol were compared for subjects who did and who did not experience occupational change during the course of the study.

G38 Willmuth, L. Ragon; Weaver, Lelon; and Donlan, Shirley: Utilization of medical services by transferred employees: Differential effect of life change on health. Archives of General Psychiatry 32:85-88, 1975.

> Subjects: 148 employees transferred to another company location and 148 fellow employees (matched for age, sex, job description) who had not been transferred in the past year.
> Method: Company medical records of subjects were reviewed for the first 12 months after transfer; control subjects' medical records were reviewed for corresponding periods. Data collected included number of visits for medical treatment and level of health care ("nurse visit" or "physician visit": health problem handled by nurse or referred to physician/psychiatrist). Health care utilization by transferred and nontransferred employees was compared and studied in relation to job description (professional vs. production and clerical employees).

RC 321 A6

SPECIFIC EVENTS:
Change in Residence, Changes in Living Conditions
(G39-G45)

G39 Bourestom, Norman, and Tars, Sandra: Alterations in life patterns following nursing home relocation. The Gerontologist 14:506-510, 1974.

> Subjects: 147 elderly patients in three nursing homes.
> Method: Subjects belonged to one of three groups: 49 in the "radical-change" group (involuntary relocation to a new physical environment with a new staff, new program, and new patient population), 49 in the "moderate-change" group (involuntary relocation to a new but neighboring building and with the same staff, program, and patient population continuing), and 49 in the control group (no relocation). Each subject was interviewed 1 month prior to relocation and at postrelocation intervals of 1, 4, 8, and 12 months to obtain data on the following: subject's perceived changes in health, in social relationships with staff and patients, and in activity patterns. Time-sample observations were made of changes in subject's level of behavioral complexity, and mortality data were collected. Outcome on all measures was compared for the radical-change, moderate-change, and control groups.

G40 Hasselkus, Betty Risteen: Relocation stress and the elderly.
American Journal of Occupational Therapy 32:631-636, 1978.
The author reviews the literature on the definition and measurement of "relocation stress," the characteristics of
people who are most vulnerable to its risks (e.g., increased
psychological problems, increased morbidity and mortality),
and the environmental factors that contribute to the "stress"
of relocation for the elderly. The author then discusses
ways in which the occupational therapist can make use of
the research findings to help modify the consequences of
relocation for older patients.

G41 Hooper, Douglas; Gill, Roger; Powesland, Peter; and Ineichen,
Bernard: The health of young families in new housing. Journal of Psychosomatic Research 16:367-374, 1972.
Subjects: 262 young families (wife under 40 years old) who
had moved to their present home within the last 2 years.
Method: Equal numbers of families were selected from
seven different housing types and areas in Bristol, England.
The wife in each family was interviewed at home; husbands
responded to similar questions in a questionnaire returned
by mail. The following data were collected: self-report
mental health of adults in past month (symptoms, untreated
complaints and problems, and problems for which treatment
was sought); adults' physical health (reports of 12 psychosomatic disorders; visiting physician in past 6 months for
physical illness; reports of serious illness, accidents, or
operations in past year); and reported behavior problems
of children in each family. Health measures were compared
and examined for differences according to the 7 housing
areas or types.

G42 Kasl, Stanislav V.: Physical and mental health effects of involuntary relocation and institutionalization on the elderly—a
review. American Journal of Public Health 62:377-384, 1972.
The author reviews the literature on involuntary relocation
and institutionalization for specific evidence of the health
consequences of those two life events for the elderly. This
extensive review (107 references) discusses research design and methods as well as findings, and the author concludes with recommendations for future research.

G43 Lawton, M. Powell, and Yaffe, Silvia: Mortality, morbidity
and voluntary change of residence by older people. Journal of
the American Geriatrics Society 18:823-831, 1970.

Subjects: 103 new tenants in an apartment building for the elderly, individually matched to 103 settled tenants in a similar building and to 103 elderly subjects living in the general community.
Method: All subjects received a medical examination by a physician and were assigned a "functional health" rating (I-VI). One year later mortality data were collected and number of deaths were compared for the three matched groups ("relocated housing," "nonrelocated housing," and "nonrelocated community") by initial functional health ratings. Twelve-month morbidity data were also collected for 77 matched pairs of relocated and nonrelocated elderly housing tenants: the medical examination was repeated and changes in functional health status were compared. Relocated and nonrelocated subjects were also compared for number of hospital admissions, number of clinic visits, and number of self-report health problems in the past 12 months.

G44 Lindemann, Erich; Fried, Marc; Satin, David; and Frieden, Elaine: Health problems of a working class population adapting to forced relocation. Psychosomatic Medicine 29:544-545, 1967. (Abstract)
Subjects: A working-class population of 10,000 persons forced to relocate because their substandard housing was scheduled for demolition in a slum-clearance project.
Method: Field observations were made by an anthropologist, and a survey was conducted to determine use of medical, social, and legal agencies. A probability sample was selected for intensive interviews to document patterns of somatic and psychiatric morbidity, coping styles and adaptive failures, and changes in social, family, and work roles of different ethnic groups (Italian, Polish, Jewish) forced to relocate.

G45 Rowland, Kay F.: Environmental events predicting death for the elderly. Psychological Bulletin 84:349-372, 1977.
The author reviews the findings of investigations of three life events as predictors of death for the elderly—death of significant other, relocation, and retirement. Methodological problems, intervention strategies, and conceptual models for future research are discussed.

SPECIFIC EVENTS:
Marriage, Separation, Divorce
(G46–G52)

G46 Bloom, Bernard L.; Asher, Shirley J.; and White, Stephen W.:
Marital disruption as a stressor: A review and analysis.
Psychological Bulletin 85:867-894, 1978.
This extensive review (168 references) evaluates the research evidence on correlates of marital disruption (psychopathology, motor vehicle accidents, morbidity, and
mortality from suicide, homicide, and disease) and the
problems on the personal, family, and community levels
for the person undergoing marital disruption. The authors
also review and discuss explanatory hypotheses for the
association of marital disruption and physical and emotional
disorders, including the "stressful life events" hypothesis.

G47 Briscoe, C. William, and Smith, James B.: Depression and
marital turmoil. Archives of General Psychiatry 29:811-817,
1973.
Subjects: 45 divorced subjects (33 women, 12 men) who
met predetermined criteria for a diagnosis of definite unipolar affective disease.
Method: Subjects were selected from 139 divorced people
interviewed in a controlled study of divorce and psychiatric
disease (see G48). These depressed subjects were administered the same structured interview for demographic and
domestic variables, and, in addition, a psychiatrist interviewed each depressed subject to obtain data on the timing,
duration, and events surrounding onset of depressive episodes before, during, and after marriage. Depressed subjects were compared by sex to nondepressed divorced subjects on demographic and domestic variables, and the temporal relationship of depressive episodes to marital disruption was examined.

G48 Briscoe, C. William; Smith, James B.; Robins, Eli; Marten,
Sue; and Gaskin, Fred: Divorce and psychiatric disease.
Archives of General Psychiatry 29:119-125, 1973.
Subjects: 139 divorced subjects (83 women, 56 men) and 61
married, never divorced control subjects (52 women, 29
men).
Method: A structured interview was conducted with all subjects to collect data on the following: demographic and domestic variables, incidence of psychiatric disorders at

RC321A66

RC321A66

time of interview (diagnosis made according to specific criteria), and history of psychiatric illness and treatment (inpatient and outpatient). Divorced subjects were compared to control subjects and to the general population (national and state census data) to identify demographic factors associated with divorce. Divorced and control subjects were compared separately by sex for incidence of psychiatric illness and history of psychiatric disorders and treatment.

G49   Chester, Robert: Health and marriage breakdown: Experience of a sample of divorced women. British Journal of Preventive and Social Medicine 25:231-235, 1971.
    Subjects: 150 divorced English women.
    Method: All subjects had petitioned for divorce between 1967 and 1970 and had been divorced for 6-36 months at time of interview. Each subject was asked an open-ended question about the effects of marriage breakdown on her health and then was specifically asked about the number, frequency, timing, and treatment of eight symptoms or behaviors (weight change, sleep difficulties, beginning/increasing smoking or drinking, concentration difficulties, crying, tiredness, tendency to self-neglect).

R35B857

G50   Felner, Robert D.; Stolberg, Arnold; and Cowen, Emory L.: Crisis events and school mental health referral patterns of young children. Journal of Consulting and Clinical Psychology 43:305-310, 1975.
    Subjects: 715 grade school children (ages 5-10) referred by their teachers to a mental health program for youngsters with significant early school adjustment problems.
    Method: Two studies were conducted, with approximately half the children in each study and using slightly modified instruments in the second study. Two rating instruments (the Teacher Referral Form and the AML) were completed by the teacher for each referred child: maladjustment scores were assigned on the basis of three factors (acting-out, moodiness and being withdrawn, and learning problems). Children were assigned to one of four groups: those whose parents were separated or divorced, those who had lost a parent by death, and two matched control groups without "parental crisis" histories. The two "crisis events" groups (separation/divorce and parental death) were compared to their matched controls and then to each other on overall adjustment scores and on specific maladjustment patterns.

BFl.J575

G51 Sheldon, Alan, and Hooper, Douglas: An enquiry into health and ill-health and adjustment in early marriage. Journal of Psychosomatic Research 13:95-101, 1969.

> Subjects: 26 young couples married from 6-12 months.
> Method: Each husband and wife was interviewed separately by an interviewer of the same sex about recent ("past month" and "since marriage") illness and health patterns: symptoms, new and chronic ailments, treatment sought, onset and course of illness, and extent of activity loss due to illness. Each subject also completed the Short Marital Adjustment Test, the Cornell Medical Index, and self-ratings of change in and satisfaction with current health status. Husbands and wives were compared for overall health and satisfaction with health, and the relationships of health, neurosis, and marital adjustment were examined for men, women, and couples.

RC52.J6

G52 Snyder, Alice Ivey: Periodic marital separation and physical illness. American Journal of Orthopsychiatry 48:637-643, 1978.

> Subjects: 48 wives of U.S. Navy submariners whose work required repetitive 3-month separations (3-months-home/ 3-months-at-sea).
> Method: During one of their regular separations from their seagoing husbands, all subjects completed three instruments: a modified Social Readjustment Rating Questionnaire (75 items, including events relevant to their cyclic marital separations and reunions, to be ranked on a 100-point scale); a modified Schedule of Recent Experience (75 events in the past year, divided according to "home" and "at sea" periods); and a health inventory (illnesses, how treated, physician visits, and medications used in past year). Life event perceptions and frequencies were examined, and the health of wives during husbands' absences was compared to their health during husbands' home-stays.

RA790.A1A5

SPECIFIC EVENTS:
Personal and Family Illness
(G53-G57)

G53 Goslin, Evelyn Roberts: Hospitalization as a life crisis for the preschool child: A critical review. Journal of Community Health 3:321-346, 1978.

The author reviews the research reported since 1965 when Vernon, Foley, Sipowicz, and Schulman published their comprehensive review of the psychological effects of hospitalization on children. This review covers the following topics: variables associated with hospitalization upset (maternal separation, age, prehospitalization personality), studies of strategies to prepare the child for hospitalization, and therapeutic intervention (with the hospitalized child and with mothers). The author then discusses theoretical formulations on which the research has been based ("anticipatory worry" and modeling theory) and proposes "crisis theory" as a useful model for future research.

G54 Kaplan, David M.; Grobstein, Rose; and Smith, Aaron: Predicting the impact of severe illness in families. Health and Social Work 1(3):71-82, 1976.

Subjects: 40 families of children with leukemia.
Method: Subjects were followed prospectively from time of confirmed diagnosis until 3 months after death of leukemic child. A social worker interviewed each family within 6 weeks of confirmed diagnosis to assess early family coping responses: each family was rated "adaptive" or "maladaptive" on the basis of three criteria. Home interviews were conducted with parents 3 months following the death of the leukemic child to collect data on the number and nature of problems (marital, sibling, health, and role functioning) experienced by surviving family members. Early coping responses of the families were examined as predictors of "stress outcome" (number of reported problems).

G55 Klein, Robert F.; Dean, Alfred; and Bogdonoff, Morton D.: The impact of illness upon the spouse. Journal of Chronic Diseases 20:241-248, 1967.

Subjects: 121 patients with chronic illness (at least 6 months in duration) and 73 spouses of patients applying to the outpatient clinic of a university medical center.
Method: A semistructured interview was administered individually to patients and spouses to collect data on reasons for applying to clinic, nature of presenting problem, and history of patient's previous medical treatment. Each subject was then administered three questionnaires concerning two time periods ("preillness" and "illness"): the Psychophysiologic Distress Index (22-item symptom inventory to indicate emotional disturbance), the Role Tension Index (14-item measure of marital integration), and an activities

questionnaire (level of work activity, time lost from work, changes in social and family activity since patient's illness). In addition, each spouse also completed the symptom inventory and role tension measures as they pertained to the patient. Preillness levels of symptoms, role tension, and work activity were compared to levels at time of application for treatment, and the relation between the patient and spouse's responses was examined.

G56 Townes, Brenda D.; Wold, David A.; and Holmes, Thomas H.: Parental adjustment to childhood leukemia. Journal of Psychosomatic Research 18:9-14, 1974.
Subjects: The parents of 8 children under treatment for leukemia.
Method: Subjects were followed for 3 years, from beginning of treatment through death of the leukemic child. At each yearly evaluation parents completed three questionnaires: the Anticipatory Fear questionnaire (rating of 12 feelings, used as indicator of acceptance of diagnosis and prognostic implications of childhood leukemia), the Semantic Differential measure of 13 concepts (scored along a 7-point scale on 4 dimensions), and the Schedule of Recent Experience (at Time 1, life change for each of the 9 years prior to diagnosis of leukemia and then for the current year; at Times 2 and 3, for past 12 months). Differences between mothers' and fathers' attitudes and their levels of anticipatory fear and of life change were compared over the three evaluation periods.

G57 Volicer, Beverly J.: Stress factors in the experience of hospitalization. Communicating Nursing Research 8:53-67, 1977.
The author reviews the development of the Hospital Stress Rating Scale, a list of events associated with the experience of hospitalization which are ranked according to the degree of "stress" they produce for the hospitalized patient. Factor analysis with varimax rotation was performed on the rank order correlation coefficients of the 49 events in the Hospital Stress Rating Scale in order to identify and distinguish eight "stress factors" in the experience of hospitalization. The author sketches future research directions to compare the relation of individual "stress factors" to illness outcome, demographic characteristics, and specific disease conditions.

SPECIFIC EVENTS:
Pregnancy and Parenthood
(G58–G62)

G58   Conone, Ruth Martha: Expectancy and first parenthood as
major life change (Doctoral dissertation, University of Wis-
consin-Madison, 1978). Dissertation Abstracts International
39:3300A–3301A, 1978.
  Subjects: 14 expectant parents from a prenatal class for
couples.
  Method: Subjects were interviewed and assessed while pre-
paring for the birth of their first child and at 1 month after
the birth. Prenatal and postnatal assessments were compared for changes in ego strength, changes in cognitive
structure, and changes in the proportion of defensive behavior to coping behavior exhibited during interview.

G59   Harkins, Elizabeth Bates: Effects of empty nest transition on
self-report of psychological and physical well-being. Journal
of Marriage and the Family 40:549–556, 1978.
HQ1.J48   This publication is based on data first reported in the
author's doctoral dissertation (see G60).

G60   Harkins, Elizabeth Bates: Stress and the empty nest transition: A study of the influence of social and psychological factors on emotional and physical health (Doctoral dissertation,
Duke University, 1975). Dissertation Abstracts International
35:7404-A, 1975.
  Subjects: 318 women who were "pre-empty nest" (youngest
child not yet graduated from high school), in the "empty
nest transition" (youngest child graduated within past 18
25053.B57 months), or "post-empty nest" (over $2\frac{1}{2}$ years since youngest child graduated from high school).
  Method: All subjects completed a mailed questionnaire
which collected data on a number of social and psychological variables (e.g., attitudes toward women's roles, employment status, marital satisfaction, other recent life
events, whether on- or off-schedule in relation to expected
timing of empty nest period) and on measures of psychological well-being (Bradburn's Affect Balance Scale) and self-
report physical well-being (modified Cornell Medical Index).
Pre-, post-, and empty nest subjects were compared in order to examine the relationship of empty nest status to
health and the effects of specific variables on that relationship.

G61 Neugarten, Bernice L.: Dynamics of transition of middle age
     to old age: Adaptation and the life cycle. Journal of Geriatric
     Psychiatry 4:71-87, 1970.

     The author reviews life cycle and adaptation studies con-
     ducted over the course of a decade by the Committee on
     Human Development at the University of Chicago. She de-
     scribes in detail a study of the effects of two "normal ex-
     pectable life events" for middle-aged women—menopause
     and children leaving home: 100 normal women, aged 43-53,
     were interviewed and tested to obtain data on a variety of
     psychological and social variables, including expectations
     and attitudes toward menopause, a checklist of menopausal
     symptoms, changes in family and nonfamily roles over the
     past 10 years, and measures of psychological well-being
     (anxiety, life satisfactions, self-concept).

G62 Taylor, Muriel K., and Kogan, Kate L.: Effects of birth of a
     sibling on mother-child interactions. Child Psychiatry and
     Human Development 4:53-58, 1973.

     Subjects: 7 working-class mothers and their firstborn
     children.
     Method: All mothers were 7-8 months pregnant with their
     second child at time of first videotaped observation; second
     observation took place about 2 months after birth of second
     child. Each mother-child pair was observed in a playroom,
     and their verbal and behavioral interaction was rated on
     three dimensions: relative status, affection, and involve-
     ment. Differences in their relationship before and after
     birth of a sibling were examined.

SPECIFIC EVENTS:
Catastrophic Life Events
(G63-G76)

G63 Arthur, Ransom J.: Extreme stress in adult life and its psy-
     chic and psychophysiological consequences. In Life Stress and
     Illness. E. K. Eric Gunderson and Richard H. Rahe (Eds.),
     pp. 195-207. Springfield, Illinois: Charles C Thomas, 1974.
     The author reviews the research about the wartime experi-
     ences and the long-term health and social problems of Nazi
     concentration camp survivors and of U.S. soldiers taken as
     prisoners of war in World War II and the Korean and the
     Vietnam wars.

G64 Bennet, Glin: Bristol floods 1968. Controlled survey of effects on health of local community disaster. British Medical Journal 3:454-458, 1970.

Subjects: Residents of Bristol, England, on the day of a major flood (July 10-11, 1968).

Method: The medical records of 209 people who had been flooded and 238 who had not been flooded were reviewed to collect pre- and post-flood health care utilization data: number of visits to physician, hospital referrals, and hospital admissions in the 12 months before and the 12 months following the flood. Interviews were conducted 2 weeks after the flood and again a year later with 197 "flooded" subjects and 231 "not flooded" control subjects to collect self-report data on general health and care-seeking in the 12 months before and 12 months after the flood, new symptoms since the flood, and bad effects on health from the flood. City registers were examined to compare mortality rates of all "flooded" vs. "not flooded" residents of Bristol in the 12 months before and after the flood; mortality data were compared by age, sex, and cause of death.

G65 Eitinger, L.: A follow-up study of the Norwegian concentration camp survivors' mortality and morbidity. Israel Annals of Psychiatry and Related Disciplines 11:199-209, 1973.

Subjects: 4,768 Norwegian concentration camp survivors (alive at liberation of German camps).

Method: Mortality data (numbers and cause of death) were collected for the years 1941-1966, and mortality rates of camp survivors were compared to expected rates (general Norwegian population) in 5-year periods from 1941. Morbidity data were collected for a representative sample of 448 former prisoners alive in 1966 and 448 matched controls (same age, sex, occupation, and health insurance program). The national health insurance records of subjects and controls were reviewed and compared for the following: number of professions, number of residences, changes in occupation, number of job changes; number of registered sick-periods and the diagnoses, number of work days lost, and number of hospitalizations and length of stay.

G66 Foster, Harold D.: Assessing disaster magnitude: A social science approach. The Professional Geographer 28:241-247, 1976.

The author uses the Social Readjustment Rating Scale of Holmes and Rahe to assign "stress values" to the deaths, injuries, and social disruptions caused by disasters. He uses those values in calculating the "event magnitudes" for disasters such as the Black Plague in fourteenth-century Europe and Asia, World War II, the 1972 flood of Rapid City, South Dakota, and the 1971 mass poisoning from fungicide-treated grain in Iraq. The Calamity Magnitude Scale compares disaster events in terms of "stress units" in order to distinguish "major catastrophes" from "catastrophes," "disasters," "tragedies," and the more common "adverse events" (jail term, parking ticket).

G67 Janney, James G.: Impact of a natural catastrophe on life style. Unpublished medical thesis, University of Washington, 1972.

Subjects: 69 earthquake victims (residents of Huaraz, Peru, a city that was 90 percent levelled in May 1970 by an earthquake) and 78 control subjects (residents of Arequipa, Peru, a city that suffered no damage from the earthquake). Method: One year after the May 30 earthquake, subjects and controls were administered a slightly modified Social Readjustment Rating Questionnaire; data were used to produce a Peruvian Social Readjustment Rating Scale for each city. Subjects and controls also completed a slightly modified Schedule of Recent Experience for two time periods: the earthquake year (June 1969-June 1970) and the post-earthquake year (June 1970-June 1971). Differences in life change magnitudes and in perceptions of life events were examined for earthquake victims and control subjects in both time periods. Cross-cultural comparisons were also made using Social Readjustment Rating Scale values from earlier studies in El Salvador, Spain, and the United States.

G68 Janney, James G.; Masuda, Minoru; and Holmes, Thomas H.: Impact of a natural catastrophe on life events. Journal of Human Stress 3(2):22-35, 1977.

This publication is based on data originally reported in the first author's medical thesis (see G67).

G69 Kinston, Warren, and Rosser, Rachel: Disaster: Effects on mental and physical health. Journal of Psychosomatic Research 18:437-456, 1974.

The authors review the literature to evaluate current knowledge of the psychiatric consequences (both immediate and long-term) of disaster for individuals and for groups. They review methodological approaches in the disaster

literature, psychological phenomena of the threat-impact-
early aftermath phases, and long-term psychological
sequelae (citing studies of war neuroses, Nazi concentration camps, and Hiroshima). They also review evidence
related to the management and prevention of psychiatric
consequences and to the planning of relief services (using
models from life events research to estimate incidence of
morbidity in disaster-struck communities).

G70 Liu, William T., and Yu, Elena S. H.: Refugee status and
alienation theory: The case of Vietnamese in U.S. Sociological Abstracts 26(3):78S08476 (ISA 1978 2069), 1978.
Subjects: 60 Vietnamese refugee families.
Method: Subjects were interviewed in May, 1975, when
they first arrived at Camp Pendleton in California and again
at 6-month intervals for the next 2 years. Data were collected on the following: basic mobility, demographic transitions, health, stress indices, and life change events [no
instruments named in abstract].

G71 McCabe, Michael S., and Board, George: Stress and mental
disorders in basic training. Military Medicine 141:686-688,
1976.
Subjects: All USAF airmen in basic training who were consecutively admitted to a psychiatric hospital during a 1-year
period (N=176).
Method: The medical charts of all subjects were reviewed
to collect the following data: sex, age, marital status,
number days completed in basic training, prior psychiatric
history, and symptoms (on the basis of which a research
diagnosis was assigned). Patients were compared to a control group (all basic airmen beginning basic training during
the same 1-year period) on sex, race, and completing
basic training or returning to active duty.

G72 Melick, Mary Evans: Life change and illness: Illness behavior of males in the recovery period of a natural disaster.
Journal of Health and Social Behavior 19:335-342, 1978.
Subjects: A probability sample of 91 working-class men
(ages 25-65) who lived in Wilkes-Barre or Kingston, Pennsylvania, during the 1972 flood.
Method: All subjects were interviewed three years after
the flood to collect data for three time periods: 1, pre-
flood (the 6 months before the flood); 2, recovery period
(the flood and subsequent $2\frac{1}{2}$ years); and 3, postflood (past

6 months). Self-report health data included physical ill-nesses, injuries, and emotional illnesses; subjects also completed Gurin's 20-item symptom checklist. Life events data for Periods 1, 2, and 3 were collected using the Sched-ule of Recent Experience. Subjects were divided into sub-groups according to flood experience (43 whose residences had been flooded in 1972 and 48 whose homes had not been flooded) and were compared for demographic characteris-tics; life change scores; number, seriousness, and mean rate of illness; and perception of current health status and effect of flood on health.

G73   Rahe, Richard H.; Looney, John G.; Ward, Harold W.; Tung, Tran Minh; and Liu, William T.: Psychiatric consultation in a Vietnamese refugee camp. <u>American Journal of Psychiatry</u> <u>135</u>:185-190, 1978.

RC321A52

<u>Subjects</u>: A random sample of 203 Vietnamese refugees (ages 13 and older) evacuated to Camp Pendleton, California, in 1975.
<u>Method</u>: Subjects were interviewed and administered three questionnaires: a modified Recent Life Changes Question-naire (with 12 new items added to reflect subjects' war and refugee experiences), the Cornell Medical Index, and Cantril's Self-Anchoring Scale (for five time periods: 5 years ago, 1 year ago, current status, 1 year in future, 5 years in future). Data were analyzed for subgroups accord-ing to age and sex and were used as representative data to assess the mental health of the refugees at large.

G74   Rogler, Lloyd H.: Help patterns, the family, and mental health: Puerto Ricans in the United States. <u>International</u> <u>Migration Review</u> <u>12</u>:248-259, 1978.
The author discusses research conducted in Puerto Rico and on the United States mainland during the past 20 years concerning how Puerto Rican families cope. Particular attention is given to the difficulties they face as migrants to a new environment ("a qualitatively new constellation of life-event changes"). The author posits membership in Puerto Rican help-giving systems as the key mediating fac-tor that enables Puerto Ricans to adapt to and to cope with minority group status in the United States.

G75   Roskies, Ethel; Iida-Miranda, Maria-Lia; and Strobel, Michael G.: The applicability of the life events approach to the problems of immigration. <u>Journal of Psychosomatic Re-</u>
RC52.J6   <u>search</u> <u>19</u>:235-240, 1975.

Subjects: 303 adult Portuguese immigrants living in Montreal, Canada.
Method: All subjects were interviewed at home by a Portuguese-born interviewer. Two questionnaires were administered verbally: the Schedule of Recent Experience (for the 2 years preceding interview) and the checklist of the U.S. National Health Survey (illnesses in the past year). Wyler's Seriousness of Illness Rating Scale was used to calculate a Severity Score for reported illnesses. The relation of life change scores to illness and severity scores was investigated, and differences between male and female scores were examined.

G76 Spradley, James P., and Phillips, Mark: Culture and stress: A quantitative analysis. American Anthropologist 74:518-529, 1972.

Subjects: 83 returned Peace Corps volunteers, 34 Chinese foreign students in the U.S., and 42 U.S. students with no intercultural experience.

MICROFILM

GN1A5

Method: A 33-item Cultural Readjustment Rating Questionnaire was developed on the model of Holmes and Rahe's Social Readjustment Rating Questionnaire. All subjects were asked to imagine themselves living in another culture for 1 year or more, and then to estimate the amount of readjustment that would be required by cultural differences (e.g., "the language spoken," "personal cleanliness of most people," "ideas about what is funny," "how parents treat children"). "Type of food eaten" was the module item with the arbitrary value of 500; each of the other 32 items was compared to the module item. Rank order correlations and geometric mean values of the 33 cultural differences were compared for the three groups of subjects.

SPECIFIC EVENTS:
Jail Term
(G77)

G77 Twaddle, Andrew C.: Utilization of medical services by a captive population: An analysis of sick call in a state prison. Journal of Health and Social Behavior 17:236-248, 1976.

Subjects: 293 inmates of a midwestern state penitentiary for men.

R11.J687

Method: The prison records of each subject were reviewed to collect demographic data (age, race, marital status, crime, length of sentence, length of time served, work assignment, number of disciplinary reports), illness history data (surgical procedures, disease types, psychiatric history, VD history, psychiatric and medical hospitalizations), and number of sick calls in a 1-month period. Differential use of services within the study population was examined, and inmate use of medical services was compared to averages for the general ("free") population and to shipboard use of sick bay in the U.S. Navy (as reported by Rahe et al.).

METHODOLOGY OF
LIFE EVENTS RESEARCH

METHODOLOGY:
Development of Life Events Research Instruments
(H1-H15)

H1   Anderson, Gail E.: College Schedule of Recent Experience.
       Unpublished master's thesis, North Dakota State University,
       1972.
            Subjects: Two samples of college students (N=103 and
            N=284).
            Method: The Schedule of Recent Experience was modified
            in order to develop an instrument appropriate for use with
            a college student population. An initial survey of 103 sub-
            jects produced a list of 47 life events for inclusion in the
            College Schedule of Recent Experience (8 original Schedule
            of Recent Experience items were dropped, 3 were revised
            or combined with others, and 15 new items were added).
            The revised life events list was used to modify the Social
            Readjustment Rating Questionnaire, which was then admin-
            istered to 284 students: subjects rated the "amount of re-
            adjustment" required by each of 46 events in comparison to
            the modulus item, "entering college" (arbitrarily assigned
            a value of 500). The college Social Readjustment Rating
            Questionnaire data (with mean scores divided by 10) were
            used to create a scale of mean values for use in scoring
            the College Schedule of Recent Experience.

H2   Antonovsky, Aaron, and Kats, Rachel: The life crisis history
       as a tool in epidemiological research. Journal of Health and
       Social Behavior 8: 15-21, 1967.

Subjects: 50 patients with multiple sclerosis and 50 individually matched control subjects (all born in Central
Europe and living in Israel).

Method: As part of a larger study of multiple sclerosis in
Israel (241 patients, 964 controls), all subjects and controls were interviewed using a "life crisis history" schedule
comprised of 30 questions about "objective experiences"
which "either imposed pain or necessitated a role transformation." Fifteen questions concerned the occurrence of
illnesses, hospitalizations, operations, and serious injuries from "birth to 15 years" and "age 15 to age at onset
of disease." The other half of the questions concerned
events or "shocks" (e.g., pregnancy, migration, death of
parents, experience in Europe during World War II) which
occurred prior to onset of disease. The 30 items were
classified into four subject areas (physical trauma, change
in general environment, changes affecting primary interpersonal relations, and changes in status) and were assigned
a "level of crisis intensity" score (1-5 points). Patients
and controls were compared using "crisis scores" calculated 6 ways. The list of 30 life crisis history items is
appended to the text.

H3   Cochrane, Raymond, and Robertson, Alex: The Life Events
Inventory: A measure of the relative severity of psychosocial
stressors. Journal of Psychosomatic Research 17:135-139,
1973.

Subjects: In Stage 1, 125 psychiatric inpatients in Edinburgh hospitals; in Stage 2, 60 psychiatrists and psychologists, 42 psychiatric patients, and 75 university students.

Method: In Stage 1, investigators administered a modified
Schedule of Recent Experience to 125 psychiatric patients
and then inquired about "any other events" in the past year.
A list of 59 new events was collected, then edited and revised in order to produce a final schedule of life events.
The Life Events Inventory (L.E.I.) documents the occurrence of 55 life events (18 Schedule of Recent Experience
items plus 37 new or revised items) in the past year;
slightly different versions are administered to "ever-
married" and "never-married" subjects. In Stage 2, the
three groups of subjects were asked to rate the "amount of
turmoil, upheaval, and social readjustment" following each
of the 55 life events on a scale of 1-100 (with "marriage"
arbitrarily assigned the value of 50). Mean life event
weightings were compared among the three groups of raters,

and rank order correlations were examined. The Life
Events Inventory, with weights from each group as well as
the total sample, is reproduced in the text.

H4 Costantini, Arthur F.; Braun, John R.; Davis, Jack E.; and
Iervolino, Annette: The Life Change Inventory: A device for
quantifying psychological magnitude of changes experienced
by college students. Psychological Reports 34:991-1000, 1974.
Subjects: Two samples of college students (N=300 and
N=523).
Method: The Schedule of Recent Experience was modified
in order to develop an instrument appropriate for use with
a college student population. Approximately 300 students
were asked to specify life events that would require readjustment of them or their fellow students, regardless of
the desirability or undesirability of the event. After testing clarity of items in various trials with small groups, the
investigators selected 50 life events for inclusion in the Life
Change Inventory (about half were original Schedule of Recent Experience items and the other half were new). In
order to develop weights for the inventory items, 523 students were asked to rate the social readjustment ("amount
and duration of change in pattern of life") required by each
life event on a scale of 0-500 ("least intense" to "most intense" change and necessary readjustment). The Life
Change Inventory items and scoring weights are reproduced
in the text. Instrument reliability data (test-retest) are
also reported along with studies of correlations of mood
and personality scores (Profile of Mood States, Eysenck
Personality Inventory, and Differential Personality Inventory) with life change scores.

H5 Dohrenwend, Barbara Snell; Krasnoff, Larry; Askenasy,
Alexander R.; and Dohrenwend, Bruce P.: Exemplification
of a method for scaling life events: The PERI Life Events
Scale. Journal of Health and Social Behavior 19:205-229,
1978.
Subjects: A community probability sample of 124 New York
City residents (stratified by sex, ethnicity, and social
class).
Method: The Psychiatric Epidemiology Research Interview
(PERI) Life Events List was developed after reviewing ear-
lier lists, consulting the researchers' own experience, and
surveying two samples of subjects living in Washington
Heights about the "last major event" which disrupted their

lives. The final list of 102 life events was classified, by consensus of four judges, according to the following: breadth of setting (universal or limited to a particular sociocultural setting), desirability (gain, loss, ambiguous), and dependence or independence of subject's physical and/or psychological condition. The 124 judges were asked to rate the "amount of change" required by each of 101 events in comparison to "marriage" (arbitrarily assigned the value of 500). Arithmetic mean values and rank orders were calculated to compare life event ratings, and the effects of sex, ethnicity, and social class (education of head of household) on life event ratings were examined. A "general decision model" was used to classify the life event ratings as "consensual" (universal agreement among raters), "status dependent" (a function of social class or other specific characteristics), or "noisy" (differences unrelated to specified characteristics). The authors discuss methodological issues raised by their experience in developing the PERI Life Events Scale.

H6   Holmes, Thomas H., and Rahe, Richard H.: Booklet for the Schedule of Recent Experience (SRE) © 1967. Four page questionnaire. [Available from Dr. Holmes, Department of Psychiatry and Behavioral Sciences RP-10, University of Washington, Seattle, Washington 98195.]

The Schedule of Recent Experience (SRE) is a printed questionnaire which asks subjects to document the frequency of occurrence of 42 life change events in four time periods (0-6 months, 6-12 months, 1-2 years, 2-3 years ago). The original SRE was developed by Hawkins and Holmes [see A119] to collect annual frequency data for a 10-year period; it was scored by simply counting the number of reported life change events. In 1966-1967 Rahe and Holmes developed the Social Readjustment Rating Scale [see H18], a ranking of life events by mean values of magnitude estimations. Since then the Social Readjustment Rating Scale has been used to score the Schedule of Recent Experience: the frequency of each reported event is multiplied by its scale value, and the sum of weighted events constitutes the subject's life change score (Total Life Change Units [LCU]). [See also A19 for a summary of the development and application of the Schedule of Recent Experience and the Social Readjustment Rating Scale.]

H7   Horowitz, Mardi; Schaefer, Catherine; Hiroto, Donald; Wilner, Nancy; and Levin, Barbara: Life event questionnaires for measuring presumptive stress. Psychosomatic Medicine 39: 413-431, 1977.

Based on life events listed in the Schedule of Recent Experience and the Paykel et al. life events interview, the authors developed a long (143 items) and short (34 items) form of the Life Events Questionnaire (LEQ). Both forms ask subjects to document the occurrence of life events in five time periods (1 week, 1 month, 6 months, 1 year, 3 years ago). To develop weightings for scoring the LEQ, three groups of subjects were asked to rate on a scale of 1-100 how "stressful" the event would be for them at present if the event had occurred at each of the five times in the past. "Presumptive stress" ratings for recent and remote events were compared for the three subject groups (119 nonpatient volunteers, 27 psychiatric outpatients, and 8 psychiatrists), and the effect of sex, age, and having experienced the event was examined within and among subject groups. The authors also review their studies of the reliability (test-retest) of life event reporting with four subject groups: 35 psychiatric outpatients, 20 medical center personnel, 112 men in a study of coronary risk factors, and 20 married couples completed the long and/or short form of the LEQ from 1-3 times and at intervals of 6 weeks to 1 year. Data on the incidence of life events were analyzed for 961 psychiatric outpatients and 107 nonpatient volunteers who had completed the short form of the LEQ: "total presumptive stress" scores were derived using four sets of weights (from the nonpatient sample of 119) appropriate to sex and age (under/over 30) of subjects.

H8   Kulcsar, Paul G.: The development and validation of a life-change checklist for juvenile delinquents (Doctoral dissertation, Utah State University, 1976). Dissertation Abstracts International 37:6335-B, 1977.

Subjects: 334 juvenile delinquents and 104 nondelinquent high school students.
Method: After analyzing case histories of 100 court-adjudicated juvenile delinquents and interviewing ten professional workers in correctional settings, the author developed a list of 58 life events observed to be "critical incidents" requiring significant readjustment in the lives of adolescents. A sample of 30 professionals (10 psychologists,

10 social workers, 10 probation officers) was administered a modified Social Readjustment Rating Questionnaire to develop weights for the 58 events: subjects rated on a scale of 1-100 the "amount of change or readjustment" required by each event in comparison to the anchor item, "birth of a brother or sister" (arbitrarily assigned a value of 50). Geometric mean values were calculated for use in computing life change scores. In the Checklist validation study, the Adolescent Social Readjustment Checklist was administered to 334 subjects and controls to collect life change data for the past year. Delinquents were compared to nondelinquents on magnitude of life change and kinds of events experienced. Delinquent subjects' court records were reviewed for offenses in the past 12 months, and the relation of life change scores to type and severity of delinquency was examined.

H9   Loop, Maj Teorell: The Seattle-King County mobile health unit: A study in child health supervision. Unpublished master's thesis, University of Washington, 1975.

Subjects: 198 mother-child pairs.

Method: As part of a pilot program that established a mobile pediatric clinic, two screening instruments were constructed and tested for their ability to identify children at high risk of illness. On the basis of a medical history questionnaire filled out by the mother and subsequently recorded diagnostic codes, each child was assigned a High Risk Score. Each mother also completed two life event questionnaires: a modified Schedule of Recent Experience for her own life changes in the past year and a 45-item inventory for the child's life changes in the past year. The child was then assigned a Life Event Score (based on the 22 Schedule of Recent Experience items, 16 items from Coddington's Schedule of Recent Experience for children, 4 items common to both, and 3 new items). The relation of mother's life change score to child's Life Event Score and health status in the past year was examined. The High Risk Score and the Life Event Score were evaluated as screening instruments.

H10   Michaux, William W.; Gansereit, Kathleen H.; McCabe, Oliver L.; and Kurland, Albert A.: The psychopathology and measurement of environmental stress. Community Mental Health Journal 3:358-372, 1967.

RA790.A1C53

The General Stress Index and the Specific Stress Index were
developed and tested for their ability to predict relapse (rehospitalization) of adult psychiatric patients in the 12 months
following hospitalization. In a larger parent study, 139
newly released patients were followed through 12 monthly
structured interviews with patient and a close informant;
the General and Specific Stress Index (total of 8 questions)
were included in those monthly interviews. Subjects and
informants were asked to indicate the occurrence in the past
month of events in the following areas of the patient's life:
general "good," general "bad" happenings (General Stress
Index); interpersonal relations, marital and sexual relations, economic and domestic affairs, occupational problems, social and recreational activities, and physical
health (Specific Stress Index of distressing events). The
interviewer certified the nature of the reported events, but
data were recorded as simple "yes or no" responses. Two
sets of subjects and their informants were selected for the
validation and cross-validation studies: 10 relapsed patients and 10 matched nonrelapsed patients (at 6 months),
and 11 relapsed patients and 11 matched nonrelapsed patients (at 12 months). Three "stress scores" were calculated for each patient (patient report, informant report,
patient-plus-informant report), and scores of relapsers
were compared to those of nonrelapsers in the first month
after release from hospital and in the prerelapse month.

H11 Morrice, J. K. W.: Life crisis, social diagnosis, and social
therapy. British Journal of Psychiatry 125:411-413, 1974.
Subjects: 266 consecutively admitted patients at a psychiatric day hospital (mental health service).
Method: The staff of a day hospital was trained to supplement conventional treatment with a psychosocial approach:
Patients were diagnosed and treated in terms of their dis-
turbed social relationships. All patients were interviewed
at admission to obtain information on the number and nature
of life crisis events which precipitated referral to psychiatric care and on the persons involved in the crises. Data
were collected on a standard form ("Day Patient Contact
and Data Summary") which is reproduced in the text. On
the basis of that information a "social diagnosis" was made
for each patient and a "social prescription" (treatment program including therapy with relatives) was planned. Data
collected by using this format with 266 patients is summarized: number of crises identified in each case, distri-

bution of crises within the patient population by nature of crisis (categories: interpersonal difficulty, antisocial behavior, financial problem, work problem, physical illness, accident, pregnancy, bereavement, other), and frequency of involvement of specified persons (e.g., mother-in-law, spouse together with another family member).

H12   Rahe, Richard H.: Epidemiological studies of life change and illness. International Journal of Psychiatry in Medicine 6: 133-146, 1975.

The author briefly reviews the development of the Schedule of Recent Experience (SRE) and the Social Readjustment Rating Scale (SRRS) at the University of Washington and then goes on to describe modified versions of the SRE used in his research from 1965-1975. The military version of the SRE was used from 1965-1968 in a variety of studies involving the U.S. Navy; in 1969 the SRE was translated into Swedish and Finnish for studies of coronary heart disease; and the military SRE was translated into Norwegian for studies involving the Norwegian Navy. In 1970 the author and his colleagues began using a revision of the SRE called the Recent Life Changes Questionnaire (RLCQ). The RLCQ is a 55-item life change inventory covering the past 2 years (at 6-month intervals). In addition to the standard SRRS Life Change Unit values used to calculate the subject's life change score, the RLCQ also uses "subjective Life Change Units (SLCU)" values. The subject is asked to rate on a scale of 1-100 the "amount of adjustment you needed to handle" each event reported in the RLCQ. Selected results from retrospective and prospective studies of life change and illness are presented. The Recent Life Changes Questionnaire is appended to the text.

H13   Sarason, Irwin G.; Johnson, James H.; and Siegel, Judith M.: Assessing the impact of life changes: Development of the Life Experiences Survey. Journal of Consulting and Clinical Psychology 46:932-946, 1978.

The Life Experiences Survey (LES) was developed and tested in studies with college student populations. The LES is a 57-item life events questionnaire which asks subjects to indicate the occurrence of events in the past year (0-6 months and 7-12 months ago). Section 1 is designed for all respondents and contains 47 life events plus 3 blank spaces for other events. Section 2 is designed for use with students and lists 10 events relevant to an academic environ-

ment. Student subjects complete both Section 1 and Section
2. Subjects are also asked to rate the desirability and impact of each reported event on a 7-point scale ("-3 = extremely negative" to "+3 = extremely positive"). Three
life change scores are calculated: positive change score
(sum of positive ratings), negative change score (sum of
negative ratings), and total change score (sum of both positive and negative ratings). The LES was evaluated in a number of studies to obtain normative data for the instrument,
to examine possible sex differences in scores, and to compare test-retest reliability. In further studies LES life
change scores (positive, negative, total) were studied in relation to a number of personality measures and measures of
psychological impairment or maladjustment (State-Trait
Anxiety Inventory, Marlowe-Crowne Social Desirability
Scale, Psychological Screening Inventory, Beck Depression Inventory, Rotter's Locus of Control Scale). Two other
studies were conducted to compare the LES and the Schedule
of Recent Experience as measures of life change. The Life
Experiences Survey is appended to the text.

H14   Timmreck, Thomas C., and Stratton, Lorum H.: The Sched-
      ule of Recent Events: A measure of stress due to life change
      events translated for the Spanish-speaking. Journal of Psy-
      chiatric Nursing and Mental Health Services 16(8):20-25, 1978.
      The Schedule of Recent Experience was modified for use as
      a tool by mental health workers in Spanish-speaking com-
      munities. A 1-year, 43-item checklist was translated from
      English into Spanish, and the clarity of the translation was
      tested by trials with Spanish-speaking subjects from differ-
      ent countries and with different social and educational back-
      grounds. The modified and translated instrument was
      named the Schedule of Recent Events. The English and
      Spanish versions of the Schedule of Recent Events are re-
      produced in the text.

H15   Volicer, Beverly J.: Perceived stress levels of events asso-
      ciated with the experience of hospitalization: Development and
      testing of a measurement tool. Nursing Research 22:491-497,
      1973.
      Subjects: A convenience sample of 216 nonpatient adults.
      Method: The author informally interviewed patients, lay
      people, nurses, and physicians to compile a list of 45
      "stressful" events experienced by hospital patients. A
      group of 216 adults was then asked to rate the amount of

"readjustment" required by 44 of the events in comparison to the module item, "emergency admission" (arbitrarily assigned a value of 50). Means scores were calculated for the items, which were then ranked from highest to lowest according to "stress values." Consensus among raters was examined by comparing rank order correlations between subgroups divided according to age, sex, education, marital status, occupation (medical vs. nonmedical), and previous hospitalization experience. This publication was the initial report in a series of studies which led to the development of an instrument called the Hospital Stress Rating Scale. [For a description of subsequent revisions and modifications, see also H53, H54, and G57.]

For development of other life events inventories, see also: For general populations, A221 (Brown and Birley interview); A364 (Schedule of Daily Experience); C22 (Myers, Lindenthal, and Pepper interview); H23 (Paykel, Prusoff, and Uhlenhuth distressing events scales); H29 (Tennant and Andrews Australian questionnaire); H103 (Hurst, Rose, and Jenkins ROLE questionnaire); and for special populations, A2 (women in religious life); A16, H36, H89 (children); B16, B17, B18, B52 (college students); B72, B73 (college athletes); B130 (geriatric subjects); G76 (people experiencing culture shock); H33, H55 (Mexican-Americans, Native Americans, and Afro-Americans); H34 (teachers); H35 (military officer candidates); H39 (pregnant women).

METHODOLOGY:
Scaling Studies—General Populations
(H16-H32)

H16 Askenasy, Alexander R.; Dohrenwend, Bruce P.; and Dohrenwend, Barbara Snell: Some effects of social class and ethnic group membership on judgments of the magnitude of stressful life events: A research note. Journal of Health and Social Behavior 18:432-439, 1977.

RII.J 687

Subjects: A systematically drawn sample (N=92) of New York City residents, stratified by sex, ethnicity, and social class.
Method: All subjects were asked by interviewers to rate the amount of "change" involved in each of 101 life events in comparison to "marriage" (arbitrarily assigned a value of 500). Investigators then isolated the 31 life events in

common between their list of 102 events and the 43 events in the Social Readjustment Rating Questionnaire, and they compared the geometric mean ratings of the New York City sample to previously published ratings of the same 31 events in 6 other samples of Americans, Europeans, and Japanese from studies using the Social Readjustment Rating Questionnaire. The New York City ratings were analyzed and compared to the other samples by sex, social class (educational level of head of household), and ethnic group membership (non-Puerto Rican white, black, and Puerto Rican).

H17   Hart, Cheryl A.; Masuda, Minoru; and Holmes, Thomas H.: Life event magnitude judgments. Psychosomatic Medicine 39: 55, 1977. (Abstract)
      Subjects: Six samples of subjects (middle-class U.S. residents, college students and football players, native Israelis, alcoholics, and heroin addicts) who completed the Social Readjustment Rating Questionnaire and the Schedule of Recent Experience in earlier studies.
      Method: Data from both the Schedule of Recent Experience and the Social Readjustment Rating Questionnaire were collated to study five components of variability in assigning magnitude estimations of the readjustment required by life events: age, sex, and social class of subjects, experience with the events, and values assigned to the reference event. The relation of event frequency (common occurrences vs. rare events) to Social Readjustment Rating Questionnaire magnitude assignments was formulated.

H18   Holmes, Thomas H., and Rahe, Richard H.: The Social Readjustment Rating Scale. Journal of Psychosomatic Research 11:213-218, 1967.
      Subjects: A sample of convenience composed of 394 U.S. adults.
      Method: All subjects completed the Social Readjustment Rating Questionnaire (SRRQ), which asked subjects to rate the amount of "social readjustment" (regardless of the event's desirability) required by each of 42 life events in comparison to "marriage" (arbitrarily assigned a value of 500). Mean scores for events were calculated, divided by 10, and arranged in rank order to produce a ratio scale, the Social Readjustment Rating Scale (SRRS). Coefficients of correlation were examined between discrete groups of raters according to age, sex, marital status, education, social class, generation U.S. residents, religion, and race. [See also H21.]

H19   Horowitz, Mardi J.; Schaefer, Cathy; and Cooney, Paul: Life
      event scaling for recency of experience. In Life Stress and
      Illness. E. K. Eric Gunderson and Richard H. Rahe (Eds.),
      pp. 125-133. Springfield, Illinois: Charles C Thomas, 1974.
         Subjects: 119 San Francisco Bay area residents (college
         students, medical center personnel, and volunteers).
         Method: All subjects completed a 34-item life events in-
         ventory, checking those events which they had experienced.
         They rated on a scale of 1-100 how "stressful" each ex-
         perienced event would be for them at present if it had oc-
         curred at each of 5 different time periods in the past (1 week
         ago, 1 month, 6 months, 1 year, and 3 years ago). And then
         subjects rated the "stressfulness" of the remaining (not ex-
         perienced) events for the same time intervals. Mean values
         were calculated for each event at the five time intervals,
         and the effect of recency vs. remoteness of events on mag-
         nitude of ratings was examined. The effect and interaction
         of sex, age, and having experienced the event was exam-
         ined by subgroup ratings. Comparisons were made with
         this scale and the Paykel et al. [H23] life event scale. [See
         also H7.]

RC49.G85

H20   Jewell, Robert W.: A quantitative study of emotion: The Mag-
      nitude of Emotion Rating Scale. Unpublished medical thesis,
      University of Washington, 1977.
         Subjects: A sample of convenience composed of 158 adults
         (87 medical students and 71 nonstudent volunteers).
         Method: All subjects completed the Magnitude of Emotion
         Rating Questionnaire (MERQ), which asked subjects to rate
         the "amount of emotion" elicited by each of 42 life events
         in comparison to "marriage" (arbitrarily assigned a value
         of 500). Means scores were calculated for each event,
         divided by 10, and arranged in rank order to produce a
         ratio scale, the Magnitude of Emotion Rating Scale (MERS).
         Arithmetic and geometric mean item values were compared
         as measures of central tendency. Rank order correlation
         coefficients and coefficients of concordance were examined
         between demographic subgroups. The Magnitude of Emotion
         Rating Scale was compared to the Social Readjustment Rat-
         ing Scale by geometric mean values and rank ordering of
         life event items.

H21   Masuda, Minoru, and Holmes, Thomas H.: Magnitude esti-
      mations of social readjustments. Journal of Psychosomatic
      Research 11:219-225, 1967.

RC52.J6

Subjects: A sample of convenience composed of 394 U.S. adults.

Method: This study presents the results of further analysis of data reported in a companion article (H18) on the development of the Social Readjustment Rating Scale. The arithmetic mean value, the geometric mean value, and the median value of Social Readjustment Rating Questionnaire item scores and item rankings were calculated, compared, and evaluated as measures of central tendency. The relationship between variability (standard error) and magnitude of item scores was analyzed.

H22　Mendels, J., and Weinstein, N.: The Schedule of Recent Experiences: A reliability study. Psychosomatic Medicine 34: 527-531, 1972.

Subjects: 187 medical students.

Method: All subjects completed the Social Readjustment Rating Questionnaire, which asks subjects to rate the amount of readjustment required by each of 42 life events in comparison to "marriage" (arbitrarily assigned a value of 500). The effect on ratings of two experimental conditions was examined: receiving vs. not receiving a gift certificate for participating in the study, and following the original Social Readjustment Rating Questionnaire instructions devised by Holmes and Rahe vs. following modified instructions. Mean item values and rank orderings for the total sample were compared to those reported in Holmes and Rahe's original Social Readjustment Rating Questionnaire study. A group of subjects was also readministered the Social Readjustment Rating Questionnaire after a 1-year interval to study the consistency of life event magnitude ratings over time.

H23　Paykel, Eugene S.; Prusoff, Brigitte A.; and Uhlenhuth, Eberhard H.: Scaling of life events. Archives of General Psychiatry 25:340-347, 1971.

Subjects: 213 psychiatric patients (inpatient, outpatient, and day patients) and 160 relatives of patients from two facilities (New Haven and Chicago).

RC321A66 Method: All subjects completed a questionnaire that asked them to rate each of 61 life events on a scale of 0-20 to show "how upsetting or distressing" the event would be for the average person. After rating the life events list, subjects marked the events they had experienced in the past year. The mean item value and standard deviation were calculated for each event, and the 61 events were ranked in descending order of magnitude to form a life events scale.

H24 Rippere, Vicky: Scaling the seriousness of illness: A methodological study. Journal of Psychosomatic Research 20: 567-573, 1976.

Subjects: 71 medical students and 38 undergraduate psychology students.

Method: In Study 1, the medical students rated the seriousness of 15 illness conditions using a questionnaire modeled on the Paykel et al. [H23] interval scaling method: subjects rated on a scale of 0-20 "how worrying it would be to be told of having" each of the 15 illnesses. Mean ratings, standard deviations, and ranks were calculated for all items, and findings using the interval scaling method were compared to the ratio scale data of Wyler's Seriousness of Illness Rating Scale [H31]. In Study 2, the psychology students each completed two 15-item rating questionnaires: the interval scaling method was the same used in Study 1, and a ratio scaling method was employed by adopting Wyler's Seriousness of Illness Rating Questionnaire directions (to rate the "seriousness" of each disease in comparison to peptic ulcer, which had been arbitrarily assigned a value of 500). Rank order correlations of interval scale ratings and ratio scale ratings were examined within and between subject groups. The relative merits of direct interval scaling and magnitude estimation are discussed.

H25 Rosenberg, Emily J., and Dohrenwend, Barbara Snell: Effects of experience and ethnicity on ratings of life events as stressors. Journal of Health and Social Behavior 16: 127-129, 1975.

Subjects: 172 students at the City College of New York.

Method: Subjects were asked to rate the "amount of readjustment" required by each of 10 life events in comparison to the modulus item, "entered college" (which all subjects had experienced). Geometric mean ratings were calculated and compared between groups of subjects divided according to ethnicity (non-Hispanic Caucasian and Asian, Black, or Hispanic) and experience (judges with experience of the event vs. judges without experience). The interaction effects of age, sex, ethnicity, and experience were examined.

H26 Ruch, Libby Olive: Scaling of life stress with direct and indirect methods. Unpublished master's thesis, University of
Hawaii, 1967.
> Subjects: 211 University of Hawaii undergraduates (mean
> age of 18 years).
> Method: All subjects completed a questionnaire concerning
> demographic characteristics and two scaling questionnaires.
> The Social Readjustment Rating Questionnaire (SRRQ) asked
> subjects to rate on a scale of 0-1000 the "amount of read-
> justment" required by each of 42 life events in comparison
> to "marriage" (arbitrarily assigned a value of 500). A
> Paired Comparisons Questionnaire asked them to underline
> the life event in 55 pairs of events that "causes the most
> change in one's usual way of life." Mean item values and
> rank orders from this adolescent sample's SRRQ data were
> compared to data from Holmes and Rahe's original sample
> of 394 American adults. The results of direct (magnitude
> estimation) and indirect (paired comparisons) scaling meth-
> ods in this adolescent sample were compared and discussed.

H27 Ruch, Libby O., and Holmes, Thomas H.: Scaling of life
change: Comparison of direct and indirect methods. Journal
of Psychosomatic Research 15:221-227, 1971.

RC52.J6
> Subjects: 211 University of Hawaii undergraduates (mean
> age of 18 years).
> Method: This publication is based on data originally re-
> ported in the first author's master's thesis (H26).

H28 Tennant, Christopher, and Andrews, Gavin: A scale to measure the cause of life events. Australian and New Zealand
Journal of Psychiatry 11:163-167, 1977.
> Subjects: 105 Australian adults (professional and non-
> professional hospital employees).
> Method: All subjects completed a scaling questionnaire
> that asked them to rate three causal components of 67 life
> events: "Chance" (uncontrollable events), "Self" (attribut-
> able to the individual's behavior), and "Other(s)" (attribut-
> able to the behavior of other individuals). For each life
> event subjects allocated 10 points among the three causes
> to indicate the proportional contribution of each factor.
> Mean values were calculated for the three components of
> each event. The list of values is appended to the text.
> [See also H29.]

H29 Tennant, Christopher, and Andrews, Gavin: A scale to measure the stress of life events. <u>Australian and New Zealand Journal of Psychiatry</u> <u>10</u>:27-32, 1976.

> <u>Subjects</u>: 151 Australian adults.
> <u>Method</u>: An inventory of 67 life events was derived from the 43 items used by Holmes and Rahe and the 61 items used by Paykel et al. Subjects were twice asked to rate each of 66 events in comparison to the same index event, "a serious personal physical illness": the first time, subjects rated the amount of life change produced by each event, and the second time they rated the amount of emotional distress produced by the events. Arithmetic mean scores were calculated for all items, and two matched scales were produced: a life change scale (Holmes and Rahe concept) and an emotional distress scale (Paykel et al. concept). Consistency of ratings on each scale among sociodemographic subgroups was evaluated using rank order correlations. The two scales were compared to the earlier scales developed by Paykel et al. and by Holmes and Rahe with American subjects. Rank order correlations between the Australian life change and distress scales were also examined. [See also H28.]

H30 Wainer, Howard; Fairbank, Dianne Timbers; and Hough, Richard L.: Predicting the impact of simple and compound life change events. <u>Applied Psychological Measurement</u> <u>2</u>(3): 313-322, 1978.

> <u>Subjects</u>: In Study 1, a community sample (randomly drawn) of 355 adult residents in El Paso, Texas, and Cuidad Juarez, Chihuahua, Mexico; in Study 2, a convenience sample composed of 33 White-American and 41 Mexican-American college students.
> <u>Method</u>: In Study 1, subjects were asked to rate 95 life events on a 7-point scale (from events requiring "least change" to events requiring "most change"). Mean ratings across four subgroups (ethnic group and city of residence) were evaluated, and 51 of the 95 items were determined to fit a Rasch model of measurement (including sample-free item calibration). A 51-item Universal Event Impact Scale was produced. In Study 2, five events were selected as representative of the range of impacts in the 51-item scale and were used to create a paired comparisons questionnaire: subjects were asked to choose which event or combination of events had the "greatest impact" of the paired items. Data from the White-American and Mexican-American

subjects were analyzed separately and compared. Impact
values from Study 1 (Rasch-type latent trait analysis) were
transformed through different procedures in Study 2 to predict the values of the impact of compound events.

H31 Wyler, Allen R.; Masuda, Minoru; and Holmes, Thomas H.:
Seriousness of Illness Rating Scale. Journal of Psychosomatic Research 11:363-374, 1968.
    Subjects: 117 physicians and 141 nonphysicians.
    Method: All subjects completed the Seriousness of Illness
    Rating Questionnaire (SIRQ), which asked them to rate the
    seriousness of 125 diseases in comparison to a modulus
    item, "Peptic Ulcer" (arbitrarily assigned a value of 500).
    Geometric mean values and rank orders were calculated
    for each disease item, and differences between subgroups
    divided according to demographic and background charac-
    teristics were examined. Data from the medical and non-
    medical groups were analyzed separately, compared, and
    then combined: a new "grand" rank order and mean were
    calculated for each disease item to produce the Seriousness
    of Illness Rating Scale (SIRS).

H32 Wyler, Allen R.; Masuda, Minoru; and Holmes, Thomas H.:
The Seriousness of Illness Rating Scale: Reproducibility.
Journal of Psychosomatic Research 14:59-64, 1970.
    Subjects: In Sample 1, 117 physicians in an earlier study;
    in Sample 2, 203 physicians who returned mailed question-
    naires.
    Method: All subjects completed the Seriousness of Illness
    Rating Questionnaire, which asked them to rate the serious-
    ness of 125 diseases in comparison to a modulus item,
    "Peptic Ulcer" (arbitrarily assigned a value of 500). Re-
    producibility of the Seriousness of Illness Rating Scale
    [H31] was tested by comparing rank order and geometric
    mean scores of disease items from Sample 1 to those in
    Sample 2. Subjects in Sample 2 were divided into sub-
    groups according to six categories of physician speciality,
    and data were analyzed to determine differences in the
    scoring of individual disease items among the six speciali-
    ties.

METHODOLOGY:
Scaling Studies—Specific Populations
(H33-H57)

H33   Brandenburg, Carlos Enrique: Validation of the Social Re-
adjustment Rating Scale with Mexican-Americans and Native
Americans (Doctoral dissertation, University of Nevada, 1978).
Dissertation Abstracts International 39:4020B-4021B, 1979.
   Subjects: 30 Mexican-American adults, 33 Native American
   adults, and 34 young adult Caucasian college students.
   Method: Researchers Brandenburg and West [see H55]
   modified the Social Readjustment Rating Scale by adding 22
   new life events with particular relevance to ethnic groups.
   Mexican-American and Native American subjects were asked
   to rate the 22 Brandenburg-West events. Rank order correlations were examined between the two ethnic groups, and
   mean scores of the Brandenburg-West items were compared
   to mean item scores in the Social Readjustment Rating Scale.
   The 22 new items were added to the Schedule of Recent Experience (SRE), and the SRE and the modified SRE were compared for predictive power in a study of life change and
   health change in the two ethnic groups. The college student
   subjects participated in a test-retest reliability study of the
   Brandenburg-West 22 items and the 43 Holmes and Rahe
   items.

25053.D57

H34   Cichon, Donald J., and Koff, Robert H.: The Teaching Events
Stress Inventory. A paper presented at the Annual Meeting of
the American Educational Research Association, Toronto,
Ontario, Canada, in March, 1978. [Reprint requests: Robert
H. Koff, Dean of the College of Education, Roosevelt University, 430 S. Michigan Avenue, Chicago, Illinois 60605.]
   Subjects: 4,934 teachers employed by the Chicago Board of
   Education.
   Method: The authors developed a list of 36 "stressful"
   events associated with teaching in elementary and secondary
   schools. Subjects completed and returned by mail a two-
   part questionnaire. Part 1 collected demographic data and
   background information (including current teaching position,
   school makeup, general health, and sick days in past year).
   Part 2 asked subjects to rate the "stressfulness" of each of
   35 teaching events in comparison to "first week of school"
   (arbitrarily assigned a value of 500). Any responses greater
   than 1,000 were reduced to 1,000, and all ratings were
   divided by 10. Mean item values and rank order were then

calculated, and the 36 events were arranged in descending order of magnitude to produce a scale called the Teaching Events Stress Inventory (TESI). Discriminant function analysis was performed between demographic subgroups to evaluate the stability of the sample's ratings. Suggestions for further research are offered.

H35   Cline, David W.: A stress-value scale for officer candidates. Journal of Psychosomatic Research 17:15-20, 1973.

RC 52. J6

Subjects: 191 cadets in training at an officer candidate school (Wisconsin Military Academy).
Method: The author interviewed officers and cadets to generate a list of 24 stressful events encountered by cadets in their daily experience at the training academy. The list was used to create a questionnaire called the Schedule of Daily Experience (SDE), which asked subjects how many times each of the 24 events had been experienced in the past 24 hours. A Stress-Value Scale (SVS) to score the SDE was created by asking 191 cadets to rate on a scale of 0-1,000 the "stressfulness" of each of 27 events in comparison to "written examination" (arbitrarily assigned a value of 500). Mean item scores (divided by 10) and rank order were calculated for all items, and they were arranged in descending order of magnitude to produce the Stress-Value Scale. Correlations of SVS ratings were examined between discrete groups in the sample. Two "total daily stress" scores were also calculated for a group of 134 cadets (daily SDE data for 2 weeks), using mean values from the SVS and also the cadet's individual stress value ratings to score the SDE data. Correlations between the two scores were examined.

H36   Coddington, R. Dean: The significance of life events as etiologic factors in the disease of children. I. A survey of professional workers. Journal of Psychosomatic Research 16: 7-18, 1972.

RC52.J6

Subjects: 131 teachers, 25 pediatricians, and 87 mental health professionals in child psychiatry divisions.
Method: The Social Readjustment Rating Questionnaire (SRRQ) was modified to determine the significance of life events for children in four age groups. Subjects were asked to use their personal and professional experience to rate the "amount of social readjustment" required of children in each age group by each life event in comparison to "birth of a brother or sister" (arbitrarily assigned a value of 500).

There were 30 life events in Coddington's SRRQ for preschool children, 36 life events for the elementary school
age group, 40 for junior high school, and 42 for senior high
school. Geometric mean item values and rank order were
calculated, and a Social Readjustment Rating Scale for each
age group was constructed by arranging life events in a descending order of mean values (Life Change Units). Rank
order correlations between discrete groups of raters (by
professional experience and demographic variables) were
examined. [See also Parts II (A16) and III (H89).]

H37 Gerst, Marvin S.; Grant, Igor; Yager, Joel; and Sweetwood,
Hervey: The reliability of the Social Readjustment Rating
Scale: Moderate and long-term stability. Journal of Psycho-
somatic Research 22:519-523, 1978.

Subjects: 159 male psychiatric outpatients and 213 male
nonpatient control subjects.
Method: A modified Social Readjustment Rating Questionnaire was administered to all subjects three times during a
2-year period. The reliability of ratings by patients and by
controls was tested by comparing rank order correlations
and stability of magnitude weights over time, for all items
and for 11 item-subgroups. Differences between ratings
by patients and by controls were examined.

H38 Grant, Igor; Gerst, Marvin; and Yager, Joel: Scaling of life
events by psychiatric patients and normals. Journal of Psychosomatic Research 20:141-149, 1976.

Subjects: 171 male psychiatric patients, a comparison
group of 181 male "normals," and 165 relatives living with
patients and normals.

Method: All subjects completed a modified Social Readjustment Rating Questionnaire (25 original Holmes and Rahe
items plus 18 new or revised items), following the original
Holmes and Rahe rating instructions. Mean item values
(divided by 10) and rank order were calculated for the total
sample and for each group of subjects; a Social Readjustment
Rating Scale was constructed for all groups. Overall reliability of life event scaling was examined by comparing rank
ordering of comparable items by (a) normals in this study
vs. the original Holmes and Rahe sample of 394 adults and
(b) this study's patients and patient relatives (N=242) vs.
Paykel's sample of 373 patients and relatives. Scaling differences between patients and controls in this sample were
examined by comparing rank ordering of events, assignment

of item magnitudes, and the effect of having experienced the event.

H39 Helper, Malcolm M.; Cohen, Richard L.; Beitenman, Edward T.; and Eaton, Louise F.: Life-events and acceptance of pregnancy. Journal of Psychosomatic Research 12:183-188, 1968.

Subjects: Six groups of women (N=129) drawn from 1 civic and 2 church groups, from a secretarial association and a class of nursing students, and from a hospital obstetric clinic.

RC52.J6

Method: Two lists were developed of life events which could affect a woman's adjustment to pregnancy: List 1 contained 21 items referring to events during pregnancy, and List 2 contained 34 items referring to events prior to pregnancy. All subjects were asked to rate "the amount of difficulty the event would create for adjustment to pregnancy" in comparison to an anchor item which had been arbitrarily assigned a value of 500. For List 1, the anchor item was "Being deserted by husband"; for List 2, the item was "Loss of mother before the age of 12." Mean item values and rank order were calculated for each of the six groups, and rank order correlations were examined between all groups. Scales of "Composite Stress Ratings" for life events during pregnancy (List 1) and prior to pregnancy (List 2) were constructed using mean item values from three groups (N=65) whose correlations were all above .60.

H40 Komaroff, Anthony L.: Magnitude estimations of life change events in two American minority subculture groups. Unpublished medical thesis, University of Washington, 1967.

Subjects: 64 blacks and 78 Mexican-Americans living in Los Angeles, California.

Method: The Social Readjustment Rating Questionnaire (SRRQ) was modified slightly before the questionnaire was completed by all subjects (wording of the 43 items was simplified and instructions for rating were explained out loud). Geometric mean item values and rank order were calculated for each group, and data from these two groups were compared to SRRQ data from Holmes and Rahe's original sample of 394 middle-class white Americans. Rank order correlations were examined, and differences in magnitude estimations between the two subcultures and the white American group were studied. An analysis of variance was performed on each of the 43 life event items rated by the three groups.

H41 Komaroff, Anthony L.; Masuda, Minoru; and Holmes, Thomas
H.: The Social Readjustment Rating Scale: A comparative
study of Negro, Mexican, and White Americans. Journal of
Psychosomatic Research 12:121-128, 1968.

    Subjects: 64 blacks and 78 Mexican-Americans living in
Los Angeles and a predominantly white sample of 394
adults in the Pacific Northwest.
    Method: This publication is based on data originally re-
ported in the first author's medical thesis (H40).

H42 Libby, Ellen Weber: Perceptions of stressful life events: A
comparison between physically disabled and non-disabled adults
(Doctoral dissertation, University of Maryland, 1977). Dissertation Abstracts International 38:3368B-3369B, 1978.

    Subjects: Severely physically disabled adults (N=unstated].
    Method: Subjects, who were clients at Maryland vocational
rehabilitation agencies, completed the Social Readjustment
Rating Questionnaire. They also completed the Acceptance
of Disability Scale, and their counselors' ratings of client
acceptance of disability were obtained through a Service
Outcome Measurement Form. Disabled adults' rank-order-
ings of life events were compared to those of nondisabled
adults (as represented by the original Holmes and Rahe
Social Readjustment Rating Scale "norms"). The effect of
age, marital status, sex, age at disability onset, and acceptance of disability on disabled subjects' perceptions of
life events were also examined.

H43 Lundberg, Ulf, and Theorell, Tores: Scaling of life changes:
Differences between three diagnostic groups and between re-
cently experienced and nonexperienced events. Journal of
Human Stress 2(2):7-17, 1976.

    Subjects: 66 myocardial infarction patients, 78 neurotic
patients, and 127 lower back pain patients plus matched
control subjects for all patients.
    Method: A list of 46 life change events was developed.
Patients and controls were divided into comparable subgroups, each of which was asked to rate the 46 life events
in different ways (magnitude estimation vs. graphical ratings) and in different terms (how much "adjustment" the
events would require vs. how "upsetting" the events would
be). Raters were told to base their responses on personal
opinion, rather than on the "average person's" experience.
Mean scale values were calculated. Differences between
estimates of "adjustment" and "upset" were examined.

Each diagnostic group's ratings were compared to its control group's ratings on both the "Upset scale" and the "Adjustment scale," and all males were compared to all females on both scales. Data on the occurrence of life events in the year prior to infarction had been obtained earlier from myocardial infarction patients and their controls. For those subjects, differences in the scaling of recently experienced and nonexperienced events were investigated.

H44 Masuda, Minoru, and Holmes, Thomas H.: Life events: Perceptions and frequencies. Psychosomatic Medicine 40: 236-261, 1978.

Subjects: 3,783 subjects in 19 studies emanating from the authors' laboratory since 1967.
Method: All subjects had completed the Schedule of Recent Experience (SRE) and/or the Social Readjustment Rating Questionnaire (SRRQ). Data from the 19 studies were collated to study the extent and source of variability in perceptions of life events (magnitude estimations) and the frequency of occurrence of life events. Geometric mean scores and rank order were used to compare the 7 SRRQ studies, and the SRE data from 12 studies were compared after calculating a "mean annual life event frequency per individual." Variables examined for their effect on magnitude estimations and/or life event frequencies included the following: age, sex, educational level, marital status, social class, race, and having experienced the event.

H45 Masuda, Minoru; Wong, N.; Felicetta, Anthony; and Holmes, Thomas H.: Magnitude estimation of current illness. Psychosomatic Medicine 37:92-93, 1975. (Abstract)

Subjects: 48 tuberculosis patients, 48 hypertension patients, and 47 depression patients, all males with a diagnosis of recent onset or exacerbation of illness.
Method: All subjects completed an abridged (23-item) version of Wyler's Seriousness of Illness Rating Questionnaire (H31). Magnitude estimations and rank ordering of the 23 illnesses by the three patient groups were compared. The effect of currently experiencing an illness on the perception of the seriousness of that illness was examined for each patient group.

H46 Miller, F. T.; Bentz, W. K.; Aponte, J. F.; and Brogan, D. R.: Perception of life crisis events: A comparative study of rural and urban samples. In Stressful Life Events: Their

Nature and Effects. Barbara Snell Dohrenwend and Bruce P. Dohrenwend (Eds.), pp. 259-273. New York: Wiley, 1974.

Subjects: A random sample of 96 adults living in a rural county in North Carolina and the Holmes and Rahe sample of 394 urban adults studied in their original Social Readjustment Rating Scale study.

Method: The Social Readjustment Rating Questionnaire was modified for use with the rural sample: three items were subdivided to make a total of 46 life events, and the method of administration was changed (instructions were presented verbally and a histogram scaled in units of 50 from 0-1,000 was used as a visual aid). Arithmetic and geometric mean item values and rank order were calculated for the rural sample, and results were compared to the Holmes and Rahe urban sample and to Komaroff's urban sample of blacks and Mexican-Americans [H41]. Rural-urban similarities and differences were investigated by rank order correlation, t-tests of differences in the distributions of means, and factor analysis of transformed individual responses.

H47   Moorehead, Nita Faye Brown: Differences between black and white students' perception of stress in life events (Doctoral dissertation, East Texas State University, 1974). Dissertation Abstracts International 35:4164-A, 1974-75.

Subjects: 140 black and 291 white college students enrolled in sociology classes.

Method: All subjects completed two questionnaires: Harris's modified Social Readjustment Rating Questionnaire for college students [see B52] and Rotter's Internal-External Locus of Control Scale. Differences in perceptions of life events (item scores) were examined in relation to race, sex, and locus of control orientation.

H48   Muhlenkamp, Ann F.; Gress, Lucille D.; and Flood, Mary A.: Perception of life change events by the elderly. Nursing Research 24:109-113, 1975.

Subjects: 8 male and 33 female members of a senior citizens' club, aged 65-84.

Method: All subjects completed a modified Social Readjustment Rating Questionnaire, which asked them to rate on a scale of 0-100 the "amount of adjustment" required by each of 42 life events in comparison to "marriage" (arbitrarily assigned a value of 50). Mean item values and rank order were calculated for all events. Results from the elderly sample were compared to mean values and ranks for the "normative" sample in Holmes and Rahe's original Social Readjustment Rating Scale study.

H49 Packard, Nancy J.: A comparison of the perceptions of life change events among low income elderly persons living in the inner-city and low income elderly persons living in the outer-city. Unpublished master's thesis, University of Washington, 1978.

Subjects: 37 inner-city and 41 outer-city residents of housing facilities for the low-income elderly.
Method: All subjects completed a 2-part questionnaire: Part 1 was a slightly modified Social Readjustment Rating Questionnaire (SRRQ) and Part 2 collected data on demographic characteristics, patterns of social contacts, self-report health status, and patterns of residence. Mean item values and rank order were calculated from the SRRQ data and were compared between the inner-city and the outer-city samples. They were also compared to SRRQ data from another elderly sample (N=41) studied by Muhlenkamp [H48] and from Holmes and Rahe's "normative" sample of 394 middle-class adults.

H50 Pasley, Suzanne: The Social Readjustment Rating Scale: A study of the significance of life events in age groups ranging from college freshmen to seventh grade. Unpublished paper submitted as part of a Tutorial in Psychology, Chatham College, 1969.

Subjects: 433 young people in four age groups (217 college freshmen, 44 eleventh-graders, 74 ninth-graders, and 98 seventh-graders).
Method: All subjects completed the Social Readjustment Rating Questionnaire (SRRQ) after wording of instructions and items had been simplified. Mean item values and rank order were calculated, a Social Readjustment Rating Scale was constructed for each age group, and data were compared to "baseline" values and ranks in Holmes and Rahe's original sample of 394 adults. Between-group consensus was analyzed, and interindividual concordance was also analyzed for each age group.

H51 Paykel, Eugene S., and Uhlenhuth, Eberhard H.: Rating the magnitude of life stress. Canadian Psychiatric Association Journal 17 (Special Supplement II):SS93-100, 1972.

Subjects: 213 psychiatric patients and 160 relatives of patients.

Method: This is the text of a paper read in October 1970 at a Research Conference on Psychiatric Crossroads held in Montreal. The data presented in this study were subsequently published in 1971 (see H23).

H52 Schless, Arthur P.; Schwartz, L.; Goetz, Christopher; and Mendels, J.: How depressives view the significance of life events. British Journal of Psychiatry 125:406–410, 1974.

Subjects: 76 consecutively admitted inpatients with the clinical syndrome of depression.

Method: All subjects completed two questionnaires at admission to the study and again at discharge from the hospital. They completed a modified Social Readjustment Rating Questionnaire (the modulus item was assigned a value of 50, and subjects were also asked to indicate which events they had experienced and when). They also completed the Beck Depression Inventory (to measure severity of psychiatric symptoms). Mean item values and rank order were calculated for patients at admission and for patients at discharge, and depressives' ratings were compared to "normative" mean values and rank order from the original Holmes and Rahe sample of 394 adults. Depressives' ratings were examined in relation to patient's age, sex, severity of depression, experience with events, and symptomatic improvement.

H53 Volicer, Beverly J.: Patients' perceptions of stressful events associated with hospitalization. Nursing Research 23:235–238, 1974.

Subjects: 47 hospital patients on surgical, medical, and cancer wards.

Method: All subjects completed an interview questionnaire that asked them to rate the "stress" produced by each of 44 events related to hospitalization in comparison to "emergency admission" (arbitrarily assigned a value of 50). Mean item values and rank order were calculated for the total sample and for each patient subgroup, and results were compared to ratings from a nonhospitalized sample (N=216) studied earlier [see H15]. Correlations were examined between the total hospital sample and the nonhospitalized sample and among the hospital subgroups (23 surgical, 13 cancer, and 11 medical patients) on "all items," "highest 23 items," and "lowest 22 items."

H54   Volicer, Beverly J., and Bohannon, Mary Wynne: A hospital
       stress rating scale. Nursing Research 24:352-359, 1975.
           Subjects: 216 medical and surgical patients at a community
           hospital.
           Method: A previously developed list of 45 events [see H15]
           was reworded and expanded to 77 items, pretested, and
           again revised to produce a final list of 49 stressful events
           associated with hospitalization. An earlier rating proce-
           dure adapted from the Social Readjustment Rating Ques-
           tionnaire was also revised: the new "card sort" procedure
           required subjects to rate the "stressfulness" of the 49
           events by first dividing 49 cards into three piles (represent-
           ing high, medium, and low stress) and then arranging the
           cards in each pile from "most" (top card) to "least" stress-
           ful (bottom card). The recombined stack of cards was then
           recorded as the subject's rank ordering of the 49 events. A
           mean rank score was calculated for each event, and final
           rank was assigned in ascending order of magnitude (Rank 1 =
           least stressful) to produce the Hospital Stress Rating Scale.
           Rank correlations were examined between subgroups by
           demographic variables and hospitalization variables (type
           of patient, length of stay, seriousness of illness) for "all
           items," "highest 25 items," and "lowest 24 items."

H55   West, John Pettigrew: The Social Readjustment Rating Scale:
       A study of life events and prediction of illness onset in the
       Afro-American (Doctoral dissertation, University of Nevada,
       Reno, 1978). Dissertation Abstracts International 39:2532B-
       2533B, 1978.
           Subjects: Afro-American and white subjects [N=unstated].
           Method: Researchers Brandenburg [see H33] and West
           modified the Social Readjustment Rating Scale by adding 22
           new life events with particular relevance to ethnic minori-
           ties. Afro-American and white subjects were asked to rate
           the 22 Brandenburg-West events, and differences in the
           numerical values they assigned were examined. The
           Brandenburg-West 22 items were added to the Holmes and
           Rahe 43 items in the Schedule of Recent Experience (SRE),
           and the SRE and the modified SRE were compared for pre-
           dictive power in a study of life change and health change in
           Afro-American subjects. A group of introductory psychology
           students rated the Brandenburg-West 22 items and the orig-
           inal Holmes and Rahe 43 items; the impact of the new items
           was compared to the impact of the other items.

H56   Wyatt, Gail Elizabeth: A comparison of the scaling of Afro-Americans' life change events. Journal of Human Stress 3(1): 13-18, 1977.

> Subjects: 40 Afro-American women in a program for parents and preschool children in South Central Los Angeles.
> Method: The Recent Life Changes Questionnaire was administered individually to each subject. For each of the 55 events, the standard event rating (Social Readjustment Rating Scale mean item values) was compared to the mean subjective ratings (personal readjustment required by event, using a scale of 1-100) of the Afro-American women who had experienced the event in the past 6 months. Ratings were compared to findings of Komaroff et al. [H41] in their study of Los Angeles blacks.

H57   Yamamoto, Kathleen J., and Kinney, Dennis K.: Pregnant women's ratings of different factors influencing psychological stress during pregnancy. Psychological Reports 39:203-214, 1976.

> Subjects: 58 low-income pregnant women.
> Method: A battery of questionnaires was administered to each subject 4-6 weeks before her delivery date: a 69-item checklist of life events (occurrence of events during "year before pregnancy" and "during pregnancy"), a life events rating questionnaire (rating "relative stressfulness" of 69 events on a scale of 1-99), a measure of coping resources, the Manifest Anxiety Scale, and the Lie Scale of the MMPI. Mean item values and rank order were calculated for the sample's life event ratings, and they were arranged in descending order of magnitude to produce a scale of "stress ratings." Life event scores were calculated three ways: using each woman's own ratings of the events, "correcting" raw scores to control for possible bias (using larger numbers), and using mean item values from the total samples' "stress ratings." The three methods were compared. The relation of life events scores to other measures was also examined.

METHODOLOGY:
Scaling Studies—Cross-Cultural Studies
(H58-H69)

H58   Boleloucky, Z.; Horvath, M.; and Kovalik, O.: Social readjustment questionnaire in a group of research workers. Activitas Nervosa Superior (Prague) 17:43, 1975.

Subjects: 141 Czech men working as scientists in engineering research.

Method: The Social Readjustment Rating Questionnaire was translated and administered to subjects. Items rated higher than the modulus item ("getting married") by this sample were compared to items marked higher than the modulus item by the Holmes and Rahe American sample. All subjects also completed the Mental Health Questionnaire (MHQ) and were divided into subgroups by high MHQ scores (N=94) and low MHQ scores (N=47). The relation of MHQ scores to rating of life events (items rated "higher than average" and "lower than average") was examined.

H59   Celdran, Harriet Hoag: The cross-cultural consistency of two social consensus scales: The Seriousness of Illness Rating Scale and the Social Readjustment Rating Scale in Spain. Unpublished medical thesis, University of Washington, 1970.

Subjects: Two samples of convenience (N=128 and N=212) composed of Spanish subjects aged 16-90.

Method: The Seriousness of Illness Rating Questionnaire [H31] was translated into Spanish, and the questionnaire was completed by 128 Spaniards. Mean item values and rank order were calculated for the 126 diseases, and the effect of sex, age, and education on magnitude ratings was examined. Spanish data were compared to mean item values and rank ordering of Wyler's American nonphysician sample of 141 [H31] and to McMahon's Irish sample of 291 [H63]. The Social Readjustment Rating Questionnaire was also translated into Spanish, and it was completed by 212 Spaniards. Mean item values and rank order were calculated for all life events, and the effect of sex, age, and education on ratings was examined. Cross-cultural consensus was examined using rank order correlations: Spanish data were compared to data from middle-class U.S. residents [H18], Japanese from two cities [H62], French-speaking Western Europeans [H60], and U.S. blacks and Mexican-Americans [H41].

H60   Harmon, David K.; Masuda, Minoru; and Holmes, Thomas H.: The Social Readjustment Rating Scale: A cross-cultural study of Western Europeans and Americans. Journal of Psychosomatic Research 14:391-400, 1970.

Subjects: A sample of convenience composed of 202 Western Europeans (90 French, 65 Belgian, and 47 Swiss) and a corresponding U.S. sample of 195 from Holmes and Rahe's original Social Readjustment Rating Scale study [H18].

Method: The Social Readjustment Rating Questionnaire was translated into French and administered to European subjects. Mean item values and rank order were calculated for each national group. Differences within national groups on the basis of sex and religion were examined. Mean item scores and rank order were compared among national groups and also between a composite European sample of 139 and the selected U.S. sample.

H61 Isherwood, Janette, and Adam, Kenneth S.: The Social Readjustment Rating Scale: A cross-cultural study of New Zealanders and Americans. Journal of Psychosomatic Research 20:211-214, 1976.

Subjects: A sample of convenience composed of 67 middle-class New Zealanders.

Method: The Social Readjustment Rating Questionnaire was completed by all subjects. Mean item values (arithmetic and geometric means) and rank order were calculated for all events. Product-moment and rank order correlation coefficients were used to compare the New Zealand data to the American SRRQ data obtained from Holmes and Rahe's sample of 394 middle- and lower-class adults [H18].

RC 52.J6

H62 Masuda, Minoru, and Holmes, Thomas H.: The Social Readjustment Rating Scale: A cross-cultural study of Japanese and Americans. Journal of Psychosomatic Research 11:227-237, 1967.

Subjects: Two Japanese samples of convenience from Hiroshima (N=55) and Sendai (N=57) and an American sample of 168 selected from Holmes and Rahe's original Social Readjustment Rating Scale study [H18].

RC 52.J6

Method: The Social Readjustment Rating Questionnaire was translated into Japanese and administered to Japanese subjects. Geometric mean item values and rank order were calculated and compared among the four Japanese subgroups (divided according to site and sex). The total Japanese sample was compared to mean item values and rank order of the selected American sample. Rank order correlations were examined, and items scored significantly different were studied.

H63 McMahon, Brian James: Seriousness of Illness Rating Scale: A comparative study of Irish and Americans. Unpublished medical thesis, University of Washington, 1971.

Subjects: 290 Irish subjects and 141 American subjects (the nonphysician sample from Wyler's original Seriousness of Illness Rating Scale study [H31]).

Method: All subjects completed the Seriousness of Illness Rating Questionnaire. Geometric mean item values and rank order were calculated for the 126 disease items, and ratings from the Irish sample were compared to Wyler's American sample. Items scored significantly different by each national group were examined, and rating differences among Irish subjects (by geographic area and age subgroups) were also studied.

H64 Paykel, E. S.; McGuiness, B.; and Gomez, J.: An Anglo-American comparison of the scaling of life events. British Journal of Medical Psychology 49:237-247, 1976.

Subjects: An English sample of 183 (113 psychiatric patients and 70 relatives of patients) and a matched American sample (selected from the 1971 Paykel et al. sample of 213 patients and relatives [H23]).

RC321B83

Method: All subjects completed a questionnaire that asked them to rate on a scale of 0-20 how "upsetting" 61 life events would be for the average person. Mean scaling scores and standard deviations were calculated for each event, corrections were made for systematic differences in levels, and the English sample was compared to the American sample. Events were grouped into a number of categories (area of activity, exits vs. entrances, desirability, and controllability) and scaling scores from the two samples were examined for significant differences. Frequency of event occurrence was compared between the English and American samples (based on reports of events in the past year).

H65 Rahe, Richard H.: Multi-cultural correlations of life change scaling: America, Japan, Denmark and Sweden. Journal of Psychosomatic Research 13:191-195, 1969.

Subjects: Four American subcultural groups (168 middle-class Caucasians, 64 lower-class blacks, 78 lower-class Mexican-Americans, and 200 native Hawaiians) and three national groups (112 middle-class Japanese, 95 Danish university students, and 75 Swedish university seniors).

RC52.J6

Method: Life change scaling data were collated from published and unpublished studies. All subjects but the Hawaiians had completed the Social Readjustment Rating Questionnaire; a modified instrument was administered to the relatively uneducated Hawaiian subjects, using a card-sort procedure to scale life events in six categories of gradation. Rank ordering of life events was compared across the seven cultural and subcultural groups.

H66 Rahe, Richard H.; Lunberg, Ulf; Bennett, Linda; and Theorell, Tores: The Social Readjustment Rating Scale: A comparative study of Swedes and Americans. Journal of Psychosomatic Research 15:241-249, 1971.

Subjects: Two Swedish samples (75 university students and 82 middle-aged men) and two matched American samples (drawn from Holmes and Rahe's original Social Readjustment Rating Scale study [H18]).
Method: The Social Readjustment Rating Questionnaire was translated into Swedish with modified scaling instructions. The younger Swedes rated life events in comparison to "marriage," which was assigned a value of 100; the older Swedes rated life events against a different modulus item, "addition of new family member," and used a different value range (1-10). Data were normalized in order to compare the Swedish and American samples. Geometric mean item values and rank orderings were compared between matched national samples. Mean item values were compared within and between national and age groups, using actual and ideal regression equations to illustrate variance between pairs of samples.

H67 Seppa, Mark Timothy: The Social Readjustment Rating Scale and the Seriousness of Illness Rating Scale: A comparison of Salvadorans, Spanish, and Americans. Unpublished medical thesis, University of Washington, 1972.

Subjects: A sample of convenience composed of 197 Salvadorans.
Method: Celdran's [H59] Spanish translation of the Social Readjustment Rating Questionnaire was completed by all subjects in El Salvador. Geometric mean item values and rank order were calculated for all events, and rank order correlations were examined between the Salvadorans, Celdran's Spanish sample (N=212), and Holmes and Rahe's original U.S. sample (N=394) [H18]. Celdran's Spanish translation of Wyler's Seriousness of Illness Rating Questionnaire was also completed by 153 Salvadorans. Mean item values and rank order were calculated for the 126 disease items, and the Salvadoran sample was compared to Celdran's Spanish sample (N=128) and to Wyler's U.S. sample (N=141 nonphysicians) [H31].

H68 Valdes, Thusnelda M., and Baxter, James C.: The Social Readjustment Rating Questionnaire: A study of Cuban exiles.
Journal of Psychosomatic Research 20:231-236, 1976.

Subjects: 117 Cuban exiles (who were at least 15 when they
left Cuba).

Method: All subjects completed a questionnaire containing
both an English and a Spanish version of a modified Social
Readjustment Rating Questionnaire (expanded to 60 items
and with a prescribed rating scale limit of 1-1,000). Arithmetic mean item values, median scores, and rank orders
were calculated for the 60 life events, and data were compared to corresponding data from the American sample
(N=394) of Holmes and Rahe's original Social Readjustment
Rating Scale study [H18]. Rank order correlation coefficients were calculated between ranks of U.S. and Cuban
mean values and between ranks of U.S. and Cuban median
scores. Significant differences in item ranking were discussed.

H69 Woon, Tai-Hwang; Masuda, Minoru; Wagner, Nathaniel N.;
and Holmes, Thomas H.: The Social Readjustment Rating
Scale: A cross-cultural study of Malaysians and Americans.
Journal of Cross-Cultural Psychology 2:373-386, 1971.

Subjects: 266 Malaysian medical students and 195 selectively matched Americans (data from Holmes and Rahe's
original Social Readjustment Rating Scale study [H18]).

Method: All subjects completed the Social Readjustment
Rating Questionnaire. Geometric mean item values and
rank order were calculated for all events. Ratings from
the Malaysian and American samples were compared, and
the Malaysian sample was also compared to an older Japanese sample studied earlier by Masuda and Holmes [H62].
Rank order correlations were examined between discrete
subgroups in the Malaysian sample (by race, religion, sex,
year of medical class, and generation Malaysian). Cross-
cultural differences and subcultural differences were examined.

METHODOLOGY:
Qualities of Life Events
(H70-H81)

H70 Chiriboga, David A., and Dean, Hannah: Dimensions of stress:
Perspectives from a longitudinal study. Journal of Psychosomatic Research 22:47-55, 1978.

Subjects: 182 adults in four age groups (high school seniors, newlyweds, middle-aged parents, and men and women facing retirement) who participated in a 5-year longitudinal study of life transitions.

Method: All subjects were interviewed in 1969, 1971, and 1974, and measures of psychosocial adjustment were administered at each interview. In 1974 subjects completed the Life Events Questionnaire (LEQ), a 138-item inventory that asked them to indicate life events experienced in the past 3 years, their feelings (positive or negative) toward reported events, and degree of current preoccupation with the event. Nine "dimensions of stress" were analyzed by classifying events into roles and activities (marital and dating, family, habits and appearance, nonfamily relationships, personal, legal, financial, work, home). LEQ data were used to calculate "negative preoccupation" scores (incidence, degree of unhappiness, and degree of intrusiveness) for each subject in each stress dimension. The distribution of the stress dimensions was compared for men and women in the four age groups. The relation of stress dimensions (negative preoccupation scores) to changes in psychosocial adjustment (measures of self-dissatisfaction, depression, psychological symptoms, self-report health, and activity scope) was analyzed using stepwise multiple regression techniques. [See also H87.]

H71 Dohrenwend, Barbara Snell: Life events as stressors: A methodological inquiry. Journal of Health and Social Behavior 14:167-175, 1973.

Subjects: A systematic sample of 124 adults.
Method: All subjects were interviewed using a checklist of 26 life events (plus an "other: explain" option) covering occurrences in the past 12 months. They were also administered Langner's 22-item index of symptoms. Four life event scores were calculated for each subject: two weighting systems for "undesirability" (losses minus gains) and two weighting systems for "amount of change entailed" (values from the Social Readjustment Rating Scale) were used. The measures of "life change" and of "undesirability" were compared. Correlations between life event measures and measures of psychological symptoms were examined.

H72 Gersten, Joanne C.; Langner, Thomas S.; Eisenberg, Jeanne G.; and Orzeck, Lida: Child behavior and life events: Undesirable change or change per se? In Stressful Life Events:

Their Nature and Effects. Barbara Snell Dohrenwend and Bruce P. Dohrenwend (Eds.), pp. 159-170. New York: Wiley, 1974.

> Subjects: 674 children and young adults living in Manhattan. Method: Mothers of subjects were interviewed at Time 1 and at Time 2 (5 years later) to collect data for 11 measures of child's psychological impairment and behavior. At Time 2 mothers also provided information about the occurrence of 25 life events in the 5 years between interviews. Researchers assigned a "desirability rating" (Undesirable, Desirable, or Ambiguous—all with a simple weight of 1) and a "social readjustment weight" (adapted from Coddington's Social Readjustment Rating Scale for children [H36]) to each of the 25 events. Six life event scoring and weighting methods were devised to compare measures of desirability and change. Correlations of the six life event measures with the 11 measures of psychological impairment and behavior change were examined.

H73   Hart, William Randall: Rheumatoid arthritis, depression, and preceding life events: A study of event desirability, anticipation, control, and coping effectiveness (Doctoral dissertation, Indiana University, 1978). Dissertation Abstracts International 39:5556B-5557B, 1979.

> Subjects: 25 subjects suffering from rheumatoid arthritis, 25 psychiatric inpatients being treated for depression, and 25 control subjects (no history of psychiatric or major physical illness).
>
> Method: Each subject was interviewed about the occurrence of 60 life events. Subjects were asked to date each reported event, and then to rate the following factors on a 5-point scale: desirability of event, degree to which it was anticipated, amount of control over event's occurrence, and the effectiveness of their coping with the event. Subject groups were compared on 18 variables including the following: life event qualities and frequencies in three time periods (5 years before illness onset, from birth to onset year, and entire life span), and scores for "average lifetime" desirability, anticipation, and control of life events.

H74   Klassen, Deidre; Roth, Aleda; and Hornstra, Robijn K.: Perception of life events as gains or losses in a community survey. Journal of Community Psychology 2:330-336, 1974.

> Subjects: A probability sample of 190 adults in Kansas City.

Method: All subjects were asked to rate a list of 40 life events as "a good thing or a bad thing for most people," marking gains with a "+" and losses with a "-." Investigators used 70% agreement as the minimum in defining events as gains and losses, and "don't know" responses were tabulated as ambiguous events. Data were compared to Dohrenwend's designated ratings of events as desirable, undesirable, or ambiguous. Ratings of the Kansas City sample were compared across discrete subgroups (age, sex, marital status, education, and race of subjects).

H75 Mond, Michael: The rating of life-events for stress in a college student sample (Doctoral dissertation, University of Wisconsin-Milwaukee, 1975). Dissertation Abstracts International 37:1443-B, 1976.
Subjects: 420 college students.
Method: All subjects completed a questionnaire which asked them to rate the "stress" of life events. Differences in ratings were studied in relation to four "concepts": "referent person" (is stress different for the average person vs. the average college student), "relevance" (could rater ever experience the event), "concern" (has rater ever been concerned about the event), and "experience" (has rater ever experienced the event). One life event was modified 27 times to test the effect of item definition (degree of information and level of desirability) on "stress" ratings.

H76 Mueller, Daniel P.; Edwards, Daniel W.; and Yarvis, Richard M.: Stressful life events and psychiatric symptomatology: Change or undesirability? Journal of Health and Social Behavior 18:307-317, 1977.
Subjects: 363 randomly selected adults in Sacramento, California.

Method: During a home interview each subject was administered two scales measuring psychiatric symptoms and distress (Langner's 22-item index and a slightly modified version of Depuy's General Well-Being Schedule). Subjects also completed a 40-item life events checklist (modified Schedule of Recent Experience) indicating the ocurrence of events in the past 30 days and designating each reported event as a desirable or undesirable experience.
Life events data were analyzed using four scoring methods (desirable events only, undesirable only, undesirable minus desirable, and all events) and two weighting systems (simple unit-weighting vs. social readjustment scores). Correlations

between the eight life events measures and the two measures of psychological status were examined. Data were compared to findings in three published studies: Dohrenwend's New York adults [H71], the Gersten et al. study of children and young adults [H72], and Vinokur and Selzer's study of male drivers [H79]. Findings from the four studies were evaluated in terms of three issues common to them all: desirability vs. change, respondent vs. investigator judgments of desirability, and weighting and scoring techniques.

H77   Ruch, Libby O.: A multidimensional analysis of the concept of life change. Journal of Health and Social Behavior 18:71-83, 1977.

Subjects: 211 University of Hawaii undergraduates.
Method: All subjects completed a modified Social Readjustment Rating Questionnaire that asked them to rate on a scale of 0-1,000 the amount of readjustment required by each of 42 life events in comparison to "marriage" (assigned a value of 500). Arithmetic mean item values (divided by 10) and rank order were calculated for all events, and results from the sample of college students were compared to Holmes and Rahe's original sample of adults. Data were also analyzed using the Guttman-Lingoes method of smallest space analysis-I for symmetrical matrixes. The unitary scaling method (magnitude estimation of life change) was compared to the nonmetric multidimensional scaling method (smallest space analysis of life change). Three life event dimensions were compared: degree of life change, desirability of life change, and area of life change.

H78   Stone, Arthur A., and Neale, John M.: Life event scales: Psychophysical training and rating dimension effects on event-weighting coefficients. Journal of Consulting and Clinical Psychology 46:849-853, 1978.

Subjects: 54 adults.
Method: Subjects were divided into subgroups to test the effects of two factors on life event ratings: psychophysical training and life event dimension. Subjects completed either the Social Readjustment Rating Questionnaire (SRRQ) or a modified SRRQ (the words "social readjustment" and "change" were replaced in the instructions by the words "stressfulness" and "stress"). Geometric mean item values were calculated for all events in both rating dimen-

sions. "Social readjustment" and "stressfulness" ratings were compared, and this sample's ratings were compared to "social readjustment" ratings from Holmes and Rahe's original sample of 394 adults. Some subjects also performed exercises using lines and numbers to represent relative magnitudes (psychophysical training) before completing the scaling questionnaires. The effect of the training on ratings was examined.

H79   Vinokur, Amiram, and Selzer, Melvin L.: Desirable versus undesirable life events: Their relationship to stress and mental distress. Journal of Personality and Social Psychology 32: 329-337, 1975.

Subjects: Two samples of male drivers: Group A (285 alcoholic drivers) and Group G (774 "normal" drivers).
Method: All subjects completed a modified Schedule of Recent Experience (for past 12 months): subjects indicated the occurrence of 46 life events, rated the "degree of pressure or adjustment" evoked by each reported event on a 4-point scale, and designated each reported event as "desirable" or "undesirable." They also completed questionnaire measures of aggression, paranoid thinking, depression, suicidal proclivity, and "stress-anxiety" physical symptoms. Three life events scoring methods were used (total number of life events, total Life Change Unit scores, total self-rating scores), and an undesirability score was calculated for each of them (by subtracting desirable events from undesirable events, resulting in a "balance" score). The relation of desirable and undesirable events to individual stress-related variables was examined and compared for Group A and Group G.

H80   Vinokur, Amiram, and Selzer, Melvin L.: Life events, stress, and mental distress. Proceedings of the American Psychological Association 8:329-330, 1973.

Subjects: 532 male drivers (274 "normal" and 258 alcoholic).
Method: All subjects completed a modified Schedule of Recent Experience (for past 12 months): subjects indicated the occurrence of 49 life events and rated the "degree of adjustment" evoked by each reported event on a 4-point scale. They also completed questionnaire measures of aggression, paranoid thinking, depression, suicidal proclivity, and physical and behavioral indications of stress. Three judges assigned the 49 events to three subdivisions: 29 undesirable events, 8 desirable events, and 12 ambiguous events.

Three life event scoring methods were used (total number of events, total Life Change Unit scores, and total self-rating scores) to calculate scores for the three subdivisions and for total responses. The relation of the three life event measures to stress-related variables was examined. [See also H79.]

H81   Zaslove, Helene Klein: Letter: Infertility as a life event. Journal of Human Stress 4(3):2, 1978.
    The writer questions the omission of two traumatic life events from the Social Readjustment Rating Scale: the problem of infertility and dealing with childlessness, and the death of a child (as an event in itself, separate from "death of family member"). Richard H. Rahe responds to explain the intentionally general wording of life event items in the research questionnaires he works with.

METHODOLOGY:
Measurement and Analysis of Data
(H82-H116)

H82   Ander, Suzanne; Lindstrom, Bodil; and Tibblin, Gosta: Life changes in random samples of middle-aged men. In Life Stress and Illness. E. K. Eric Gunderson and Richard H. Rahe (Eds.), pp. 121-124. Springfield, Illinois: Charles C Thomas, 1974.
    Subjects: 406 Swedish men selected by random sampling of three age groups: 52-year-olds (N=241), 62-year-olds (N=84), and 65-year-olds (N=81).
    Method: Rahe and Theorell's Swedish translation of the Schedule of Recent Experience was modified. Subjects were asked to report the occurrence of 43 life events in the past year, and to rate the intensity of reported events on a 5-point scale of severity (1=minor change, 5=total change of one's entire life situation). The frequency of life changes (total group) and the distribution of severity scalings (for each event) were studied. Mean number of reported life changes was calculated and compared for each age group. A life change scoring formula was developed to correct for age differences in life change reporting.

H83   Beach, Lee Roy; Beach, Barbara H.; Carter, William B.; and Barclay, Scott: Five studies of subjective equivalence. Organizational Behavior and Human Performance 12:351-371, 1974.

Five separate studies were conducted and compared to evaluate factors that influence the equivalence interval (EI), the "range of acceptable error" within which subjective judgments about numerical values are deemed correct or essentially the same. In each study, subjects were asked to set intervals around a different kind of numerical value (historical dates, proportions, people's ages, seriousness of diseases and life events, and money values of inheritances and gifts). In Study 4, 17 college students were provided with background information about the development and meaning of the Social Readjustment Rating Scale (SRRS) and the Seriousness of Illness Rating Scale (SIRS). They were then given a questionnaire which listed seven life events with their SRRS values and seven diseases with their SIRS values. Subjects were asked to write in an upper limit and a lower limit for each value, to indicate "how different the average for one disease or life event has to be from the average for another for us to regard them as actually different in seriousness." Mean EI's were calculated for each disease and each life event, and the effects of two task variables on EI's were examined and compared.

H84   Brown, George W.: Meaning, measurement, and stress of life events. In Stressful Life Events: Their Nature and Effects. Barbara Snell Dohrenwend and Bruce P. Dohrenwend (Eds.), pp. 217-243. New York: Wiley, 1974.

The author discusses what he sees as the central problem in life event research: how to control the meaning of life events to avoid systematic error and invalidity from direct contamination, indirect contamination, and spuriousness. He critiques the Schedule of Recent Experience and some of the research that uses its measurement system. Based on his London studies of schizophrenia and depression, the author discusses ways to control the meaning of life events, and he reviews the development of contextual measures of threat.

H85   Caplan, Robert D.: A less heretical view of life change and hospitalization. Journal of Psychosomatic Research 19:247-250, 1975.

The author responds to Wershow and Reinhart's criticisms of Schedule of Recent Experience (SRE) research [A70]. He discusses three areas of controversy: use of "normed" Life Change Unit values vs. use of ratings for special populations and self-ratings; qualities of life events (desirable vs.

undesirable, category or area of activity); and research design (retrospective vs. prospective studies, statistical techniques, theory of causality). He concludes his discussion with a six-point outline of proposed refinements and directions for future research using the SRE and similar life events instruments.

H86 Casey, Robert L.; Masuda, Minoru; and Holmes, Thomas H.: Quantitative study of recall of life events. Journal of Psychosomatic Research 11:239-247, 1967.

Subjects: 54 medical students.

Method: All subjects completed a 10-year, 40-item version of the Schedule of Recent Experience at Time 1 and again 9 months later at Time 2. The stability of the questionnaire was tested by calculating correlation coefficients (based on total Life Change Unit scores for each subject in three separate years) for Time 1 and Time 2. Differences between subjects' Time 1 and Time 2 scores were examined, and four factors affecting consistency of recall were studied (saliency of life event item, item qualifiers, item phraseology, and amount of life change of the individual at time of questionnaire administration).

RC 52.J6

H87 Chiriboga, David A.: Life event weighting systems: A comparative analysis. Journal of Psychosomatic Research 21: 415-422, 1977.

Subjects: 189 men and women, evenly distributed in two age groups (21-43 and 44-72 years old).

Method: All subjects completed a 48-item life events inventory (covering past 3 years). For each reported event subjects also indicated their "feelings about the event when it occurred" (very happy/somewhat happy/somewhat unhappy/very unhappy) and how much they "still think about the event" (not at all/some/a lot). Subjects also completed measures of a number of criterion variables (indicators of psychosocial functioning and adaptation such as self-report health status, psychiatric symptoms, locus of control, morale, self-concept). Seven life event weighting systems were used to calculate scores for three time periods: recent past (past year), distant past (2-3 years ago), and combined past (1-3 years). Intercorrelations were examined among the seven weighting systems (Social Readjustment Rating Scale values, Horowitz's presumptive stress ratings, simple frequency of occurrence, negative events, positive events, negative preoccupation, positive preoccu-

RC 52.J6

pation), and correlations with criterion variables were
also examined.

H88   Cleary, Patrick J.: Life events and disease: A review of
methodology and findings. Report No. 37, Laboratory for
Clinical Stress Research. Stockholm: Karolinska Institute,
1974. [Available from the Documentation Department,
Laboratory for Clinical Stress Research, Box 60205, S-104 01
Stockholm, Sweden.]
       This review of the literature discusses the following topics:
selection of life event items, rating of items, reporting of
life events, Life Change Unit (LCU) scoring and summation,
and correlation of LCU scores with illness indices. The
author's conclusions are followed by an extensive bibliography. [See also H102.]

H89   Coddington, R. Dean: The significance of life events as
etiologic factors in the diseases of children. II. A study of
a normal population. Journal of Psychosomatic Research 16:
205-213, 1972.
       Subjects: 3,526 healthy children in four age groups (pre-
school, elementary, junior high, and senior high).
       Method: Older subjects and mothers of younger subjects
completed a version of Coddington's life events record for
children (for past year). The frequency of all life events
was calculated for each age group. The average number of
life events was also computed and compared by age, sex,
race, and social class of children. The average amount of
social readjustment required of each age group was calculated using life event weights from Coddington's Social Readjustment Rating Scale for children [H36], and average
Life Change Unit (LCU) scores were compared by sex,
race, and social class of children. An age-related curve
of average social readjustment scores was constructed
and compared to a growth curve. [See also Part I (H36)
and Part III (A16).]

H90   Dailey, Charles A.: Psychotherapy and the life history.
Psychotherapy and Psychosomatics 25:239-242, 1975.
       The author proposes use of the Schedule of Recent Experi-
ence to measure outcome in psychotherapy (measuring
changes in the patient's "course of life" by analyzing rate
of change and timing of life events before and after psychotherapy). In a pilot project to develop "norms" on life
events experienced by the general, nonpsychiatric popula-

tion, "street-corner" interviews were held with subjects recruited in public places around Boston. The author reports sample findings concerning duration of "stress" for men and women, rate of life change and types of life events associated with different age groups, and correlations of stress to drinking, aggression, and antisocial behavior.

H91 Dohrenwend, Barbara Snell, and Dohrenwend, Bruce P.: A brief historical introduction to research on stressful life events. In Stressful Life Events: Their Nature and Effects. Barbara Snell Dohrenwend and Bruce P. Dohrenwend (Eds.), pp. 1-5. New York: Wiley, 1974.

BF575.S75
C6411973

Citing the work of W. B. Cannon, Adolf Meyer, and Harold G. Wolff, the editors review the historical development of the general hypothesis that links the work of all the contributors to this collection, "that stressful life events play a role in the etiology of various somatic and psychiatric disorders." The editors also identify two central research issues addressed in this book: What distinguishes "more stressful" from "less stressful" life events, and what are their pathological effects?

H92 Dohrenwend, Barbara Snell, and Dohrenwend, Bruce P.: Overview and prospects for research on stressful life events. In Stressful Life Events: Their Nature and Effects. Barbara Snell Dohrenwend and Bruce P. Dohrenwend (Eds.), pp. 313-331. New York: Wiley, 1974.

3F575.S75
C6411973

The editors review and discuss the evidence presented by contributors to this volume in terms of two major issues. They discuss the following topics under the first heading, "Effects of Stressful Life Events": variety of correlates, magnitude of risk, seriousness of effects, mediating factors, and alternative hypotheses. Under the second heading, "Conceptualization and Measurement of Stressful Life Events," they discuss defining "possibly stressful life events," devising procedures to sample selected life events, and using perceptions of life events as measures of stressfulness. They conclude with five proposals for the direction and design of future research.

H93 Dohrenwend, Barbara Snell, and Dohrenwend, Bruce P.: Some issues in research on stressful life events. Journal of Nervous and Mental Disease 166:7-15, 1978.

RC321.J83

The authors review and discuss three methodological issues: defining populations of life events (to distinguish

events which are independent of the subject's physical
health and psychiatric condition from dependent events),
measuring the magnitude of life events (scaling procedures,
use of group-specific ratings, scaling for different properties of life events), and choosing appropriate research de-
signs (case-control vs. cohort studies). They also propose
a systematic investigation of a neglected substantive issue,
the study of situational factors that mediate the "stress" of
life events.

H94 Dohrenwend, Bruce P.: Problems in defining and sampling
the relevant population of stressful life events. In Stressful
Life Events: Their Nature and Effects. Barbara Snell Dohrenwend and Bruce P. Dohrenwend (Eds.), pp. 275-310. New
York: Wiley, 1974.

Subjects: 528 New York City adults, aged 21-64 (67 community leaders, 257 heads of families, 118 psychiatric outpatients, 62 psychiatric inpatients, and 24 convicts in city
prisons).
Method: All subjects participated in a larger methodological study concerned with the measurement of psychopathology and role functioning over time. All were interviewed
by a psychiatrist and rated for severity of psychiatric disorder (well, some symptoms but no disorder, and mild,
marked, or severe disorder). As part of the interview
schedules, subjects were asked to name, date, and describe
the "last major event in your life that, for better or for
worse, interrupted or changed your usual activities." They
also completed a 26-item checklist of life events (past 12
months). Types of major life event elicited by the open-
ended question were examined and compared to categories
of events reported in the checklist by the five subject groups.
The relation of severity of psychiatric disorder to types of
reported events was also examined and compared among the
leaders, community sample, patients, and convicts.

H95 Fairbank, Dianne T., and Hough, Richard L.: Reply to
Roberts and Starr. Journal of Health and Social Behavior 18:
440-441, 1977.

The authors reply to comments by Roberts and Starr (H114)
on their 1976 article, "Problems in the Ratio Measurement
of Life Stress" (H99).

H96 Finkel, Norman J., and Jacobsen, Catherine A.: Significant
life experiences in an adult sample. American Journal of
Community Psychology 5:165-175, 1977.

Subjects: 45 adults, aged 30-60.

Method: All subjects completed a booklet asking them to name, date, and describe in detail their "significant life experiences." A follow-up interview was held with each subject to categorize each reported experience as a "stren" (health-promoting experience), a "trauma" (a crisis event), a "trauma converted into a stren" (a cognitive reevaluation that resolves the crisis and thereby enhances personality), or "other." The prevalence and frequency of occurrence of strens (S), traumas (T), and trauma-converted events (T-S) was examined, and findings were compared to data collected previously from a sample of undergraduates. Adult and undergraduate subjects were also compared on the following: timing of events (age differences), types of significant events, and changes in the patterns of experience of those subjects who had experienced a conversion vs. those who had not. Event type, age of subject, and previous conversion experience were examined for their effect on the conversion (T-S) process.

H97 Gersten, Joanne C.; Langner, Thomas S.; and Simcha-Fagan, Ora: The power of time. Journal of Health and Social Behavior 19:345-346, 1978.

RII.J687

The authors respond to Bruce G. Link's methodological critique (H105) of their 1977 article, "An Evaluation of the Etiologic Role of Stressful Life-Change Events in Psychological Disorders" (C10).

H98 Grant, Igor; Sweetwood, Hervey; Gerst, Marvin S.; and Yager, Joel: Scaling procedures in life events research. Journal of Psychosomatic Research 22:525-530, 1978.

Subjects: 357 male psychiatric outpatients and 250 male nonpatient controls.

RC52.J6

Method: All subjects completed a slightly modified Schedule of Recent Experience (SRE) and a correspondingly modified Social Readjustment Rating Questionnaire (SRRQ). They also completed a 67-item symptom checklist (frequency in past 2 months of symptoms commonly associated with psychiatric illness). Four life change scoring methods were used: (1) simple count of life events; (2) Life Change Unit (LCU) scores using "normative" weights (mean item values from control group's SRRQ data); (3) calculating patient SRE scores from patient group's Social Readjustment Rating Scale (SRRS) and control SRE scores from control group's SRRS; and (4) scoring individual SREs using each subject's

SRRQ ratings. Correlations between symptom scores and each of the four life change scores were examined and compared for patients and controls.

H99   Hough, Richard L.; Fairbank, Dianne Timbers; and Garcia, Alma M.: Problems in the ratio measurement of life stress. Journal of Health and Social Behavior 17:70-82, 1976.

R11.J687

The authors critique the Social Readjustment Rating Scale developed by Holmes and Rahe. Their discussion of methodological limitations covers three main issues: problems in instrument construction and administration (selection of items, questionnaire vs. two card-sort modes of administration, order of item presentation); cultural variability (use of "norms" vs. use of group-specific ratings); and problems in analysis (use of control variables, use of ratio scales, fitting data to appropriate model, and appropriate techniques for ratio measurement). The authors illustrate their discussion with data from their own experiments in administering a modified Social Readjustment Rating Questionnaire (63 items) to some availability samples (undergraduates at the University of Texas at El Paso). [See also H114 and H95.]

H100   Hudgens, Richard W.; Robins, Eli; and Delong, W. Bradford: The reporting of recent stress in the lives of psychiatric patients: A study of 80 hospitalized patients and 103 informants reporting the presence or absence of specified types

RC321B856X

of stress. British Journal of Psychiatry 117:635-643, 1970.

Subjects: 80 newly admitted psychiatric inpatients and 103 relatives.

Method: Subjects and informants were interviewed separately about the occurrence of 11 types of stressful events in the year prior to patient's admission to hospital. For each reported event, the following data were also collected: chronology of event, frequency of occurrence, and relationship to present illness. Matched sets of patient responses and informant responses were compared to study reliability of event reporting and level of agreement in estimating relationship between events and illness.

H101   Hull, Diana: Life circumstances and physical illness: A cross-disciplinary survey of research content and method for the decade 1965-1975. Journal of Psychosomatic Research 21:115-139, 1977.

RC52.J6

The author conducted an archival survey of the primary literature, represented by 19 journals, for research articles published during the period 1965-1974. A total of 329 articles were selected based on content (the social, psychological, and life event antecedents of physical illness), and then articles were classified by method of research. Articles were analyzed using a 10-factor scheme (including discipline of author and traditional interest of journal as well as content and method of article). Cross-tabulation and trend analysis were performed. The relation of author's discipline to research content (specific illness, types of antecedents) and research method was examined.

H102   Hurme, Helena: Life event research: Findings and methodological problems. Report No. 215. Jyväskylä, Finland: University of Jyväskylä, Department of Psychology, 1978.
This extensive review is divided into two parts. In Part 1 the author presents a "synthesis of what is presently known about the consequences of life events on individuals," complementing this discussion with a review of the research findings on predisposing and mediating factors related to life events. In Part 2 the author discusses the major methodological issues in life events research, particularly those issues that have developed since the publication in 1974 of Cleary's review of life events methodology (H88). A 165-item bibliography follows the text.

H103   Hurst, Michael W.; Jenkins, C. David; and Rose, Robert M.: The assessment of life change stress: A comparative and methodological inquiry. Psychosomatic Medicine 40:126-141, 1978.
Subjects: 416 air traffic controllers participating in a larger study of health change in their profession.
Method: All subjects were administered the Review of Life Experiences (ROLE) questionnaire using a video display terminal linked to a computer. The ROLE is a life events inventory which asks subjects to indicate the occurrence of 130 life events in the past 2 years (0-6 months and 7-24 months ago). The subject was also asked to rate each reported event twice using a scale of 1-99: first, to rate the amount of "adjustment" the event required, and second, to rate the amount of "distress or discomfort" caused by the event. Mean "adjustment" ratings and mean "distress" ratings were calculated for each ROLE event

(using ratings assigned by subjects who had experienced the event), and those mean subjective ratings were compared to "normative" ratings of adjustment (Holmes and Rahe's Social Readjustment Rating Scale) and "normative" ratings of distress (the Paykel et al. scale). Four life change scores were calculated for each subject using both "normative" and the individual's ratings of adjustment and distress (two adjustment scores based on the 39 ROLE items in common with the Schedule of Recent Experience, and two distress scores based on the 52 ROLE events in common with the Paykel et al. inventory). The four assessment methods were compared to investigate the effect of using individual vs. normative ratings on total life stress, and the effect of using weighted ratings vs. simple counts of life events. Psychometric characteristics of the Schedule of Recent Experience and the Paykel et al. inventory are discussed and compared to the ROLE.

H104   Kellam, Sheppard G.: Stressful life events and illness: A research area in need of conceptual development. In Stress-ful Life Events: Their Nature and Effects. Barbara Snell Dohrenwend and Bruce P. Dohrenwend (Eds.), pp. 207-214. New York: Wiley, 1974.

The author discusses the research design of the studies reported in the three chapters preceding his (see H72, C19, and C24). He outlines several concepts to develop and strengthen life event inventories in future research. Inventories based on "more theoretically meaningful categories of stressful life events" (1) would be appropriate for the subject's "stage of life," (2) would reflect differences between "fateful events" and "personal failure events," (3) would "sufficiently and coequally" sample both good and bad events, and (4) would take into account the subject's "social organizational hierarchy from broad societal to familial." The author illustrates his proposals for further conceptual development by describing an "elaboration" in research design that he developed with colleagues, a concept called the "life course-social field concept."

H105   Link, Bruce G.: On the etiologic role of stressful life-change events. Journal of Health and Social Behavior 19:343-345, 1978.

The author critiques the method used by Gersten et al. (C10) to assess direct causal significance of life events in their 1977 study. He traces their "faulty use of method" to what Gordon called the "partialling fallacy." (See H97 for a reply by Gersten et al.)

H106   McDonald, Blair W.; Pugh, William M.; Gunderson, E. K. Eric; and Rahe, R. H.: Reliability of life change cluster scores. British Journal of Social and Clinical Psychology 11:407-409, 1972.

F1 B723

Subjects: 663 U.S. Navy enlisted men serving aboard a carrier at sea.
Method: All subjects completed the military version of the Schedule of Recent Experience (SRE), a 42-item inventory covering the past $2\frac{1}{2}$ years (in five 6-month periods). Six months later, subjects again completed the military SRE. Test-retest reliability of the SRE was examined by comparing total SRE scores and scores in four clusters of life change events (9 personal and social items, 4 work, 11 marital, 3 disciplinary) for each of the four overlapping 6-month periods in life event reports and for combined 12-month periods. Suggestions are offered for increasing reliability of life event measures.

H107   Mechanic, David: Some problems in the measurement of stress and social readjustment. Journal of Human Stress 1(3):43-48, 1975.

The author critiques the Holmes and Rahe Social Readjustment Rating Scale, discussing the following problems: The instrument fails to distinguish the effects of favorable events from those of adverse events on the occurrence of illness; the wording of its life event items is ambiguous; and its use may confound dependent and independent variables (e.g., illness or injury) and thus contaminate the research measures.

H108   Nelson, Philip; Mensh, Ivan N.; Hecht, Elizabeth; and Schwartz, Arthur N.: Variables in the reporting of recent life changes. Journal of Psychosomatic Research 16:465-471, 1972.

RC52.J6

Subjects: Four samples of veterans in the same hospital facility (50 males in an extended care setting, 28 males in residential status, 33 female veterans, and 6 males who recently served in Vietnam).
Method: All subjects completed the Recent Life Changes Questionnaire (RLCQ), a 42-item inventory covering three time periods (0-6 months, 7-12 months, and 1-2

years ago). They also completed a shortened version of
Rotter's Internal-External Locus of Control Scale, the
Gordon Survey of Interpersonal Values (support, conformity, recognition, independence, benevolence, lead-
ership), and a 12-item Biographical Data form. Weighted
life change scores and simple item counts were calculated
for each subject in four areas of experience (health, work,
home and family, other social and personal adjustments).
Correlations among questionnaire measures were examined within subject groups. Differences in life change reporting were examined in relation to age, education, sex,
hospital status, ethnic origin, recency of military experience, and the questionnaire measures of values,
locus of control, and biographical characteristics.

H109   Pugh, William M.; Erickson, Jeanne; Rubin, Robert T.;
       Gunderson, E. K. Eric; and Rahe, Richard H.: Cluster
       analyses of life changes: II. Method and replication in Navy
       subpopulations. Archives of General Psychiatry 25:333-339,
       1971.
       Subjects: 2,025 U.S. Navy enlisted men serving on an
       aircraft carrier and a battleship.
       Method: This study replicated an earlier study in which
       all subjects completed the military Schedule of Recent
       Experience (for past 18 months). Subjects in the replica-
       tion study were divided into four subgroups according to
       site (carrier vs. battleship) and pay grade ("rated" vs.
       "unrated" personnel). A cluster analysis (the Iterative
       Intercolumnar Correlational Analysis technique) was per-
       formed to identify life event item clusters which demon-
       strated the greatest stability across all subgroups. This
       report provides detailed descriptions and illustrations of
       the techniques involved in cluster analysis of life change
       events. [See also Part I (H113).]

H110   Rahe, Richard H.: Editorial: Life change measurement
       clarification. Psychosomatic Medicine 40:95-98, 1978.
       The author briefly reviews the development of instruments
       for measuring and scaling recent life change since the
       Schedule of Recent Experience (SRE) was first devised in
       1957. He explains the differences between the SRE and
       the Recent Life Changes Questionnaire (RLCQ), between
       LCU (Life Change Units) and SLCU (Subjective Life Change
       Units), and between the Social Readjustment Rating Ques-
       tionnaire (SRRQ) and the Social Readjustment Rating

Scale (SRRS). He discusses the problems associated with attempts to assess the quality of life events (e.g., positive vs. negative, desirable vs. undesirable) in addition to measuring their quantity.

H111 Rahe, Richard H.: The pathway between subjects' recent life changes and their near-future illness reports: Representative results and methodological issues. In Stressful Life Events: Their Nature and Effects. Barbara Snell Dohrenwend and Bruce P. Dohrenwend (Eds.), pp. 73-86. New York: Wiley, 1974.

The author outlines his conceptualization of the pathway between exposure to life change and near-future illness reports. He uses selected findings to illustrate the relationship between the six "filters" or intervening variables: subject's past experience, psychological defenses, physiological reaction, coping abilities, symptom formation and illness behavior, and illness reports. He also discusses three methodologic issues: positive vs. negative events, use of Life Change Units vs. simple counting of events, and validity and reliability of the Schedule of Recent Experience.

H112 Rahe, Richard H.; Jensen, Phyllis D.; and Gunderson, E. K. Eric: Regression analysis of subjects' self-reported life changes in an attempt to improve illness prediction. Report No. 71-5, U.S. Navy Medical Neuropsychiatric Research Unit. San Diego: Naval Health Research Center, 1971. [Available from Naval Health Research Center, P.O. Box 85122, San Diego, CA. 92138.]

Subjects: A validation sample of 2,378 enlisted men from three U.S. Navy cruisers and a cross-validation sample of 1,085 enlisted men from a battleship.
Method: All subjects completed the military Schedule of Recent Experience at the beginning of their ships' cruises. At the end of the cruise, illness data (number of reported illnesses) were abstracted from each subject's medical record during the 6- to 8-month cruise. Subjects in the validation sample were divided into five subsamples according to age and marital status and compared for mean number of illnesses. Regression analyses were performed on life change (year prior to cruise) and illness data from the five subsamples and the total validation sample to determine significant life change events, their regression coefficients, and correlations with illness.

Multiple regression equations (separate subsample and total sample equations) were developed for the prediction of illness. They were tested by using the validation sub- samples' equations to predict illness in corresponding subgroups in the cross-validation sample. Cross-valida- tion coefficients were compared to correlations using standard Life Change Unit scoring method.

H113   Rahe, Richard H.; Pugh, William M.; Erickson, Jeanne; Gunderson, E. K. Eric; and Rubin, Robert T.: Cluster analyses of life changes: I. Consistency of clusters across large Navy samples. Archives of General Psychiatry 25: 330-332, 1971.

Subjects: 2,678 U.S. Navy enlisted men.
Method: All subjects completed the military Schedule of Recent Experience (SRE) for the 18 months prior to be- ginning sea duty. Life change data were scored either as occurring ("1") or not ("0") in the 18-month period. A cluster analysis technique (the Iterative Intercolumnar Correlational Analysis) was used to identify groups of life events with high intracluster and low intercluster correlations. Response rates of events in the identified clusters were compared to response rates of the remain- ing noncluster events. [See also Part II (H109).]

H114   Roberts, Alden E., and Starr, Paul D.: Problems in "Prob- lems in the ratio measurement of life stress." Journal of Health and Social Behavior 18:440, 1977.

The authors comment on Hough, Fairbank, and Garcia's 1976 critique (H99) of the Social Readjustment Rating Scale. They discuss the properties of a ratio scale, and they suggest two alternatives—an inductive curve fitting method and multiple regression analysis—for assessing the life change-illness relationship. (See H95 for a reply by Fairbank and Hough.)

H115   Schless, Arthur P., and Mendels, Joseph: The value of in- terviewing family and friends in assessing life stressors. Archives of General Psychiatry 35:565-567, 1978.

Subjects: 117 outpatients and 117 "significant others" (family member or friend of patient).
Method: Patients and their informants were interviewed separately about the occurrence of life events in the pa- tient's life (using either the authors' Inventory of Discrete Events or a version of the Dohrenwends' PERI question-

naire). Differences in life event reports were analyzed to assess the contribution ("percentage of information added") of the significant other, both in number of events reported and in types of events. A "knowledgeable third party" was also interviewed to test the validity of reports by some patients and their significant others. Sources of disagreement between patients, significant others, and third parties were investigated by holding conjoint interviews after the initial separate interviews.

H116   Weinman, Maxine; Justice, Blair; Lorimor, Ronald J.; and McBee, George W.: Sex differences in perception of life events using self-weights. Perceptual and Motor Skills 47: 1227-1230, 1978.

Subjects: 36 male and 35 female psychiatric patients newly admitted to the inpatient service.

Method: All subjects completed the Recent Life Changes

BF311 P36 Questionnaire (RLCQ) and three measures of psychological and social functioning (Taylor Manifest Anxiety Scale, Denver Community Mental Health Questionnaire, and the MMPI Mini-Mult). One-year and 2-year life change data were scored two ways: using standardized weights (Life Change Units) and subject's self-weights (Subjective Life Change Units). Sex differences in the number of reported life events and in the two types of scoring systems were assessed in relation to the psychological measures. One sex differential was found, between patient-weighted events (SLCU) and the L (social desirability) scale of the Mini-Mult. Regression analysis was performed to determine the independent contributions of sex and social desirability to variance in subjective perceptions of life events.

USE OF
LIFE EVENTS INVENTORIES IN
THE HEALTH CARE SETTING

I1   Bird, H. Waldo, and Schuham, Anthony I.: Meeting families'
     treatment needs through a family psychotherapy center. Hos-
     pital and Community Psychiatry 29:175-178, 1978.
          The authors describe a five-phase evaluation program used
     at a St. Louis family therapy center. A panel of evaluators
     uses the information to recommend the appropriate type of
     family therapy and the staff therapist. In Phase 2 of the
     evaluation, family psychosocial data are collected by ques-
     tionnaires, including modified versions of the Schedule of
     Recent Experience and Coddington's Schedule of Recent Ex-
     perience for children.

I2   Blankenship, Larry Lee: Computer-conducted assessment of
     life-change psychological stress (Doctoral dissertation, Uni-
     versity of Illinois at Urbana-Champaign, 1976). Dissertation
     Abstracts International 37:2495-B, 1976.
          Subjects: 30 male and 30 female volunteers.
          Method: An on-line real-time computer program was de-
     signed and tested. It included the Schedule of Recent Ex-
     perience, an anxiety test, two cognitive tasks, and ques-
     tions to assess subject's attitude toward being interviewed
     by computer. "Hardware" limitations of computer-con-
     ducted assessment were analyzed. The computer-adminis-
     tered Schedule of Recent Experience was evaluated as a tool
     to assess "psychological stress" vs. "physiological stress."

I3   Caldwell, Laura Ryan: Use of the Social Readjustment Rating
     Scale combined with the P.O.R. in a college health service.
     Nurse Practitioner 3:24-26, 1978.

The author describes the use of a modified Schedule of Recent Experience with the Problem Oriented Record (P.O.R.) by health center staff to counsel patients and to involve them in the planning and carrying out of individual programs of preventive health care.

I4   Clark, Ewen M.: A non-automated multiphasic health testing program in a student health service. <u>American Journal of Public Health</u> 63:610-618, 1973.

The author describes the development of a polyphasic health testing program at the Student Health Service of the University of Florida, designed to provide routine medical examinations to large numbers of students every year. A life change events questionnaire (modified Schedule of Recent Experience) is administered in addition to a machine-readable medical and family history form as part of the "History" section of the program.

I5   Cross, Harold D.: Psychiatric screening in general practice. <u>Lancet</u> 1:913, 1976.

The author discusses the benefits resulting from the use of three instruments to screen patients in a clinic as part of a comprehensive health evaluation: a standardized health questionnaire, an index of depression, and a life change scale (modified Schedule of Recent Experience).

I6   Gordon, Richard E.: Psychiatric screening through multiphasic health testing. <u>American Journal of Psychiatry</u> 128: 559-563, 1971.

The author describes the procedures and uses of automated multiphasic health testing (AMHT). He discusses his work with colleagues at the University of Florida to develop a battery of effective, brief psychiatric screening instruments for use in AMHT. The screening questions under investigation relate to psychiatric symptoms, life events, and upsetting developmental experiences. The paper-and-pencil measures are complemented by psychophysiological measurements, blood chemical testing, and somatopsychic tests.

I7   Gordon, Richard E.; Bielen, Leslie; and Watts, Anne: Psychiatric screening with automated multiphasic health testing in the VA admission procedure. <u>American Journal of Psychiatry</u> 130:46-48, 1973.

<u>Subjects</u>: 241 veterans applying for admission to a VA hospital.

Method: While subjects were undergoing the standard admitting process at a VA hospital, they were also tested by automated multiphasic health testing and services (AMHTS). The AMHTS included the following psychiatric screening tests: modified Leighton Scale (psychiatric symptoms), modified Schedule of Recent Experience (life change), and modified Selective Service Questionnaire (personal and familial psychiatric history). Admitting physicians sent 52 subjects to the psychiatry service for evaluation and then decided whether to admit (N=28) or not admit (N=24) them to the hospital. The AMHTS data for the 52 were then analyzed to see "whether AMHTS can simulate the physician's decisions in the admitting office." Medical records were reviewed to evaluate sources of disagreement between the AMHTS analyses and the physician's decisions.

I8   Harrington, Robert L.; Koreneff, Constantine; Nasser, Sarah J.; Wright, Colin; and Englehard, Curtis: Systems approach to mental health care in a HMO model: Three-year Report, Project MH 24109. March, 1977. [Copies available through National Institute of Mental Health, Washington, D.C.]
The authors report their progress toward developing a systems approach to mental health care and integrating it into the program at Kaiser/Permanente (Santa Clara and San Jose, California). One of the program objectives is the early detection of psychosocial risk factors and subsequent specific intervention for those at high risk. Patients regularly complete a set of psychosocial questionnaires (dubbed the "Golden Rod"): the Schedule of Recent and Anticipated Experiences (modified Schedule of Recent Experience), an Assessment of Current Life Conditions (for self and spouse), the Schedule of Social Functioning (a version of Heimler's Scale of Social Functioning), and a Background Information and Demographic Data form. Data collected during the first 3 years of the ongoing project are reported.

I9   Raft, David; Davidson, Jonathan; Toomey, Timothy C.; Spencer, Roger F.; and Lewis, Ben F.: Inpatient and outpatient patterns of psychotropic drug prescribing by non-psychiatrist physicians. American Journal of Psychiatry 132: 1309-1312, 1975.
Subjects: 128 medical and surgical inpatients and 100 outpatients from the same hospital's outpatient clinic.
Method: Subjects were selected after a review of pharmacy records identified them all as receiving psychotropic medication. All outpatients were administered two depression

scales (Zung Self-Rating Scale and Beck Depression Inventory) and a modified Schedule of Recent Experience, and most outpatients were clinically evaluated by one of the investigators. In addition, outpatients' physicians were interviewed about their choice of psychotropic medications for the patient. Patterns of psychotropic drug use in treatment were investigated for inpatients and outpatients: correlations were examined between prescription of psychotropics and demographic characteristics of patient; presence or absence of depression; magnitude of life stress; minor vs. major tranquilizer choice; and physician's speciality.

I10   Schuman, Stanley H.; Curry, Hiram B.; Braunstein, Mark L.; Schneeweiss, Ronald; Jebaily, Gerard C.; Glazer, Howard M.; Cahn, Jack R.; and Crigler, William H.: A computer-administered interview on life events: Improving patient-doctor communication. Journal of Family Practice 2:263-269, 1975.

The authors describe the development of CAI-LEV (computer-administered interview on life events) and its use in a model family practice unit at the Medical University of South Carolina, Charleston. Patients spend 15-30 minutes using a computer terminal in the waiting room to answer questions about life events in 16 areas (e.g., habits, finances, work). For each reported event, the patient also indicates when it happened; whether it was expected; a large or small change; a good/neutral/bad change; whether patient needs help coping with it, and if so, from whom and what kind of help; and whether patient thinks the event will have a positive/neutral/negative effect on health. A computer printout is available to the physician within minutes. Case histories are presented to illustrate the uses and benefits of CAI-LEV to both patients and doctors.

I11   Seime, Richard J.; McCauley, Roger L.; and Madsen, Robert K.: Comparing interview impressions and test results: A new test interpretation format and procedure. Professional Psychology 8:199-205, 1977.

The authors describe a new format and procedure adopted to enhance psychological testing and patient evaluation in a university hospital's adult psychiatry outpatient clinic. All new patients are administered three questionnaires: the MMPI, the Minnesota-Briggs History Record, and a Life Changes Checklist (modified Schedule of Recent Experience). The new format allows recording of the test results and interpretations for comparison with the impressions noted by the clinical interviewer.

AUTHOR INDEX

311

314

SUBJECT INDEX

Abortion, elective, 102, 105

Absenteeism, 9, 19, 129-31, 133-34, 141

Academic performance of students, 127, 129-35, 137-38, 260

Accidents, 112-14, 130-45; 14, 32, 88, 117, 150, 159, 275, 290

Acupuncture, 24, 25

Adjective Generation Technique (AGT) word list, 197

Adjustment, psychological, 2, 44, 127, 166, 180, 187, 190-91, 194, 197, 203, 204, 228, 285

Adolescent Behavior Rating Scale (Devereux), 136

Adolescent Social Readjustment Checklist (Kulcsar), 257

Adolescent subjects, 8, 41, 42, 51, 55, 71, 105, 131, 134, 136, 142, 144, 147, 149, 169, 189, 199, 257, 267, 271, 277, 285-86, 294

Age differences in life event reporting: see Frequency of life events and separate listings for age groups (Children, Adolescent subjects, College students, Older adults)

Age identity, 200

Alcohol consumption, 10, 69, 73, 95, 103, 147, 158, 180, 214, 216

Alcohol treatment programs, outcome of, 158

Alcoholism, 69-75; 32, 48, 142-44, 150, 186, 214, 224, 226, 263, 275, 290

Amenorrhoea, secondary, 99

American subcultures: see separate listings (Black Americans, Mexican Americans, Native Americans, Native Hawaiians, Italian-Americans) and Ethnic and racial differences in life event perceptions and reports

Amphetamine addiction, 69

Angina, 90, 91

Anorexia nervosa, 42

Anticipated vs. unanticipated life events, 11, 55, 123, 168, 198, 287, 310

Anxiety, 192-94; 50, 77, 81, 102, 104, 112, 118, 181, 196, 202, 224, 246, 280

Anxiety, manifest: see Pittsburgh Manifest Anxiety Scale and Taylor Manifest Anxiety Scale

Anxiety, state-trait: see State-Trait Anxiety Inventory (STAI)

Appendicitis/appendectomy, 22, 95

Arrests and "trouble with the law," 70, 73, 142-43, 147, 257

Arthritis: Osteoarthritis of the hip, 108; Polyarthritis, 62, 107; Rheumatoid arthritis, adult, 109, 287; Rheumatoid arthritis, juvenile, 5, 107, 109

Asthma, 2, 10, 93, 94, 121

Athlete Schedule of Recent Experience (Bramwell), 139

Athletes, 125, 139, 161-62, 211, 263, 275

Athletic injuries, prediction of, 139

Autonomic balance, relative, 210

Ballistocardiography, 89

Basic military training, 68, 117, 286

Berle Index, 93, 156

Bipolar affective illness, 55, 56, 58, 62

Birth of child/gaining new family member, 134-36; 28, 45, 48, 96, 111, 257, 271, 284

Black American subjects, 62, 139, 146, 175-76, 192, 273-76, 279, 280-81, 283

Blindness, 2

Blood pressure, 10, 18, 161, 209, 212, 236

Breast tumors, 36-40

Bronchitis, 35, 94

Brown and Birley life events interview method, 65; 43, 44, 46, 47, 53, 54, 62-64, 66, 72, 77, 83, 92, 120, 124, 140, 292

Burn patients, 2, 112, 142, 277

Calamity Magnitude Scale, 247

Cancer, 35-46; 22, 28, 100, 278

Cantril's Self-Anchoring Scale, 250

Cardiac disease, 77; 15, 32, 90

Cardiovascular changes during hospitalization: see Hospitalization, cardiovascular changes during

Menstrual cycle changes, 99, 101
Mental deterioration in elderly women, 160, 161
Mental Health Questionnaire (MHQ), 280
Mexican American subjects, 261, 268, 270, 273-75, 281, 283
Middlesex Hospital Questionnaire, 100, 226
Migration, 2, 6, 16, 40, 96, 166, 172, 250, 251
Military subjects, 3, 5, 12-18, 68, 83, 88, 117, 124-26, 128-29, 138, 141, 161, 189, 211, 212, 242, 249, 260, 271, 301-4
Minnesota Multiphasic Personality Inventory (MMPI) and the Mili-Mult, 16, 19, 24, 25, 39, 45, 52, 72, 76, 86, 99, 102, 107-9, 115, 117, 118, 152, 156, 167-70, 175, 192, 280, 305
Minor health changes (signs and symptoms), 3, 7, 32, 111, 124, 166, 168, 178, 220, 234
Miscarriage, incidence of, 103
Missouri Children's Picture Series, 202
Mobility, organizational, 6, 81
Mobility, residential: see Residence, change in
Mobility, sociocultural, 91
Mononucleosis, infectious, 35
Mood Adjective Checklist, 101
Mood and lithium in drinking water, 174
Mortality rates: General, 214, 220, 224, 231, 237-39, 247; Heart disease, 81, 213, 214; Infant and maternal, 213
Mother-child interaction, 140, 155, 192, 246
Multiple Affect Adjective Checklist, 3
Multiple sclerosis, 109, 253
Myers, Lindenthal, and Pepper life events inventory, 65; 67, 68, 157, 158, 167, 172, 173
Myocardial infarction, 77-89; 91, 274
Myocardial infarction, adjustment after, 79, 80, 83, 86

Nationality of subjects: Australia, 2, 97, 148, 159, 165, 176, 177, 227, 267, 268; Belgium, 281; Canada, 10, 19, 165-67, 172; Colombia, 172; Cuba, 285; Czechoslovakia, 280; Denmark, 20, 52, 283; El Salvador, 248, 275, 284; Finland, 83-86; France, 281; Great Britain, 46, 53-55, 62, 64, 65, 72, 140, 174, 193, 226, 228, 229, 231, 234, 241, 247, 283; Greece, 28; Holland, 1, 47, 99; Ireland, 281, 282; Israel, 39, 76, 180, 253, 263; Japan, 275, 281-83, 285; Malaysia, 275,

285; Mexico, 118; New Zealand, 282; Norway, 13, 247; Peru, 248; Portugal, 16, 250; Scotland, 146, 151, 254; South Africa, 95; Spain, 248, 275, 281, 284; Sweden, 18, 52, 78, 82, 84, 87-89, 99, 100, 283-84, 291; Switzerland, 281; United States: passim; see also American subcultures; Vietnam, 249, 250; West Indies, 63, 166
Native American subjects, 147, 270
Native Hawaiian subjects, 283
Natural disasters: General, 25, 247, 248; Earthquake, 248; Flood, 247, 249
Neighborhood contexts, self-perceived, 172, 220
Neurologic illness in children, relation of economic depression to, 216
Neurosis and neuroticism, 42, 46-49, 52, 60, 61, 63, 81, 88, 137, 176, 177, 224, 242, 274

Obesity treatment modes, long-term outcome of, 157
Occupations of subject groups: Air traffic controllers, 16, 299; Ambulance paramedics, 131; Blue-collar workers/plant closure, 187, 207, 209, 233, 234; Brewery workers, 19, 134; Case workers, 11; Classical composers, 136; Computer operators, 235; Construction workers, 18, 88; Counselor trainees, 129; Executives and managers, 132, 137, 174, 236, 237; Firefighters, 115, 131; Government employees, 9; Hospital employees, 34, 141; "Large working place" employees, 9, 237; Medical students, 7, 18, 19, 265, 266, 275; Military: see separate listing for Military subjects; Nursing students, 35, 111; Peace Corps volunteers, 251; Petroleum servicing company workers, 251; Pharmacy students, 8; Physicians, 147, 269; Pilots, 138, 141, 145; Prisoners/convicted criminals, 148, 159, 214, 251, 296; Religious life, women in, 1; Research scientists, 280; Security guards, 168; Smelter and mine workers, 95; Students: see separate listings for Children, Adolescent subjects, and College students; Teachers, 129, 130, 133, 270; Telephone company employees, 6, 81; Transferred employees, 236-38
Older adults (as subjects), 121, 134, 136, 160, 161, 163, 167, 175, 176, 196, 198, 200, 229, 233-35, 237-39, 276, 277, 291, 293

Osteoarthrosis, 109
Ovarian cancer, 38

Pain: Chronic pain, 24-25; 108; Facial
pain, 96; Head pain: see separate listing for Headache; Low back pain, 108,
112, 274; Reports of pain by hospitalized patients, 22
Parental adjustment to childhood illness,
111, 183, 208, 243, 244
Paykel et al. life events interview/scaling,
60, 265; 49, 57, 58-63, 65-68, 74, 75,
95, 97, 122, 145, 150, 157, 158, 169,
178, 179, 188, 264, 272, 277, 283, 299
Perceived health status, 4, 22, 115, 118,
120, 174, 178, 237, 242, 249
Perceptions of life events—scaling studies:
Cross-cultural studies, 280-85; 248,
251, 262; General populations, 262-69;
6, 49, 59, 254, 255, 257, 261, 272,
289; Specific populations, 270-80; 1, 24,
35, 59, 71, 73, 74, 82, 85-87, 89, 139,
235, 242, 253, 254, 257, 292, 295, 297,
299, 305
Perceptions of life events, subjective: see
Subjective perceptions of life events
Perceptual motor dysfunction, 2
PERI Life Events Scale (Dohrenwends),
255; 304
Personal construct systems, 197
Personality inventories: Boston University, 120, 121, 127, 175; Edwards, 86,
139; Eysenck, 11, 36, 38, 45, 108, 110,
159, 255; Maudsley (and Short Maudsley),
37, 57, 60-63, 127; MMPI: see separate listing for Minnesota Multiphasic
Personality Inventory (MMPI) and Mini-
Mult; Omnibus, 4, 196; Psychological
Screening Inventory, 195, 260; Others,
46, 47, 74, 90, 99, 105, 110, 147, 155,
195, 196
Physiological changes and measures, 207-
12; 10, 12, 16, 18, 83, 88, 93, 131,
156, 161, 187
Pittsburth Manifest Anxiety Scale, 196
Poisoning, 113, 145
Poliomyelitis, 183
Prediction of accidents, 190, 193, 194
Prediction of illness, 4, 7, 11, 12, 14, 16,
35, 39, 92, 117, 125, 129, 139, 174,
196, 201, 215, 279, 303
Prediction of personnel success, 129, 137
Prediction of physician suicide, 147
Prediction of relapse (rehospitalization) of
psychiatric patients, 258

Pregnancy, 101-5, 280-82; 14, 15, 48, 55,
96, 108-11, 194, 213, 273, 275, 280
"Presumptive stress" questionnaire (Horowitz), 257; 198, 293
Prevention/intervention strategies, 28-30,
41, 50, 51, 86, 131, 185, 195, 202, 216,
264, 265, 267, 271, 239, 248, 296, 307,
309
Prison incarceration, 159
Prisoner of war camp, 6, 246
Problem Oriented Record (P. O. R.), use
with the SRE, 307
Profile of Mood States (POMS), 19, 90, 93,
157, 195, 255
Prognosis of illness, 4, 38, 44, 50, 60, 63,
64, 95, 104, 153, 186
Prospective studies, 3-8, 11-19, 21, 26,
32, 35, 40, 42, 47, 50, 55, 58, 72, 87-
89, 99, 100, 103, 115, 117, 123, 125-27,
139, 141, 142, 161, 162, 168, 201, 224,
243, 244, 260, 292, 303
Prostatectomy, 22
Prostatic hypertrophy, benign, 100
Pruritic skin disease, 106
Psoriasis, 105
Psychiatric diagnosis: Changes over time,
43; Cross-national differences in, 67;
Use of SRE as screening instrument in,
308, 310
Psychiatric disorders, maintenance treatment for, 61, 65, 66
Psychiatric hospitalization: see Hospitalization, psychiatric
Psychiatric illness (general), 42-52; 2, 15,
18, 22, 53, 54, 66, 69, 99, 117-19, 125,
127, 128, 140, 150, 152, 167, 169, 170,
172, 173, 178, 179, 181-83, 188, 192,
216, 219, 220, 232, 239, 240, 250, 254,
257, 259, 265, 272, 277, 283, 296, 297,
305
Psychiatry, child, 5, 50
Psychogenic illness, mass outbreaks of,
45
Psychological distress, 25, 122, 123, 143,
144, 158, 165, 169, 170, 172, 177, 179,
203, 238, 290, 293
Psychological impairment, 8, 42, 157, 158,
165, 166, 168, 176, 190, 202, 220, 230,
286, 299
Psychotherapy, 26, 121, 204, 294
Pulmonary symptoms and function, 10, 93-
95
Purdue Elementary Problem Solving Inventory, 184
Pyloric stenosis, infantile, 109, 110

328

Qualities of life events, 285-91; 9, 44, 49, 59, 60, 65, 145, 146, 150, 172, 183 272, 283, 292, 295, 296, 302. See also separate listings for Anticipated vs. unanticipated life events, Controllable vs. uncontrollable life events, Desirable vs. undesirable life events, Entrance-related vs. exit-related life events, Internal vs. external life events, Losses vs. gains (life events), and Upsetting/distressing life events

Quality of life, ratings of, 180

Race: see Ethnic and racial differences and American subcultures

Ratio measurement, problems in, 289, 296, 298, 304

Reactive psychoses, 67

Reading achievement, 133

Recall of life events, reliability of, 49, 167, 293, 298, 301, 304

Recency vs. remoteness in time of experienced event, 3, 13, 15, 48, 171, 257, 264, 265, 285, 293, 297

Recent Life Changes Questionnaire (RLCQ), 260; 11, 37, 44, 69, 76, 79, 83, 159, 179, 280, 287, 301, 302, 305

Recent Life Events questionnaire (Schless et al.), 18

Recidivism among drinking drivers, 70, 158

Refugee subjects, 6, 249, 250, 285

Regional enteritis, 96, 97

Regional ileitis, 99

Regression analysis, advantages of, 303, 304

Reliability, test-retest, 7, 116, 117, 255, 257, 260, 265, 270, 272, 293, 301, 303

Religious behavior, 157, 180

Religious life, women in, 1

Relocation, involuntary, 228, 229, 237-39

Relocation, residential: see Residence, change in

Renal failure, chronic: see Hemodialysis, adjustment to

Repression-sensitization scales, use of, 176, 181

Research content and method, a cross-disciplinary survey of, 298

Research design, discussions of, 8, 13, 32, 36, 43, 44, 49, 52-55, 62, 78, 87, 124, 187, 209, 219, 238, 260, 275, 292, 294-304

Research instruments, use of: see separate listings by name of instrument

(e.g., Life Events Inventory, Recent Life Changes Questionnaire)

Residence, change in, 237-39; 10, 91, 113, 124, 149, 172, 194, 228, 236, 237

Respiratory illness, 92-95; 20, 120, 121, 156

Retirement, 232-35; 161, 186, 198, 239, 246, 285

Review of Life Experiences (ROLE) questionnaire (Rose, Hurst, and Jenkins), 16, 299

Risk-taking behavior, 132, 142, 144

Rumination as a cognitive strategy, use of, 185

Rural subjects, 10, 113, 144, 167, 275

Sample size, effect of, 47, 116

Scaling methods, comparisons of: Direct vs. indirect scaling of life events, 267; Interval vs. ratio scaling of the seriousness of illness, 266; Unitary vs. multidimensional scaling of life events, 289

Schedule of Daily Experience (SDE) [T. S. Holmes], 7, 111

Schedule of Daily Experience and Stress-Value Scale for Officer Candidates (Cline), 271

Schedule of Recent Experience (SRE): Development of, 6, 28, 34, 256, 260, 302; Use of: passim; Version for children and adolescents: see Coddington's Schedule of Recent Experience for Children and Adolescent Social Readjustment; Checklist (Kulcsar); Verson for college athletes: see Athlete Schedule of Recent Experience (Bramwell); Version for college students: see College Schedule of Recent Experience (Anderson) and Harris's Social and Collegiate Readjustment Rating Scale; Version for large social units (macroscopic level): see Index of Changes in Social Activities; Version for older adults: see Geriatric Schedule of Recent Experience

Schedule of Recent Life Events for the Elderly, 175

Schizophrenia, 63-69; 42-44, 48, 49, 52, 53, 224, 292

School, beginning/returning to, 28, 139, 183, 194, 253, 266

School drop-outs, 129, 130

Scoring procedures, differences in, 16, 17, 21, 22, 116, 125, 138, 141, 144, 146, 173, 191, 260, 280, 286, 288, 290-94, 297, 299, 301, 303

Seat belts, safety restraints, use with children in cars, 154
Self-concept, 2, 37, 70, 103, 137, 153, 175, 199, 204, 246, 293
Self-derogation, 199
Self-description, 197, 200
Self-empowerment construct, 131
Self-esteem, 19, 116, 122, 123, 165, 174, 177, 195
Selye theory of stress, 29-31, 33
Sensation seeking, 201, 203
Seriousness of illness, 3, 4, 6, 15, 19, 23, 105, 115, 119, 121, 123, 124, 201, 212, 249, 269, 279
Seriousness of Illness Rating Scale (SIRS) [Wyler], 269; 1, 2, 4-6, 19, 23, 25, 28, 32, 71, 74, 119, 134, 200, 250, 266, 275, 281, 282, 284, 291
Serum uric acid, 10, 41, 88, 161, 207, 209-12
Sex differences in life change reporting: see Frequency of life events and Female subjects
Sex, psychological (homosexual and non-homosexual populations), 204
Sexual identification, feminine, 104
Sexual identification, masculine, 159
Shipley Institute of Living Scale, 167
Sick role tendency, 8, 19, 32, 34
Skin disease, 105-7; 15
Sled dog racers, Alaskan Iditarod Race, 162
Sleeping habits, change in, 47, 209, 241
Smallest-space analysis, use of, 289
Smoking, 10, 38, 77, 91, 95, 103, 156, 157, 216, 241
Social and Athletic Readjustment Rating Scale (SARRS) [Bramwell], 191
Social Assets Scale (Luborsky, Todd, and Katcher), 35, 94, 201
Social change, 6, 26, 119, 151, 192, 193
Social class, 2, 9, 53-55, 62, 140, 142, 166, 169, 173, 175, 176, 185, 219, 220, 236, 262, 263, 275, 294
Social desirability, 118, 200, 202, 260, 305
Social integration, 173, 177
Social integration of refugees, 249
Social interest, 190
Social mobility, 81, 91, 172, 176
Social Readjustment Rating Questionnaire (SRRQ), use of, 263; 1, 6, 24, 52, 71, 73, 74, 242, 246, 248, 253, 262-65, 271-85, 289, 291, 297, 299, 302

Social Readjustment Rating Scale (SRRS): Development of, 263; 6, 28, 256, 260, 302; El Salvador version, 284; Finnish version, 85, 86, 260; Japanese version, 282; Malaysian version, 285; New Zealand version, 282; Spanish version, 281; Swedish version, 78, 87, 260, 284; Western European version, 281
Social Readjustment Rating Scale for Women in Religious Life, 1
Social role performance, 45, 116, 122, 123, 152, 170, 172, 174, 192
Social services, use of, 116, 119, 121-23, 239
Social supports, 186-89; 2, 8, 11, 16, 22, 45, 48, 92, 103, 104, 116, 122-25, 152, 165, 167, 182, 185, 207, 208, 220, 223, 225, 227, 234
Socioeconomic status, 9, 57, 95, 155, 169, 172, 177, 214, 277
Somatotyping, 159
Spastic colon, 98
Specificity theory vs. non-specificity theory, 27, 31, 53, 59, 80
Spina bifida, 110
State-Trait Anxiety Inventory (STAI), 9, 11, 24, 25, 76, 80, 94, 102, 109, 123, 129, 191, 260
State-Trait Anxiety Inventory (STAI) for Children, 2, 184
Stimulus screening, 9
Stress Ratings of Life Events Occurring During/Prior to Pregnancy (Helper), 273; 280
Subarachnoid haemorrhage, 92
Subjective equivalence, five studies of, 291
Subjective perceptions of life events, 52, 78, 82, 111, 123, 143, 144, 161, 168, 175, 179, 191, 260, 274, 280, 285, 290-93, 297, 299, 300, 302, 305
Sudden death, 78, 79, 84, 85, 86
Suicide and suicide attempts, 145-52; 32, 49, 59, 63, 214, 216, 217, 231, 240
Surgery, recovery from, 22, 98, 181
Surgical patients, 5, 22, 23, 98, 181, 212, 275, 278, 279
Symptom Checklist 90 (SCL-90), 47, 72, 75, 98, 122, 127, 158, 202
Symptom configuration, 68, 178
Symptom intensity, 178, 179
Symptoms and moods, reporting of, 95, 120, 174, 200, 241

Symptoms, questionnaire measures of, 165-80; see also separate listings by name of instrument (e.g., Langner's 22-item index, Cornell Medical Index)

Taylor Manifest Anxiety Scale, 76, 86, 190, 192, 193, 280, 305
Teacher performance, 129, 130, 133, 270
Teaching Events Stress Inventory (Cichon), 270
Temperature range, daily life events and, 111
Temporomandibular joint (TMJ) clinic patients, 96
Tennant and Andrews life event inventory and scales, 267, 268; 2, 97, 165, 176, 177, 188
Thyroid conditions, recovery from surgery for, 181
Time, effect of: see Recency vs. remoteness in time of experienced event; Recall of life events, reliability of; and Reliability, test-retest
Tonsillectomy, 109
Total Adaptive Potential for Pregnancy Score (TAPPS) [Nuckolls], 103, 104
Tranquilizer effectiveness, 112
Tranquilizer prescribing, 309
Tranquilizer use, 158, 225
Transactional Analysis, 150, 153
Transcendental meditation, 150
Tuberculosis, 15, 32, 34
Twins, studies of illness- or death-discordant, 36, 78

Type A behavior pattern, 80, 81, 86, 91, 236

Ulcerative colitis, 95-98
Ulcers (gastric, peptic, duodenal), 22, 27, 32, 88, 95, 97, 98
Underwater demolition team training, 125, 161, 211, 212
Unemployment: see Job-related life events
Universal Event Impact Scale (Wainer, Fairbank, and Hough), 268
Urban mental health (Yorklea Study), 165-67
Upsetting/distressing life events, ratings of, 49, 82, 123, 178, 265, 268, 274, 277, 283
Urinary retention, acute, 100
Uterine cancer, 38, 39

Values orientation: see Gordon Survey of Interpersonal Values
Violent vs. non-violent behavior, 148, 159
Vulnerability hypothesis, 204

Weighting of life events, 16-18, 55, 82, 191, 257, 260, 263, 265, 266, 272, 274, 277, 283, 286, 288-90, 292, 293, 294, 297, 298, 299, 303, 304, 305
Well-being, psychological, 11, 80, 125, 170, 171, 174, 175, 185, 200, 245, 246, 251
Work, 232-37; see also separate listings for Job-related life events and Occupations of subject groups

ABOUT THE EDITORS

THOMAS H. HOLMES is Professor of Psychiatry and Behavioral Sciences at the University of Washington, Seattle, Washington. He joined the faculty of the School of Medicine in 1949.

Dr. Holmes has published widely in the areas of psychosomatic medicine, psychophysiology, and life change events research. His articles have appeared in the <u>Journal of Psychosomatic Research</u>, <u>Psychosomatic Medicine</u>, and <u>Archives of General Psychiatry</u>.

Dr. Holmes holds an A.B. from the University of North Carolina and an M.D. from Cornell University Medical College.

ELLA M. DAVID is Research Publications Editor in the Department of Psychiatry and Behavioral Sciences, University of Washington.

Ms. David has worked in Dr. Holmes's psychosocial laboratory since 1978. She is a member of the American Medical Writers Association.

Ms. David holds a B.A. from Scripps College and an M.A. in English from the University of Washington.

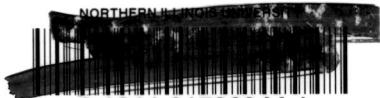